THE DOCTORS BOOK®
of
WEIGHT-LOSS REMEDIES

THE DOCTORS BOOK®
of
WEIGHT-LOSS REMEDIES

The latest findings on the power of food
and exercise to prevent health problems,
plus doctor-recommended remedies
for fast, safe weight loss

LAURA ROBERSON and the Editors of **Prevention**®

RODALE®

© 2013 by Rodale Inc.

All rights reserved. No part of this publication may be reproduced or transmitted in any form or by any means,
electronic or mechanical, including photocopying, recording, or any other information storage and retrieval system,
without the written permission of the publisher.

Prevention is a registered trademark of Rodale Inc.

Printed in the United States of America

Rodale Inc. makes every effort to use acid-free ⊗, recycled paper ♻.

Photographs on pages 306–314, 316–325, 341–345, 425–428, 430, 431–433 ©Beth Bischoff;
page 313, top right (Split Squat) ©Thomas MacDonald; page 432, top left (Reverse Fly) ©Karen Pearson

Book design by Carol Angstadt

Library of Congress Cataloging-in-Publication Data is on file with the publisher.

ISBN 978-1-60961-519-2   direct hardcover

2   4   6   8   10   9   7   5   3   1   hardcover

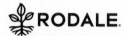

We inspire and enable people to improve their lives and the world around them.
For more of our products visit **prevention.com** or call 800-848-4735

To Mom and Paul

Contents

Part 2
YOUR BRAIN

Part 3
YOUR DIET

SPECIAL SECTION

Part 4
YOUR FITNESS

Part 5
YOUR PLAN

Introduction

Your Weight-Loss Companion

There are books that you read one week and forget the next. Or books you give to a friend when you're finished reading. This isn't one of those. This is a book you'll keep in a handy spot because you'll find yourself returning to it again and again. This is a book whose pages you'll dog-ear and highlight with fluorescent markers and flag with those sticky papers. Go ahead and scribble notes in it. Start with your name. So no one swipes it!

The Doctors Book of Weight-Loss Remedies is a user's guide to a healthier, fitter, leaner body. It's a book that'll give you your money's worth—and then some—because in it you'll find tons of practical tips and hints that you'll use every day of your life. How many diet books can you say that about?

In most diet and weight-loss books, you get the advice of one person about one way to lose weight. But is there just one way that really works? And will it work for everyone? We're all different. We all have different metabolisms, different life schedules, different tastes in food and preferences for exercise. What works for one person may not work for a woman like you or a man like you. Maybe that's why all those one-size-fits-all fad diets fail about 2 or 3 months after the initial 10-pound loss of water weight.

Not here. *The Doctors Book of Weight-Loss Remedies* is bursting at the seams with choice pearls of wisdom from hundreds of doctors, nutritionists, trainers, and other experts. These are people on the front lines of the war on obesity, diabetes, and heart disease in this country. They've seen it all, and they know what works for the very different people who walk through their doors looking for help in losing weight and improving their health. They also know that fad diets of extreme denial and quick fixes don't work for sustained weight loss. You know that, too, because, like us, you've tried them.

No diet should feel like a hunger strike. Rather, your weight-loss plan should be one that you can stick to for weeks, months, even years to come. It should quickly feel natural and become rote. Just a part of normal life. That's what this book will help you accomplish. You don't have to banish your favorite foods from your diet to lose weight—you just have to learn how to practice moderation and smartly offset your indulgences with waistline-friendly foods and exercise. What you *will* have to do is banish some really bad nutrition habits, if you have them. Bad habits mean regular, daily overindulgences in foods that have no redeeming qualities other than they taste good—like a box of chocolate chip cookies or six fudge brownies as a TV snack. There's just no losing weight if you don't have the sense and the willpower to knock off that kind of behavior. But this book contains hundreds of strategies that will help you do just that: Strengthen your willpower, cheat the right way (yes, there *is* a right way), and keep the weight off once you've met your goal.

What makes this book different is that it doesn't just give you a single plan. It guarantees your success by anticipating every roadblock you may encounter on your journey. If you struggle with cravings, there's a section for that. If you can't kick your soda habit, there's a whole list of expert-approved solutions. Do you need to lower your cholesterol? Find 12 natural doctor-approved suggestions beginning on page 15. Or if you feel hungry constantly—you guessed it—there's a section for that, too. You'll even find easy better-for-you recipes that taste every bit as delicious as the foods you already enjoy.

The other crucial part of a new healthy lifestyle is exercise. Don't worry if you're a beginner. In Part 5, you'll find an exercise plan—the Ultimate 4-Week Fat-Burning Exercise Workout—that's suited for both newbies and seasoned exercisers. (You're in control; you decide how easy or difficult to make it.) We've also included walking-workout progressions that will help you gradually build strength and endurance without soreness and fatigue. Your new fitness plan is accompanied by hundreds of tips to make exercise fun, boost your weight loss, and track your progress.

We're not going to sugarcoat something so important to living a healthy and long life. Losing weight and maintaining a healthy body take effort to change deeply ingrained lifestyle habits. They require dedication to a new approach toward moving your body and fueling it right, but you're not alone. Over the next few months, this book will become your ultimate weight-loss companion—your nutrition bible, your personal trainer, your supermarket shopping buddy, main motivator, and accountability partner, all rolled into one. It's almost like having a weight-loss doctor on call 24/7. There's literally no weight-loss question *The Doctors Book of Weight-Loss Remedies* can't answer, and no struggle it can't help you defeat. All that's left is your decision to accept the challenge and achieve your goal.

Your weight-loss journey begins with one simple word: *yes.* Yes, I commit to eating the foods that will help me live the life I want. Yes, I can live a more active life—not just tomorrow, but for years to come, using the advice of the doctors featured in this book. Yes, I can achieve the body I desire.

Good for you! Your journey starts here.

Part 1
YOUR BODY

How to reshape your body and boost your health—at the same time

There are lots of metaphors used to describe the human body: a machine. A work of art. A temple. All of those things are true—and important—but there's a less poetic way you can describe your body: healthy. Sure, shedding weight (especially through your midsection) is about looking good. Who doesn't want to hit their physical peak? But dropping pounds is also a means to keeping what's on the inside of your body in tip-top shape. A lower number on the bathroom scale has a big impact on controlling cholesterol, triglycerides, blood sugar, and blood pressure, as well as taming hormones that can affect your weight and revving up your internal fat-burning furnace. In this section, you'll find expert-approved strategies for taking control of your health—and your waistline.

Abdominal Fat

15 effective ways to banish the belly

Belly fat, beer gut, tummy—you can call it what you like, but it's all the same dangerous fat. The excess, often firm fat around your middle is what doctors call "visceral fat." And it's not just a threat to the button of your jeans. Abdominal fat is more metabolically active than the other types of fat in your body (like the padding around your hips), meaning it releases hormones and chemicals, called adipokines. Adipokines include compounds that raise your risk of high blood sugar, diabetes, arterial inflammation, and high blood pressure. "Having a hard [protruding] belly is like having a ticking time bomb in your body," says Jean-Pierre Després, PhD, a professor in the department of social and preventive medicine at Laval University.

As your waistline expands, individual fat cells inflate, which can lead to lower HDL "good" cholesterol and higher levels of triglycerides, a type of fatty acid in the blood linked to heart disease. Visceral fat may also work its way into your liver—the organ responsible for clearing toxins from your blood—so it can compromise

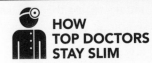

HOW TOP DOCTORS STAY SLIM

"I try to eat as much protein as possible, and I rarely eat bread. My carbs are the fruit and whole grains I eat in the morning: Barbara's Oats with blueberries, blackberries, and strawberries."

—**NICHOLAS DAVIDSON, MD,** a professor of medicine at Washington University in St. Louis your entire circulatory system. It's no surprise that people with thick midsections are more prone to developing heart disease, diabetes, and even cancer.

Men tend to gain their weight in their bellies throughout life, but for women, it's not until middle age that their midsections become the hot spot for weight gain. As women's estrogen levels decline with age, their testosterone levels increase, causing them to shift to the male pattern of abdominal weight gain. Regardless of gender, you naturally accumulate more fat as you age, often due to loss of muscle mass and a more sluggish metabolism. But that doesn't mean you should sit idly by and let the fat infiltrate your midsection. Use the following strategies to banish your belly fat for good.

■ **TARGET YOUR FAT CELLS** Here's the great news about fat that sits around your middle: It pays attention when you exercise. "Abdominal fat cells may have different amounts of metabolic enzymes than other parts of your body, causing them to be more responsive to exercise," explains Tongjian You, PhD, the author of a Wake Forest University study on how belly fat is metabolized. He and other researchers found that people who diet *and* exercise shrink their abdominal fat cells twice as much as those who only diet—even if they lose the same amount of total weight. (You'll find many wonderful tips and suggestions for adding exercise to your day in this book. Check out pages 424–433 for specific belly-fat burning routines.)

■ **HIT THE GROUND RUNNING (OR WALKING)** Studies show that the easiest way to shed your spare tire is by logging at least 30 minutes of moderate-intensity aerobic exercise every day. What does "moderate intensity" mean? It's not a casual stroll. To be effective, you need to huff and puff a bit and break a sweat. And, no, that doesn't mean you have to sprint like a track star. Brisk walking is fine. Whether you're walking, running, or cycling, just make sure that you're exercising at 50 to 70 percent of your maximum heart rate. The math is easy to calculate. First, find your maximum heart rate by subtracting your age from 220 (Example: 220 - 40 = 180). Then multiply your max heart rate by 0.5 (180 x 0.5 = 90). Repeat the calculation, this time multiplying by 0.7 (180 x 0.7 = 126). The two numbers represent your target range in heartbeats per min-

HOW MUCH BELLY FAT ARE YOU WEARING?

You don't have to visit a high-tech lab to determine the amount of abdominal fat weighing you down. You just need a simple tape measure. Determining your waist-to-hip ratio can help indicate your level of visceral fat, according to George Blackburn, MD, PhD, a professor of medicine at Harvard University. To measure your waist, wrap the tape around your body at the midpoint between your lowest rib and your hipbone. Then to determine your hip circumference, measure the widest part of your hips and butt. Now divide the first number by the second. Women should have a waist-to-hip ratio no higher than 0.8, and the target for men is 0.95 or lower.

ute. Make sure you're hitting your max during exercise. Check your rate manually by counting pulse beats on your wrist for 10 seconds and then multiplying by 6. Even easier, use a heart-rate monitor, such as the Polar RS300X.

■ **TRY INTERVAL TRAINING** Even better than a half-hour run is speed interval training, which involves short, intense bursts of exercise followed by brief "rest" periods of moderate effort. You can do interval-style training with any type of exercise. Walking is a great way to start. In a Canadian study, exercisers who completed 30-minute interval workouts lost three times as much fat over 15 weeks as those who performed easier workouts at a steady pace for 45 minutes. Another study found that exercisers who did short, intense workouts experienced a 20 percent drop in visceral fat after 3 months. Those who did longer workouts at a more moderate pace saw no such change.

You should perform intervals at an intensity where you can speak no more than a few words at a time. This helps you burn more calories while you exercise, but the real benefit comes afterward. The harder your workout, the longer it takes for your body to return to normal. The effect: You keep burning calories long after you leave the gym. Start by supplementing your normal workouts with two or three interval sessions per week. Some simple suggestions: Slip in your earbuds during your run and speed up during every other song. Or walk or jog quickly to the top of hill, then walk back down to recover. (For more on intervals, see Interval Training on page 326.)

■ **USE THE RESISTANCE-TRAINING SECRET** Muscle burns calories even when it isn't engaged in lifting groceries or propelling you up a long set of stairs. It's more metabolically active than fat is, requiring more calories just to sustain itself on your skeleton. The secret to staying lean as you age is to build muscle through resistance training. We're not talking about bulging bodybuilder muscles. Just firm, toned, attractive muscle. You can do it by using body-weight-only exercises or exercise bands or by lifting weights. Studies have shown that total-body resistance training actually targets visceral fat. In one study at Skidmore College, scientists found that people who performed a high-intensity resistance routine along with their cardio lost more than four times as much belly fat as cardio-only exercisers. (The weight-training group also increased their protein intake.)

■ **GO SLOW** When doing resistance training, mix up your workout by adding what's called a "tempo exercise" to boost the fat-burning benefits of the routine. Tempo exercises, where you lift weights using slow, steady movements, condition your body to burn more fat, according to a study in the *Journal of Strength and Conditioning Research*. How to do it: Lower the weight for 3 seconds, then take 3 seconds to press it up, without pausing in between. This can help boost your number of mitochondria—the parts of your cells that use fat to create fuel. The more mitochondria you have, the more belly fat you'll burn. Make sure to target all of the major muscle groups: arms, legs, shoulders, chest, back, hips, and core using this technique at least once a week.

■ **DRINK IN MODERATION** There's a reason it's called a "beer belly." Beer is loaded with carbohydrates, but any alcohol—wine, wine spritzers, fruity cocktails, even straight vodka or whiskey—will inflate your waistline. That's because alcohol impairs your body's ability to burn fat; one study found it does so by as much as 36 percent. What's more, as your body breaks down the alcohol, it starts making fat from a chemical by-product of the process—a double whammy for your belly. A University of Buffalo study found that men who drink only once or twice every 2 weeks, but imbibe more than four drinks at a time, have more belly flab than those who down two alcoholic drinks a day. To limit alcohol's belly-expanding effects, women should limit themselves to a single serving of alcohol per sitting; men should stop at two.

■ **KEEP YOUR COOL** When you're stressed out, your body releases a flood of cortisol, a hormone that encourages your body to store belly fat. The explanation: The fat around your middle has a higher number of cortisol receptors and a greater blood supply, so the hormone can travel there quickly. (For simple ways to slash stress, see page 85.)

■ **SIP ON GREEN TEA** The benefits of this beverage just keep adding up—green tea has been shown to help fight cancer, make your skin glow . . . and shrink belly fat! In a recent study in the *Journal of Nutrition*, exercisers who downed about four cups of green tea per day for 3 months shed eight times more abdominal fat than those who drank another caffeinated beverage. Green tea is loaded with weight-loss-promoting compounds called catechins, including epigallocatechin gallate (EGCG), which has been shown to accelerate fat burning. If you can't stand the stuff, try taking a green tea extract supplement that contains at least 200 milligrams of EGCG.

■ **TURN IN EARLIER** A poor sleep schedule doesn't just make you grumpy. Like stress, a lack of sleep spikes your cortisol levels, causing you to store more abdominal fat. According to Canadian researchers, people who average just 5 to 6 hours of sleep per night tend to be 60 percent heavier around the middle than those who sleep 7 to 8 hours. Keep in mind, the "more is better" approach has its limits. Another study showed that people who sleep too much also have thicker midsections, since time in bed can cut into your exercise schedule. The ideal: Set a bedtime that permits 8 hours of sleep, and stick with it, day in and day out.

■ **JOIN THE CALCIUM CLUB** Milk isn't the only dairy that deserves real estate in your fridge. A University of Tennessee study found that overweight people who ate three servings of any type of calcium-rich dairy a day for 6 months lost more belly fat than dieters who consumed less. The calcium may decrease the likelihood that fat will flock to your stomach. Aim for one serving with every meal: a glass of milk with breakfast, a slice of cheese with lunch, and yogurt as an after-dinner treat, for example. Calcium supplements probably won't have the same effect, since proteins in dairy enhance the fat-burning effect of calcium.

■ **EAT MORE HEALTHY FATS** Fat doesn't make you fat. Some people haven't gotten the message. Even saturated fats like those in beef and butter can help you lose weight because they are satiating. But monounsaturated fats are the best because they are heart healthy as well as satiating, and they may actually help trim your waistline. A recent study found that insulin-resistant people who ate a diet high in monounsaturated fats had less belly flab than those who loaded up on carbohydrates or saturated fats. Top sources of the healthy fats include macadamia nuts, hazelnuts, pecans, almonds, peanut butter, and olive oil.

■ **HAVE YOUR WHEY** Whey protein—the kind that's found in dairy—can help zap abdominal fat, according to a study in the *Journal of Nutrition*. Ideally, you'll take in most of your whey protein from foods like yogurt and cheese. However, when you're in a pinch, a whey protein smoothie or meal-replacement bar can provide a substantial hit of the belly-blasting stuff. Try storing one of the bars in your glove box in case you need an emergency pick-me-up. (For a protein bar buying guide, see page 230. For delicious whey protein smoothie recipes, see page 416.)

■ **ELIMINATE REFINED CARBS** If you see "enriched flour" in a food's ingredient list, you've fallen victim to refined carbs, which have been stripped of their fiber, vitamins, and minerals. Switching to whole-grain versions of bread, pasta, rice, and cereal not only provides you with a payload of nutrients, but it can also target harmful belly fat. In a Penn State study, dieters who ate whole grains lost twice as much belly fat as those who ate refined carbs. (For whole-grain versions of your favorite foods, see pages 291–293.)

■ **GET MORE VITAMIN D** Research suggests that vitamin D partners with calcium to stamp out cortisol, the stress hormone that can increase your belly-fat storage. Also known as the "sunshine vitamin," vitamin D is produced by your skin when it's exposed to sunlight. Unfortunately, few of us produce enough vitamin D through sun exposure alone. That means you need to eat D-rich foods, such as salmon, swordfish, rainbow trout, tuna, or fortified cereals. Consider taking a vitamin D_3 supplement for extra insurance.

■ **DON'T FALL FOR DIET SODA** You may think switching to diet soda is a smart move for your waistline. Wrong—the only smart move is cutting out soda entirely. In 2009, University of Texas researchers found that people who drink one diet soda a day have larger waists than those who rarely drink any soda. If you crave fizz and flavor, sip on spritzers—carbonated water with a shot of fruit juice—instead.

Basal Metabolism

6 strategies to raise your resting metabolism

Even the most serious fitness fanatics expend no more than 30 percent of their daily calories at the gym. You burn most of your calories slowly—at a constant simmer—to fuel the processes that keep you alive, such as breathing, contracting the muscles in your heart, and repairing damaged tissue. These calories make up your basal metabolic rate (also called your resting metabolism), which represents about 60 to 70 percent of the daily calories you burn. It's the number of calories your body would burn, say, if you had nothing to eat and stayed in bed all day.

Your basal metabolism is highly related to your body mass, explains Jeff Volek, PhD, RD, an exercise and nutrition scientist at the University of Connecticut. In other words, the heavier you are, the higher your basal metabolism is. So, inevitably, as you lose weight, you burn fewer calories a day—generally, about 2 to 10 calories per pound you drop. So if you lose 20 pounds, you need to eat 40 to 200 fewer calories per day just to maintain your new slimmer figure (not factoring in exercise). The good news: You can take measures to elevate your resting metabolism even as you lose weight.

■ **EAT MORE DAIRY** Maintaining muscle as you lose weight can keep your resting metabolic rate from slipping. The secret: loading up on dairy. According to recent Canadian research, milk, yogurt, and cheese can help you slim down *and* gain muscle. In the study, overweight people who exercised every day and followed a calorie-controlled diet rich in protein and dairy lost about 10 pounds of fat and gained 1½ pounds of muscle after just 16 weeks. (Dieters who ate less dairy and protein still lost weight, but they also lost muscle.) Dairy can help keep your appetite in check, while its whey protein can fuel muscle growth.

■ **DON'T CRASH DIET** If you take in too few calories, you'll burn fewer calories every day. That's because drastic dietary measures—say, limiting yourself to 900 calories a day—stifle your resting metabolism and cause you to lose muscle mass. Instead, aim to trim a reasonable 250 calories per day, and then burn another 250 through exercise. That way, you'll be more likely to retain your muscle as you lose your fat, and you should drop about 1 pound per week.

■ **SPEED THINGS UP** Don't just slog through a few miles on the elliptical, then call it a day. If you push yourself—*really* push yourself—during your cardio workout, you may be able to boost your resting metabolism for an hour after you stop moving. Your goal should be to exercise at moderate to high intensity. To gauge your level of effort, use what exercise scientists call "the talk test": At moderate intensity, you will be able to talk, but not sing, and at high intensity, you will only be able to say a few words before gasping for breath.

■ **LIFT WEIGHTS THREE TIMES A WEEK** Regular resistance exercise can raise your resting metabolism. As you pack on muscle, you burn more calories even while you're resting, since muscle is more metabolically active than fat. In fact, a study in *Medicine & Science in Sports & Exercise* found that after 6 months of lifting weights 3 days a week, people boosted their basal burn by 7 percent! (For a primer on resistance training, see page 330.)

■ **MUNCH ON PEANUTS** Peanuts may be high in fat and calories—but they won't necessarily make you gain weight. In a recent Swedish study, people who snacked on peanuts every day for 2 weeks experienced a boost in resting metabolism. Limit yourself to one handful per sitting, and always opt for unsalted.

■ **DRINK MORE WATER** You've heard it a million times: Drinking water is a free and effective weight-loss strategy. Not only does it fill your belly and stifle cravings, but staying hydrated can also keep your metabolism humming. German researchers found that downing six cups of cold water per day can raise your daily burn by about 50 calories—which could help you lose an extra 5 pounds per year! Make it a policy to drink a glass of ice-cold water before every meal and snack.

Bloat

11 ways to beat that "fat day" feeling

HOW TOP DOCTORS STAY SLIM

"I rarely weigh myself. Instead I check my strength-to-weight ratio by doing 20 chinups daily. The ease or difficulty tells me how I'm doing. My goal is to hover around 160 pounds, my high school graduation weight, because that's close to the optimal weight for many guys."

—DAVID KATZ, MD, MPH, director of the Yale-Griffin Prevention Research Center

Even if you're dropping weight, you may still feel bloated—that sense of being overly full or uncomfortably gassy. There may be sneaky reasons behind your bloat. Target them with these smart food swaps and bloat-relieving strategies.

■ **AVOID EXCESS SALT** Sodium loves water. Eating too much of it is like hitting the "inflate" button on your body—the more sodium in your bloodstream, the more water you retain. Even if you aren't heavy-handedly sprinkling every meal with salt, you may still be taking in more than your daily allowance of 2,300 milligrams (1,500 milligrams if you're middle age or have diabetes or hypertension). Eliminate sneaky sources of sodium in your diet, such as salad dressing, Parmesan cheese, smoked salmon, salami, bacon (especially the turkey kind), anchovies, and teriyaki sauce. And watch out: Many "diet" foods are high in sodium to compensate for lower fat and calories.

■ **AVOID SUPERSALTY COCKTAILS** Margaritas are loaded with tequila and sodium, both of which make your retain water. If you must have your 'rita or Bloody Mary, sip a glass of water as you imbibe to dilute all that sodium.

■ **LIMIT BROCCOLI AND CAULIFLOWER** On a normal day, cruciferous vegetables—broccoli, Brussels sprouts, cauliflower, cabbage—are a wise addition to any meal. They're loaded with fiber and the cancer-fighting compound sulforaphane. But if you're about to bare all in your bikini, steer clear of this class of veggies, as they contain raffinose. Your body can't break down this complex sugar, causing excess gas to build up in your digestive tract. Steaming your cruciferous vegetables can cook off some of the raffinose, or you can simply opt for produce that contains lots of water, such as watermelon or cucumbers, instead.

■ **PACK IN THE POTASSIUM** You can help counteract salt's negative effects by eating foods that are rich in potassium (see the table below). Aim to consume 4,700 milligrams of potassium every day.

■ **DRAIN CANNED BEANS** The same compound in cruciferous vegetables is also behind beans' gassy reputation. But you don't have to eliminate the legumes entirely. Draining the liquid from canned varieties, then rinsing them with water, can help remove raffinose. Another strategy: Mix a serving of beans with a teaspoon of baking soda.

■ **EXERCISE YOUR BOWELS** Thirty minutes of daily exercise will give you the best bloat-reducing results, but even a 10-minute walk is enough to move things along in your digestive tract, says Christine Lee, MD, a gastroenterologist at the Cleveland Clinic. In fact, a recent Swedish study found that running helps food move more quickly through your bowels and can loosen stools.

■ **DRINK MORE WATER** Carbonated beverages can inflate your belly. Artificial sugars in diet soda compound the effect. Drinking more water, on the other hand, can actually help ease bloat. If you're dehydrated, your body will

WHERE TO FIND THE POTASSIUM

FOOD	POTASSIUM (MG)	CALORIES
Baked sweet potato	694	131
Beet greens (½ cup, cooked)	655	19
Baked white potato	610	145
Canned white beans (½ cup)	595	153
Canned clams (3 oz)	534	126
Plain low-fat yogurt	531	143
Green soybeans (½ cup, cooked)	485	127
Yellowfin tuna (3 oz)	484	118
Lima beans (½ cup, cooked)	484	104

hang on to water to make sure it has enough for your kidneys to function properly, explains Elisa Zied, MS, RD, a former spokesperson for the Academy of Nutrition and Dietetics. Make it your goal to drink a glass of water before and with every meal.

■ **STEER CLEAR OF FAKE FIBER** As a filling, low-calorie nutrient, fiber is a crucial element of any weight-loss plan. But not all fiber is created equal. Foods that boast "added fiber"—Fiber One bars, for example—often contain inulin, a type of fiber made from chicory root that may be used to replace fat. Inulin isn't bad—it's found naturally in bananas, garlic, and asparagus—but it can cause tummy troubles. To avoid bloat, fulfill most of your fiber needs with fruits, vegetables, whole grains, nuts, and legumes, rather than "added fiber" granola bars and cereals.

■ **SNACK ON PINEAPPLE** The juicy yellow fruit is loaded with bromelain, an enzyme that helps break down protein and promotes digestion. Add pineapple chunks to your salad, or try grilling pineapple rings for a tasty sandwich topper.

BONUS BENEFIT!

Studies show that the bromelain in pineapple may speed muscle repair and fight swelling. Plus, since it's a digestive enzyme, it may also help ease indigestion.

■ **SIP ON TEA** Drinking a cup of peppermint or chamomile tea may relax your digestive muscles. This decreases the amount of gas in your belly and helps speed up digestion.

■ **WATCH YOUR WHEAT** If you feel bloated after eating wheat, you may have a gluten sensitivity. Other signs include stomach cramps and diarrhea. If you're concerned, talk to your doctor, and consider switching to gluten-free grains, like barley, millet, and oats, to see if your symptoms ease up.

Body Mass Index

How to calculate—and interpret—your BMI

Body mass index, or BMI, is simply a measure of fatness used to determine whether your weight is in the appropriate range. By itself, body weight doesn't tell you much about your body composition, but because BMI considers both weight *and* height, it can be used to more accurately assess whether or not you're lugging too much lard. The formula is fairly straightforward: Your weight (in pounds), divided by your height (in inches), squared. Then that number is multiplied by 703 for your BMI. So, for example, if you weigh 190 pounds and stand 6 feet tall, your calculation would be:

$$[190 \div (72)^2] \times 703 = 25.8$$

From there, you can determine your weight status.

BMI	WEIGHT STATUS
Below 18.5	Underweight
18.5 to 24.9	Normal
25.0 to 29.9	Overweight
30 or higher	Obese

HOW TOP DOCTORS STAY SLIM

"I don't count my calories—I just eat lots of fruits and veggies. I am lucky to live in California, where I have year-round access to beautiful, reasonably priced fruits and vegetables. Whenever I can, I shop at farmers' markets and stock the fridge with seasonal fruit. I also make lots of smoothies with fruits and vegetables."

—NAOMI STOTLAND, MD, a doctor at the Center for Obesity Assessment, Study, and Treatment at the University of California, San Francisco

Having a high BMI has been linked to everything from diabetes to high blood pressure to sleep apnea. However, there's one problem with using the number as an indicator of health: When you calculate your BMI, you can't account for muscle. In other words, a fit guy who is 5 foot 10 and 180 pounds has the same BMI as an equally tall, 180-pound man with a gut. In fact, according to the CDC, people who have a BMI that technically falls in the overweight range may not always be fat—bodybuilders and highly trained athletes tend to have higher BMIs, even though their body fat is low. "BMI doesn't distinguish whether a large body is due to muscle mass or obesity," says Anne E. Sumner, MD, an obesity researcher for the National Institutes of Health.

The link between BMI and fatness can also vary by gender and age. Women tend to carry more body fat than men at the same BMI, and older people generally have a higher amount of body fat than younger people at the same BMI, say CDC experts.

That said, you *can* assume you're in trouble when your BMI enters the obese range, regardless of how muscular you are. Your best bet is to track several numbers: your BMI, waist-to-hip ratio (see "How Much Belly Fat Are You Wearing?" on page 4), weight, and body fat, as well as your cholesterol and blood pressure. If you see a significant change for the worse in any one number, you may need to reevaluate your exercise and diet plan.

In addition, consider tracking a new mea-sure of fatness called the body adiposity index (BAI). BAI is calculated using your height and hip circumference (both are linked to body-fat percentage)—and may be a more reliable measure of fatness than BMI, according to a recent study in the journal *Obesity*. (Note: The accuracy of BAI hasn't yet been confirmed for all races. Continue tracking other numbers, too.) The formula is complex, so use an online calculator, like the one on the Texas State University Web site (www.campusrecreation.txstate.edu/programs/ fitness/personal-training/calc.html). Not sure how to judge your hip circumference? Measure around the most pronounced part of your buttocks, positioning the tape at a uniform height around your body. From there, you can gauge your weight status.

AGE 20 TO 40	
BAI Male	Weight Status
< 8	Underweight
8 to 18.9	Healthy
19 to 25	Overweight
> 25	Obese
BAI Female	Weight Status
< 21	Underweight
21 to 32.9	Healthy
33 to 39	Overweight
> 39	Obese
AGE 41 TO 60	
BAI Male	Weight Status
< 11	Underweight
11 to 21.9	Healthy
22 to 27	Overweight
> 27	Obese
BAI Female	Weight Status
< 23	Underweight
23 to 34.9	Healthy
35 to 40	Overweight
> 40	Obese

Cholesterol: 12 Drug-Free Ways to Improve Your Numbers

Cholesterol is one of those words you've probably heard doctors throw around, but you may have little idea of what it *actually* is or why you should watch it. A quick primer: Cholesterol is a waxy, fatlike substance that helps your body manufacture hormones, vitamin D, and chemicals needed to digest foods. The problem is, a certain type of cholesterol, called low-density lipoproteins, or LDL, can dangerously accumulate in your arteries, increasing your risk of heart disease. When your doctor tells you to lower your cholesterol, it's probably because your LDL levels are high—which, according to national guidelines, means your LDL is above 160 milligrams/deciliter. Borderline high is in the 130–159 mg/dl range, while the optimal level is below 100 mg/dl. For more numbers, check out the chart:

IS YOUR CHOLESTEROL ON TARGET?

LDL "BAD" CHOLESTEROL		TOTAL CHOLESTEROL		HDL "GOOD" CHOLESTEROL	
<100	Optimal	<200	Desirable	<40	Low (above 40 is desirable)
100–129	Near optimal/above optimal	200–239	Borderline high	40–60	Desirable
130–159	Borderline high	240+	High	60+	High
160–189	High				
190+	Very high				

What's your response to doctor's orders? Order an egg-white omelet, since scrambled eggs will inevitably end up in your arteries. Right? One problem: The idea that dietary cholesterol—the stuff found in eggs, butter, and ricotta cheese—translates to high blood cholesterol is a nutritional myth. In fact, one study found that men who ate three eggs a day experienced a 20 percent increase in their HDL "good" cholesterol, which actually helps shuttle cholesterol out of your body. If you eat a six-egg omelet, your body responds by simply producing less of its own cholesterol. So rather than purging your refrigerator of all things dairy, try these 12 strategies to keep your cholesterol in check.

1 MUNCH ON PECANS

Stash a jar of pecans at your desk for an afternoon snack. Eating about ¾ cup of the nuts can lower your levels of one form of LDL "bad" cholesterol by up to 33 percent, according to Loma Linda University researchers. Why pecans? They contain a type of antioxidant called gamma-tocopherols, thought to slash levels of oxidized LDL, a harmful form of cholesterol that can inflame your arteries. Regularly eating pecans may also lower total cholesterol, other studies suggest.

2 POP A PISTACHIO

In a recent Penn State study, people who ate two servings of pistachios a day cut their bad cholesterol by an average of 13 percent. "Phytosterols in nuts act almost like a drug—they bind cholesterol in the GI tract and block its absorption," says Paul Ziajka, MD, PhD, a clinical lipidologist with the Southeast Lipid Association. Pistachios pack a higher concentration of phytosterols than any other nut, according to a study from Virginia Tech.

3 AVOID FAST FOOD

It's not just fast food's sky-high calorie counts that do you in. Perfluoroalkyl acids—chemicals found in grease-resistant packaging, such as Chinese take-out containers, pizza boxes, and burger wrappers—have been linked to high LDL cholesterol among teens. "The control of cholesterol is uniform throughout our lives," says John Elefteriades, MD, chief of cardiothoracic surgery at the Yale School of Medicine. "So this would likely translate to adults."

4 RETHINK YOUR GRAINS

Fiber was originally popularized as a cholesterol-lowering nutrient in the 1960s. Recent research, however, suggests that not all fiber packs the same LDL-fighting punch. In a 2011 Italian study, men who ate foods enriched with beta-glucans for 4 weeks experienced a nearly 9 percent drop in LDL levels, compared to only 1 percent in those who ate foods enriched with rice bran. Unlike rice bran, beta-glucan is a soluble fiber, so it turns gummy, binds with cholesterol, and drags it out of your body. Make barley and oatmeal high-priority grains.

5 ADD BEANS TO YOUR PLATE

There's a reason that beans have a heart-healthy reputation. Consuming ½ cup of pintos every day may cut your LDL cholesterol by 8 percent, according to a study done by Arizona State University scientists. Like barley, pinto beans contain cholesterol-fighting beta-glucan. For a quick, fiber-filled veggie dip, pulse a cup of pinto beans, 2 tablespoons of olive oil, a dash of red-pepper flakes, and a tablespoon of chopped fresh parsley in a food processor until chunky.

6 EAT A GRAPEFRUIT A DAY

Grapefruit has often been touted as a weight-loss food. But it turns out that it's also a heart-saving fruit. Recent Israeli research reveals that eating a daily red grapefruit can lower your cholesterol by 20 percent. (If you're taking cholesterol-lowering medication—or any prescription drug for that matter—don't follow this advice, as grapefruit can compound the drug's negative effects.) If you hate the citrus fruit's tartness, try adding a little honey to your grapefruit, sprinkle it with cardamom, then stick it under the broiler for 2 to 3 minutes. For a savory twist, try stirring grapefruit wedges into your stir-fry after everything else is cooked.

7 . . . OR TWO APPLES

Apples really do keep the doctor away. In a study from Florida State University, women who snacked on dried apples (the equivalent of about two fresh apples) every day for a year experienced a 23 percent drop in bad cholesterol. Apples are rich in pectin, a type of soluble fiber that reduces your absorption of cholesterol, says study author Bahram Arjmandi, PhD, RD. Opt for raw apples—they have the same cholesterol-lowering benefit but are more filling than dried fruit.

8 PUMP UP YOUR TIRES

Get on your bike and ride! Women who bicycled for an hour three times a week saw a significant increase in HDL "good" cholesterol in a recent Lithuanian study. (They also lost weight!) Try hitting the trails: That way, you can ride without stopping for traffic, allowing you to maintain a consistently fast pace.

9 STOCK UP ON LEAN MEAT

Despite the heart-damaging reputation of meat, lean cuts may actually help lower your LDL cholesterol. Johns Hopkins University researchers recently found that a diet in which roughly 25 percent of the calories came from lean protein helped lower people's blood pressure, bad cholesterol, and triglycerides more effectively than a higher-carb diet. Make sure to work protein into every meal and snack—it also boosts satiety, so you eat less and stay fuller longer!

10 BAN SODA FROM YOUR FRIDGE

You don't have to drink soda for years to experience its negative effects. In a recent study, people who guzzled one high-fructose corn syrup–sweetened drink per meal for only 12 days saw a 17 percent increase in their LDL cholesterol. Your best bet is, of course, water, but you can also swap in coffee, seltzer water sweetened with juice, or tea.

11 SWITCH YOUR SPREAD

Why settle for sugary jelly on your toast? Research suggests that spreads that contain sterols, a compound from plants, may lower your LDL cholesterol by as much as 15 per-cent. Two tasty options: Smart Balance HeartRight Light (1.7 grams of sterols) and Promise Activ Light (1 gram of sterols). Unlike other vegetable spreads, they contain no hydrogenated oils, a source of heart-clogging trans fats. Shoot for 2 grams of sterols every day.

12 DISCOVER BLACK GARLIC

Unlike standard supermarket cloves, black garlic has been fermented, which gives it a sweet, caramel-like flavor (no bad breath!) and doubles its antioxidant content. These powerful compounds may help lower your cholesterol, says Janet Helm, MS, RD, of NutritionUnplugged blog. Try stirring black garlic into fondue or pasta sauce, or use it as a topping for homemade pizza.

Diabetes

16 simple ways to lower blood sugar

Diabetes is a devastating disease that is reaching epidemic levels worldwide. In the United States, more than 25 million people are living with the disease. Fifty-four million people may have the precursor to type 2 diabetes, called prediabetes or metabolic syndrome. Some experts believe both of those figures may be on the low side because many people have not been tested for diabetes.

Prediabetes and type 2 diabetes are caused primarily by dietary choices that raise blood sugar. After you finish eating a meal, your digestive system starts breaking down complex carbs—whole wheat bread, spinach, beans—into a simple sugar called glucose. As these glucose molecules rush into your bloodstream, the hormone insulin ushers them to cells throughout your body, a process that generally takes 3 to 4 hours. So far, so good: You fed your body whole grains, vegetables, and legumes, and your insulin transported the energy to your cells. But what happens when you eat white bread instead of whole wheat? Or a candy bar instead of a sensible salad?

The simple carbs in these junky foods immediately bombard your body with a hefty dose of glucose, causing your blood sugar to skyrocket and your insulin levels to rapidly rise. This totally depletes your bloodstream of glucose, so you eventually crash—and crave more junk to bring your blood sugar back up. In the long term, if

HOW TOP DOCTORS STAY SLIM

"Chronic inflammation plays a role in many serious illnesses. I try to eat more anti-inflammatory foods, such as salmon and sardines, which are rich in omega-3 fatty acids; antioxidant-dense fruits, vegetables, and nuts; and garlic, ginger, and turmeric."

—JEFFREY BLUMBERG, PhD, director of the antioxidants research laboratory at Tufts University you regularly eat high amounts of simple carbs, your cells may begin refusing to accept the glucose that insulin delivers. This is what doctors call "insulin resistance," or prediabetes.

When you're prediabetic, your pancreas stops making as much insulin, so sugar stays in your bloodstream longer. This can lead to chronically high blood sugar, and eventually full-blown diabetes. When it comes to dieting (and staying healthy), it's all about keeping your blood sugar levels steady—not too high, not too low. Although balanced blood sugar isn't a magic fat-blasting bullet, it does help stifle cravings, tame your hunger, and make you feel better overall as you lose.

■ **DRINK DECAF** If you're worried about your blood sugar, you may need to tame your coffee addiction. In a Canadian study, people who drank coffee after a big meal had 32 percent higher blood sugar levels for 8 hours than those who drank decaf. Blame the caffeine overload—it may disrupt glucose processing, causing your blood sugar to spike. Habitual elevations could increase your diabetes risk, so hold the repeated refills or switch to decaf.

■ **EAT MORE BLUEBERRIES** The little blue fruit may lower your blood sugar, according to Canadian researchers. In their study, overweight men who drank a cup of wild blueberry juice every day for 3 weeks experienced a roughly 10 percent drop in blood sugar. The pigments, called anthocyanins, that make the berries blue may help your pancreas do its job—that is, regulate your blood sugar levels. Frozen wild blueberries offer the same benefits as juice, the scientists say.

■ **GO FISH** The omega-3 fatty acids in fatty fish—wild salmon, tuna, sardines—can improve your body's ability to respond to insulin. Shoot for at least one serving of fatty fish per week. Try adding canned fish to your omelets or salads, or cook a fillet for dinner instead of red meat or chicken.

BONUS BENEFIT!

Omega-3 fatty acids may also reduce the dangerous effects of high blood pressure, according to a recent study review in the *British Journal of Nutrition*. The fatty acids are thought to ease stiffness in your arteries, allowing blood to flow more freely.

■ **TAME IT WITH CINNAMON** Cinnamon does more than warm up the flavor of your food. The antioxidants in the spice can help lower your blood sugar, according to a study by the USDA's Beltsville Human Nutrition Research Center. These compounds are thought to make your cells more responsive to insulin, effectively controlling the level of glucose circulating through your body. Your move: Sprinkle cinnamon on your frozen yogurt or oatmeal to slow the rush of carbs.

■ **SNACK ON HEALTHY FATS** About half an hour before a big meal, eat a small piece of cheese or a spoonful of peanut butter. Even a little fat can constrict the valve at the outlet of your stomach, slowing your rate of digestion and preventing a sudden blood sugar spike when you eat a major meal.

■ **EAT EARLY AND OFTEN** Never skip breakfast! You may think you're saving calories, but really, you're only setting yourself up for a blood sugar roller coaster the rest of the day. When your body is deprived of calories, your blood glucose shoots up when you do decide to eat—exactly the response you *don't* want. By contrast, if you supply your body with a steady stream of calories, you'll avoid a high insulin response come mealtime. (To keep your calorie intake under control, limit your meals to 500 calories or less, and snacks to fewer than 200.)

■ **SWITCH TO BROWN RICE** Thanks to its payload of fiber and magnesium, brown rice causes your blood sugar to rise less rapidly after a meal than white rice does. Hate the taste? Blend the two varieties until you become accustomed to the healthier grain. In a study in the *Archives of Internal Medicine,* swapping ⅓ cup cooked brown rice for white every day was linked to a 16 percent lower risk of diabetes.

■ **CUT TRANS FATS** Trans fats aren't just harmful to your heart—they can also raise your blood sugar levels. Even if a food's nutrition panel says "0 g trans fat," there may still be small but harmful amounts of the fats lurking inside that box (or tub of margarine). So scan the ingredient list instead of relying on the nutrition panel. Do you see any "hydrogenated" or "partially hydrogenated" oils? Shelve

it—those are all sources of the blood sugar–spiking fats.

■ **FUEL UP THE RIGHT WAY** Thirty to 90 minutes before you exercise, grab a healthy-carbohydrate-rich snack, such as a slice of whole grain bread or a piece of fruit, and pair it with a little protein. This helps you avoid an exercise-induced blood sugar drop, which makes you feel ravenous and prone to overeating afterward.

■ **REV UP YOUR CARDIO** High-intensity interval training—short, repeated bursts of aerobic exercise, followed by brief recovery periods—may lower your blood sugar response to food you eat later in the day, according to a 2012 McMaster University study of people with type 2 diabetes. Try the workout used in the study: On a stationary bike, cycle as hard as you can (ideally 80 to 100 rpm) for a minute, then rest for 60 seconds. Repeat 10 times. Try to work in two or three of these interval sessions per week.

■ **GET NUTTY** A recent study in the journal *Diabetes Care* found that people with type 2 diabetes who ate a handful of nuts every day had more stable blood sugar than those who ate whole-wheat muffins instead. Swapping carbs for healthy fats (like those in nuts) may keep your blood sugar in check—and even stave off diabetes, says study coauthor Cyril Kendall, PhD. Remember, nuts are still high in calories, so keep it to a palmful. More easy fat-for-carb swaps: a small amount of butter instead of jam on toast; bacon instead of potatoes; milk instead of a sports drink.

■ **BE A CARB SNOB** Make sure the carbs you do eat are loaded with fiber—think fruit, vegetables, legumes, and whole grains. The rough stuff slows the absorption of sugar into your bloodstream. "The more carbohydrates you eat, the more fiber becomes important to help minimize the wide fluctuations in blood sugar levels," says Jeff Volek, PhD, RD, a nutrition researcher at the University of Connecticut. Grab a banana: The yellow fruit contains "resistant starch," a type of fiber that your body digests more slowly, helping to keep your glucose stable longer.

■ **SWAP SODA WITH TEA** It's no secret that soda is loaded with sugar. And unlike fruit, which contains fructose and fiber, the liquid calories in soft drinks come from fructose and glucose. Glucose is a simple sugar that notoriously sends your blood sugar skyrocketing and deploys a rush of insulin, a fat-storing hormone. Ready to cut the junky drinks? Cut back gradually: If you rely on a midafternoon soda, say, drink it—but resist more random cravings throughout the day. Eventually, replace your afternoon hit with black, green, or oolong tea; these beverages have been shown to lower blood sugar.

■ **KEEP CALM** When your body senses stress, it releases hormones that increase blood sugar. Regular meditation or listening to calm music can help keep your stress—and blood sugar—under control. (For more about stress, see page 85.)

■ **EMBRACE BEANS** One study found that eating beans every day helped diabetic people keep their blood sugar under control. Credit the legumes' incredible load of fiber, a nutrient that slows your body's absorption of carbs. Try to work them onto your plate at least five times per week.

■ **SIP ON MILK** Adding low-fat dairy to your diet—a glass of 1% milk, a smoothie made with low-fat yogurt—could help preserve your cells' sensitivity to insulin. That means your body more efficiently mops up sugar from your bloodstream. In a 10-year study, overweight people who regularly consumed dairy were 70 percent less likely to develop insulin resistance than those who avoided it. "The lactose, protein, and fat in milk all have the potential to improve blood sugar," says researcher Mark Pereira, PhD. "Milk sugar [lactose] is converted to blood sugar at a relatively slow rate, which is good for blood sugar control. Protein helps fill you up. And fat may keep you feeling satisfied, too."

Fatigue

13 strategies for better sleep and faster weight loss

What could your hours tucked in bed—the only time you *can't* eat or exercise—possibly have to do with weight loss? Everything, actually. If you don't log enough shut-eye, your body cranks out more ghrelin, the appetite-triggering hormone, and less leptin, the appetite-suppressing hormone. The result: You feel less satiated by food and hungrier overall. Research shows that can lead you to consume as many as 300 extra calories each day! And even when sleep-deprived people do manage to drop weight, only a quarter of it is due to fat loss, compared to 50 percent in dieters who sleep longer.

That may be because a lack of sleep raises your levels of the stress hormone cortisol, which has been linked to belly fat storage. "There's a definite association between lack of sleep, increased stress hormones, and weight gain," says Michele Olson, PhD, an exercise researcher at Auburn University. During deep sleep, your brain secretes growth hormone, which tells your body how to break down fat for fuel. Without enough rest, you don't manufacture enough of the hormone to do the job.

Not only are you hungrier and more prone to fat storage, but you're also more likely to cave to temptation when you skimp on sleep. One study found that sleep-deprived folks reported more

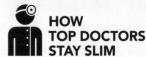

HOW TOP DOCTORS STAY SLIM

"Sleep deprivation simultaneously lowers your levels of the appetite-suppressing hormone leptin while boosting the appetite stimulant ghrelin. If you're tired and feel a craving for a Snickers bar, it's not because you're hungry but because you're sleepy. Knowing this has helped me understand the importance of being well rested when I need to shed some pounds."

—W. CHRISTOPHER WINTER, MD, medical director of the Martha Jefferson Hospital Sleep Medicine Center in Virginia intense cravings for salty snacks and sweets. Plus, after just 6 nights of sleep restriction, you may begin to show signs of insulin resistance, so you struggle to mop up sugar from your bloodstream, according to University of Chicago researchers. Luckily, you can break the sleep-fat cycle with strategic eating and lifestyle changes.

■ **CALCULATE YOUR HOURS** Too much or too little sleep can tack on extra pounds. In a Wake Forest University study, people under age 40 who slept 5 hours or less each night packed on nearly 2½ times more abdominal fat than those who logged 7 hours. However, sleeping too much was also linked to inflated waistlines. The reasons are obvious: People who sleep too little have more opportunity to eat, while those who sleep longer than 8 hours a night may be less active. The classic advice is your best bet: Aim for 7 to 8 hours per night.

■ **DEVELOP A PRESLEEP RITUAL** If you struggle to switch off at night, you may need a nightly habit to help you banish the day's stresses. Try meditating for 10 minutes before bed, or write down your plans for the next day. This can help you avoid late-night hours spent worrying about tomorrow—and hitting up the pantry.

■ **KEEP YOUR LAPTOP ON THE DESK** Your bed is not your office. "If you work in bed, you associate the bed with wakefulness and activity, not with sleep and relaxation," says Mark Rosekind, PhD, a former sleep scientist at NASA. Plus, the glow of your laptop's screen can disrupt your secretion of the sleep hormone melatonin. (Same goes for your smart-

phone.) Rather than messing with electronics, do something calming—read or take a bath, for example—in dim light before bed. That way, you'll nod off shortly after hitting the sheets.

■ **CLOSE THE CURTAINS** Light that leaks through your shades—from street lamps or the sunrise—can dampen your secretion of the sleep hormone melatonin. Try hanging room-darkening shades over your windows to maximize your melatonin. You can also wear a sleep mask to block out unwelcome light.

■ **RISE AND SHINE** If you miss the *Today* show, you may be at greater risk of weight gain. And it has nothing to do with Matt Lauer. Late risers consume more calories—nearly 200 more at dinner and 375 after 8:00 p.m.—and make poorer food choices than people who wake up around 8:00 a.m., according to a recent Northwestern University study. Specifically, people who wake up late eat more fast food and fewer servings of fruits and vegetables and drink more soda than early risers. Your goal: Set your alarm for the same time (ideally 8:00 a.m. or earlier) every day—even on the weekends. A consistent schedule can improve the quality of your sleep.

■ **EAT WITHIN AN HOUR OF YOUR ALARM** Your body interprets sleep as hours of starvation. That means you enter energy-conservation mode, burning only about 1.2 calories a minute. At the same time, your levels of leptin and insulin drop—both of which affect how fast your body converts food into fuel. It's up to you to shut off these sleep-induced changes come morning. The solution is simple: Eat breakfast without delay. If you chow down immediately after waking, you'll spike your leptin levels, notifying your body that your recent fast isn't a famine.

But don't just down a couple of Toaster Strudels and call it a morning. A sugar-packed breakfast will only lull your metabolism back to sleep. Your ideal meal is one that results in a slow, steady increase in insulin, rather than an immediate spike (which is inevitably followed by a crash). Whip up a breakfast rich in protein and fiber, such as cottage cheese topped with berries or scrambled eggs stuffed into a whole-wheat pita.

■ **MAKE DINNER YOUR SMALLEST MEAL** Americans have a tendency to cap off their day with a giant-size dinner. But, really, dinner should be your smallest meal. Since your metabolism slows to a crawl while you sleep, you don't need to load up on energy right before bed. Make breakfast your biggest meal, and gradually decrease your intake as the day goes on. Aim to stop eating 3 hours before you go to bed.

■ **SNACK WISELY BEFORE BED** If you're cutting calories throughout the day, you may find yourself hungry before bed. Nothing deters sleep like a growling tummy, and once you do doze off, you may wake up frequently, since hunger pangs can rouse you. If you need the occasional bedtime snack, choose one that's rich in belly-filling protein while offering a dose of healthy carbs. (Nighttime carbs can help trigger melatonin secretion.) Perfect night bites: an apple and cheese, or a thin turkey sandwich. Avoid spicy or high-fat foods, which can make it harder to fall asleep.

■ **SET YOUR THERMOSTAT FOR SLEEP** If you're too warm in bed, your internal alarm assumes it's time to rise, so sleep becomes fitful. A bedroom temperature between 68° and 74°F is ideal for solid slumber, says Tracey Marks, MD, a psychiatrist, sleep specialist, and author of *Master Your Sleep*. Still wake up sweating? Try outfitting your bed with 400-thread-count sheets, which are breathable but soft.

■ **CUT OFF THE CAFFEINE** The caffeine in coffee and tea is a natural metabolism booster. However, guzzling the stuff after 4:00 p.m. can prevent you from falling asleep at night.

■ **EXERCISE IN THE A.M.** Morning workouts are great—especially if you head outside. The early-morning light helps your body reset itself to a healthier sleep/wake cycle, plus pre-breakfast exercise can help you burn fat more efficiently. The caveat: You have to hit the sack by 10:00 p.m. Skimping on sleep even in order to make it to the gym can still elevate your risk of weight gain. If you live for the morning endorphin rush, but struggle to get to bed on time, keep it to three or four times per week.

■ **TAKE A QUICK NAP** Instead of hitting the vending machine at 3:00 p.m., find a quiet place for a siesta. (Hint: your car.) Just 15 to 20 minutes is enough to energize your body without affecting your ability to sleep come bedtime.

■ **TIME YOUR DRINKS** If you love a glass of wine with dinner, make sure to dine before 7:00 p.m. Drinking too late can delay dream (REM) sleep, so you wake up frequently during the night.

Hormones

How to harness your body's chemical messengers to shed pounds

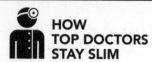

HOW TOP DOCTORS STAY SLIM

"As a dean, I have an all-you-can-eat job—it's packed with lunches and breakfasts. But those breakfast scones are 600 calories! So I've had to learn to say no. But every now and then I'll treat myself to a bite instead of having the entire thing."

—ALLEN LEVINE, PhD, dean of the College of Food, Agricultural and Natural Resource Sciences at the University of Minnesota

Every time you eat, you experience a rush of hormones that determine how full you feel. And in between meals, another set of hormones takes over, prompting you to eat certain foods. Add stress, sex, and thyroid hormones—all of which have been shown to affect which foods you reach for—to the mix, and it becomes clear: Your body is largely at the mercy of whichever hormones are circulating through your bloodstream. Luckily, you have some say in the matter—and can even harness your hormones to help you lose weight. Let's explore your hormones and how you can use them to your advantage.

THE FULLNESS HORMONES

■ **LEPTIN** Leptin, your primary fullness hormone, is released into your bloodstream from your fat cells. As it circulates through your body, it sends your brain information about the status of your body's energy stores. "When leptin signals to the brain, it triggers the production of a family of molecules called melanocortins," says Giles Yeo, PhD, a researcher for the Institute of Metabolic Science at the University of Cambridge. "These reduce appetite and therefore reduce food intake." Leptin may also increase your calorie burning, according to a 2006 study review in *Obesity*. Unfortunately, consistently overeating can cause your body to become resistant to leptin.

■ **CHOLECYSTOKININ (CCK)** Cholecystokinin controls the rate at which nutrients are delivered to your small intestine. Unlike leptin, it doesn't communicate directly with your brain. Rather, it stamps out your appetite and prevents food from exiting your stomach, a 2012 British study review reports. Your intestines release CCK primarily in response to fat and protein; your levels remain elevated for about 5 hours after a meal.

■ **PEPTIDE YY (PYY)** Like CCK, peptide YY is a hormone released by your intestinal cells to help control both your appetite and intake of fat, while making you feel satisfied after a meal. (It may also boost your calorie burning and help you break down fat.) Your levels of the hormone generally peak 1 to 2 hours after a meal, then remain high for several more hours. The problem: When you're obese, you not only have a lower baseline level of PYY, but your body may also release less of it after you eat, British scientists say. That means you miss out on the full potential of its appetite-squashing effects.

■ **GLUCAGON-LIKE PEPTIDE-1 (GLP-1)** Between 5 and 15 minutes after you eat, your levels of glucagon-like peptide—a gut hormone—rise according to the number of calories you consumed. This stimulates the release of insulin (which mops up sugar in your blood) while blocking the release of glucagon (see below), the British review says. GLP-1 has been shown to promote weight loss and may also help you feel full and satisfied.

■ **GLUCAGON** This hormone tells your liver to break down stored carbs into glucose, or sugar, to keep your blood sugar steady. Glucagon is a good thing, unless your liver is unhealthy. When you have a fatty liver, the glucagon in your body may mishandle sugar, so your blood sugar rises unnecessarily.

■ **PANCREATIC POLYPEPTIDE (PP)** Secreted primarily from your GI tract, pancreatic polypeptide is thought to reduce your food intake by directly communicating with your brain. Studies suggest that obese people may have lower levels of PP, as is the case with other appetite-regulating hormones.

■ **OXYNTOMODULIN** This is yet another hormone that helps you set down the fork. It's released from your intestines about 5 to 10 minutes after a meal and peaks after half an hour, according to a review in the *Journal of Human Nutrition and Dietetics*. When British researchers injected overweight people with oxyntomodulin three times a day for a month, the people ate 250 fewer calories per day and dropped 5 pounds over the course of the study.

How to Trigger Your Fullness Hormones

■ **SNACK ON SUNFLOWER SEEDS** A 2008 study from Denmark found that when men were given oleic acid (a type of monounsaturated fat), their levels of GLP-1 shot up and remained high for 5 hours. Luckily, there are foods that naturally contain the healthy fat: almonds, olive oil, olives, sunflower seeds, dark chocolate, and even steak.

■ **SAVOR YOUR FOOD** Taking half an hour to eat can raise your levels of PYY and GLP-1, according to Alexander Kokkinos, MD, PhD, of the University of Athens Medical School. In his research, he found that men who scarfed a bowl of ice cream in 5 minutes had lower levels of the fullness hormones than guys who devoted 30 minutes to their treat.

■ **PACK IN PROTEIN** Protein is one of the primary nutrients that trigger the release of fullness hormones. Plus, as a slow-digesting substance, protein ensures that you have a steady supply of the hunger-fighting chemicals. Make sure to choose lean sources of protein, such as chicken breast, tuna, or eggs.

For more fullness enhancers, see Protein on page 229.

THE HUNGER HORMONES

■ **GHRELIN** As the "hunger hormone," ghrelin is leptin's nemesis. When your belly starts rumbling, you're feeling the effects of ghrelin, which is secreted primarily from your stomach (but also from your pancreas). The effect: It prevents leptin from doing its appetite-suppressing job, according to the *Obesity* review. When your belly is empty, your ghrelin levels shoot up; when it's full, your ghrelin levels decline. Think of ghrelin as a dinner bell—when it floods your bloodstream, you head to the table.

■ **NEUROPEPTIDE Y (NPY)** Once ghrelin reaches your brain, it stirs up neuropeptide Y, a stress hormone that makes you crave carbs, awakens your appetite, and lowers your metabolic rate. It's particularly active in the morning, making you susceptible to the call of Krispy Kreme. New research suggests that NPY is manufactured by visceral fat—the dangerous blubber that congregates around your midsection.

■ **GALANIN** Around lunchtime, the hunger hormone galanin wakes up and levels rise until the evening, when it peaks. It's produced in your brain and sends signals to make you crave fat (and possibly alcohol).

How to Harness Your Hunger Hormones

■ **EAT HEALTHY CARBS FOR BREAKFAST** Grab a slice of whole-wheat toast or nuke a packet of instant oatmeal. A dose of early-morning carbs will help keep neuropeptide Y quiet. Make sure to eat within an hour of waking up—otherwise, your body will only pump out more "feed me" hormones.

■ **THINK THIN** As soon as you wake up, tell yourself, "I will eat right today." Just thinking about healthy foods may suppress a ghrelin tsunami. In a Yale University study, people who considered drinking a "sensible" milkshake had lower levels of the hunger hormone than those who were told the shake was "indulgent."

■ **SNACK STRATEGICALLY** A couple of hours before lunch, your ghrelin levels begin to creep up. Stifle them with a snack. The perfect midmorning munchie is one that combines healthy carbs and protein, both of which help quiet ghrelin. Your go-to nibble: low-fat Greek yogurt with fresh blueberries.

■ **DON'T EAT TAKEOUT FOR LUNCH** Although galanin, the fat-craving hormone, spikes at lunchtime, trying to calm it with a fatty meal won't do you any favors. In fact, it will only cause your body to release *more* galanin, so you crave *more* fat. It's a vicious cycle. At lunchtime, your ghrelin is also rising. Although protein has been shown to suppress ghrelin most effectively over a 6-hour period, complex carbs have a stronger effect in the shorter term. So to stamp out both hormones, fill up on protein and complex carbs at your midday meal. Chicken-vegetable soup or black bean chili should do the trick.

■ **AVOID A SUGAR HIGH** Foods that are loaded with sugar—ice cream, cake, dough-nuts—raise your levels of ghrelin. And once you awaken this hormone, you'll have trouble stopping at just one bite. If you can't cut out sweets altogether (or struggle to stop after a few spoonfuls), buy single-serve treats so your portions are controlled for you.

■ **CATCH UP ON SLEEP** When you're sleepy, your gut produces more ghrelin, so you're driven to indulge in sugary foods. "It causes your body to seek quick energy from food to try to keep you awake," says W. Christopher Winter, MD, medical director of the Martha Jefferson Sleep Medicine Center in Virginia. (In an unfair double whammy, a lack of sleep also reduces your levels of leptin, the appetite-suppressing hormone.) Lie down for a quick power nap—even if it's in your car in the parking lot outside of your office. Just 10 minutes of shut-eye can ward off fatigue (and boost your brainpower), according to Australian researchers. You should also make sure to avoid caffeine within 8 hours of bedtime.

■ **STAY ACTIVE** Don't worry: Exercise won't cause you to eat more later in the day, British research suggests. In the study, men who hit the treadmill for 90 minutes consumed just as many calories over the next 24 hours as they did on days they skipped the gym. The reason: Physical activity may suppress your secretion of ghrelin, the scientists say. To maximize the hunger-dampening effect of exercise, make your cardio workout more intense by adding intervals—that is, quick bursts of speed with short periods of rest in between.

■ **EAT HEALTHY FATS FOR DINNER** In the early evening, your levels of ghrelin and galanin begin to creep up again. Now is the time to incorporate some good-for-you fats. Look for monounsaturated and polyunsaturated fats. (Hint: You'll find them in olive oil, nuts, and fatty fish, such as salmon and mackerel.) Eat an early dinner, since dining after 8:00 p.m. has been linked to weight gain.

THE STRESS HORMONE

■ **CORTISOL** Cortisol is released from your adrenal glands in response to danger or stress. The effect: Your heart begins to race, oxygen pumps into your brain, and you seek sweet and fatty foods for instant energy. If your body is perpetually plagued by cortisol, you may begin to store more fat in your belly.

How to Control Cortisol

■ **AVOID ALCOHOL** Drinking excessive alcohol ramps up your body's levels of cortisol, driving your body to squirrel away fat. Eliminate alcohol altogether or limit yourself to one or two drinks per occasion.

■ **FUEL UP AFTER EXERCISE** When you exercise, you experience a rush of cortisol—it's what gives you that extra push, even when you're starting to wear out. (Surprisingly, it's also been shown to play a part in the antidepressant-like effect of exercise.) However, if the stress hormone lingers too long, it prevents muscle repair and kicks your body into fat-storage mode. The key is noshing on protein—a hard-cooked egg or low-fat yogurt, for example—within half an hour of an intense workout. If you're making a smoothie, throw in a handful of blueberries or strawberries. A shot of vitamin C can also dampen the effects of cortisol, according to German scientists.

■ **SNACK ON WALNUTS** If you're feeling the heat at work, grab a handful of walnuts. They're a rich source of omega-3 fatty acids, shown to keep your cortisol in check in a recent National Institutes of Health study. Other ways to eat them: chopped up in oatmeal, mixed into casseroles, or even ground up in smoothies.

(For more ways to control cortisol, see Stress on page 85.)

THE THYROID HORMONES

■ **THYROID-STIMULATING HORMONE (TSH)** Your pituitary gland, located at the base of your brain, pumps out thyroid-stimulating hormone. When your levels of TSH are low, it's a sign that your thyroid gland is underactive; this may lead to unexpected or sudden weight gain.

■ **THYROXINE (T4)** Once TSH is released, your thyroid gland produces thyroxine—the major form of thyroid hormone that circulates through your body. If your levels of T4 are low, you may have hypothyroidism—or underactive thyroid.

■ **TRIIODOTHYRONINE (T3)** Once inside your cells, T4 is converted to triiodothyronine, or T3, which directly regulates your energy levels and every aspect of your metabolism, from your heart rate to the number of calories you burn. If you're lacking in either T4 or T3, your metabolism slows down (hypothyroidism).

■ **REVERSE T3 (RT3)** In response to stress (or selenium deficiency), your body may raise its levels of reverse T3. Elevated rT3 usually indicates hypothyroidism.

How to Control Your Thyroid Hormones

■ **VISIT YOUR DOCTOR** This is one problem you don't want to leave unchecked. If you detect warning signs of thyroid trouble—say, you've been feeling unusually tired or have gained unexplained weight—ask your doctor to administer a thyroid-stimulating hormone test. This simple blood test can help determine whether your thyroid function has gone awry. You can also request that your T4 and T3 levels be tested.

SELF-TEST: IS YOUR THYROID MAKING YOU FAT?

Hypothyroidism, or underactive thyroid, is when your thyroid fails to crank out enough of its hormones. This can lead to weight gain, even if you're eating all of the right foods, according to the National Institutes of Health. Take this quiz to find out if your thyroid may be slacking off.

1. Do you frequently have to turn up the heat in your house?
2. Are you often constipated?
3. Have you felt unusually weak during your normal workouts?
4. Does your face look puffy?
5. Is your hair dry and thinning?
6. Women only: Are your menstrual periods unusually heavy or irregular?

If you answered yes to any of these questions and have unexplained weight gain, ask your doctor to test you for hypothyroidism.

■ **CHECK YOUR NECK** Every 2 months, perform a thyroid self-check. If the gland is swollen, you may be pumping out too much or too little thyroid hormone, according to the American College of Endocrinology. Step 1: Hold a mirror in front of you and zero in on the lower front area of your neck (right above your collarbone and below your Adam's apple). Step 2: Tilt your head back, moving the mirror along with you. Step 3: Take a medium-size sip of water. Step 4: As you swallow, watch your thyroid area. See any unusual bulges? Go see your doctor.

■ **MONITOR YOUR IODINE INTAKE** Iodine is essential to your thyroid—it helps the gland regulate your body's use of energy and control your metabolism. So, without enough of the element, you may begin to feel lethargic or gain weight. (Left untreated, iodine deficiency may even cause thyroid cancer.) The problem is, one of the best sources of iodine is table salt (i.e., iodized salt), which most nutritionists will tell you to avoid.

Instead of sprinkling salt on every meal, take a daily multivitamin that contains iodine plus other thyroid-supporting nutrients such as selenium, says Angela Leung, MD, an assistant professor of medicine at Boston University. Make sure the iodine in your multi comes from potassium iodide, rather than kelp, and keep it to a dose of 150 micrograms. Overloading on iodine (1,100 micrograms or more per day for adults) can actually hurt your thyroid.

■ **WAGE WAR ON BPA** Bisphenol A (BPA), the chemical embedded in certain types of plastics, may disrupt your thyroid function, according to physician Rashel J. Tahzib, DO, of Advance Health Integrative Medicine in Los Angeles. Protect yourself with the strategies beginning on page 46.

THE FEMALE SEX HORMONE

■ **ESTROGEN** The female sex hormone may increase sensitivity to leptin (the fullness hormone) while quieting neuropeptide Y (the hormone that makes you crave carbs), according to a 2010 study review in the journal *Brain Research*. The hormone may also protect against deep, dangerous visceral fat, which concentrates around your middle. Unfortunately, estrogen is also associated with accumulation of subcutaneous fat—the kind that's just below the surface. As women's ovaries secrete less estrogen with age, they may gain weight due to the side effects of declining estrogen, such as disrupted sleep, and begin packing on the pounds around their middle.

How to Regulate Estrogen

■ **EAT A WHOLE-FOODS DIET** The right diet doesn't just help you lose weight. "Cruciferous vegetables like cabbage and cauliflower, citrus fruits, and whole grains are crucial for regulating estrogen," says ob-gyn C. W. Randolph, MD, of the Natural Hormone Institute in Jacksonville, Florida. Cut out processed junk, and fill up on foods like kale, spinach, oranges, and brown rice.

■ **MONITOR YOUR MEATS** Avoid buying fatty foods, like meats, that are packaged in plastic wrap. Synthetic chemicals that mimic estrogen are often embedded in PVC, a material found in the plastic wrap that supermarkets use. These scary chemicals may trick your body into storing fat. (Your plastic wrap at home is safer, since it's made from more benign polyethylene.)

■ **EMPHASIZE HEALTHY FATS** Dietary fat helps your body produce estrogen. So if you eat too little of the stuff, your estrogen levels may dangerously drop. Just make sure your calories come from poly- and monounsaturated fats, found in foods like olive oils, nuts, and avocados.

THE MALE SEX HORMONE

■ **TESTOSTERONE (T)** The male sex hormone plays the same role in men and women: It helps build muscle, revs up your libido, and boosts your metabolism. Weight gain can cause your testosterone levels to dip.

How to Boost Testosterone

■ **LIFT WEIGHTS SLOWLY** Weight training raises testosterone—and the right technique can increase the T-boosting benefit. When you lift weights, do it slowly, taking 6 seconds per rep (3 up, 3 down). This increases your body's T production more than lifting faster does, according to a recent Japanese study.

■ **DRINK WHILE YOU GRUNT** Lifting weights while you're dehydrated can dampen the release of testosterone while ramping up the release of fat-storing cortisol, a study in the *Journal of Applied Physiology* found. Make sure to guzzle a glass of water before you hit the bench, especially if you exercise in the morning (when you're more likely to be dehydrated), and take water breaks periodically during your workout.

■ **MAKE ROOM FOR MONOUNSATURATED FATS** Trimming dangerous lard from your diet can help you stay lean. But eliminating all fat can cause your T levels to plummet. A study published in the *International Journal of Sports Medicine* found that men who consumed the most fat also had the highest testosterone levels. To protect your heart and preserve your T, focus on foods high in healthy monounsaturated fats, such as nuts, fatty fish, and olive oil.

■ **SLEEP FOR 8 HOURS** It's not just bedroom thrills that impact your T levels. The amount of time you spend asleep between the sheets also plays a role in regulating your testosterone. Research shows that a shortage of shut-eye can interfere with your production of the hormone. The best sleep schedule is one that's consistent—pick a bedtime that allows for 8 hours of sleep, and stick with it.

THE PANCREATIC HORMONE

■ **INSULIN** This is the hormonal "key" that opens the door for glucose to move from your blood into your cells, where it's either burned or stored. Insulin resistance occurs when your body no longer responds to the hormone, allowing sugar to linger in your bloodstream, possibly causing hunger, overeating, and plummeting energy levels. When your body stops responding to insulin, you may churn out even more insulin, and that can cause your body to store fat. Eventually, insulin resistance can develop into full-blown diabetes.

How to Make Insulin Efficient

■ **MAKE MUSCLE** Adding lean muscle to your frame may help insulin do its job in your body, according to a study in the *Journal of Clinical Endocrinology and Metabolism*. The researchers found that for every 10 percent increase in muscle mass, people's risk of prediabetes dropped by 12 percent. Incorporate 3 days of lifting into your workout plan, resting 1 day in between sessions.

■ **FIBER UP** Fiber prevents postmeal blood sugar spikes by slowing the flow of glucose into your bloodstream. If you have a sweet-tooth attack, curb it with fruit instead of dessert. Although fruit contains sugar, it also packs a serious fiber punch to slow down the absorption of the sugar. A word of caution: Exercise portion control when it comes to canned, dried, and tropical fruits like pineapple and mango, which are concentrated with sugar and calories.

■ **ADD A DASH** Sprinkling cinnamon on your food may reduce your blood sugar levels. That's because the spice contains a specific type of antioxidant that helps insulin do its job in your body. Try adding it to your oatmeal, yogurt, or coffee.

(For more ways to tame your blood sugar, see Diabetes on page 19.)

Hunger

28 ways to keep the pangs at bay

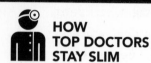
If anything dooms a diet, it's hunger. The longer your stomach growls, the more dangerous it becomes: With every passing minute, you grow crankier—and the call of the drive-thru or the bag of chips becomes harder to ignore. You know you have to eat to feel full, or, as scientists call it, satiated. The tricky part is determining what exactly flips that fullness switch.

It isn't merely a matter of loading up your plate. Rather, it's about choosing foods that trigger the release of fullness hormones, chemicals that rush into your bloodstream when you eat. Think of these hormones as signals to your brain that you're full and to your body that you should stop eating. One of the most important fullness hormones is leptin, which is released from your fat cells. It acts as your primary appetite suppressor and signal of satiety. The key to keeping your calorie intake in check is harnessing these hormones through what you eat, when you eat it, and even where you dine. Here's how:

■ **LOSE WEIGHT GRADUALLY** Although severely cutting calories may help you lose weight quickly, you'll most likely gain it all back once you resume a more normal diet. The reason: Extremely calorie-restrictive diets reduce your levels of leptin, encouraging you to eat more. To keep your leptin in balance, aim to lose weight at a slow, steady pace—about 1 to 2 pounds per week. To do that, trim about 500 calories from your daily diet (or cut 250 calories and burn another 250 through exercise).

■ **PACK IN THE PROTEIN** Make sure to eat a serving of protein—skinless chicken breast, eggs, chunk light tuna—at every meal. Protein has been shown to raise satiety hormone levels, helping you stay full and satisfied longer. This means you're less likely to overeat. In a Purdue University study, dieters who ate 30 percent of their calories from protein reported feeling more satisfied and less hungry than those who ate only 18 percent of their calories from protein. If you're a vegetarian, prioritize hearty, protein-rich vegetables like portobello mushrooms and eggplant.

■ **FILL UP ON FIBER** Like protein, fiber helps you feel full faster, longer. Your body breaks down fiber-rich foods more slowly, plus the rough stuff helps put the brakes on glucose and other nutrients as they enter your bloodstream (so you enjoy a steady stream, rather than a momentary rush).

Foods high in fiber also tend to be high in volume, so they fill you up for fewer calories. To maximize your intake, choose whole grains over refined and fruit over fruit juice, and add more beans to your diet. Try tossing the legumes into your salad, or add them to your soup or stew.

■ **FRONTLOAD YOUR CALORIES** Skipping meals is never wise—but forgoing breakfast is especially detrimental to your diet. What you eat in the a.m. sets the tone for the rest of your day. A recent study in the *British Journal of Nutrition* found that people who ate more fat, protein, and carbs in the morning stayed satisfied and ate less later than those who made lunch or dinner their largest meal. Studies show that eggs are particularly effective at staving off midmorning hunger pangs. However, if time is an issue, portion out some Greek yogurt and slice up fruit before you go to bed at night, or stash instant oatmeal, such as Quaker Weight Control, and ground flaxseed at your desk.

■ **EAT A BORING DIET** Ever wonder why you overeat at buffets? One word: *variety*. Eating a range of foods skews your body's fullness detectors. Each new flavor—sugary salad dressing, salty french fries, savory meats—fires up your appetite, even if you've had enough. But if you remove the novelty of new foods, you'll pay attention to how each item on your plate fills your belly rather than how it tastes on your tongue. You don't have to eat the same exact meal every day. Rather, establish a routine, such as eating a soup-and-salad combo for lunch every day.

■ **GUZZLE GREEN TEA** Coffee fires you up, but green tea fills you up. According to a 2010 study in *Nutrition Journal*, people who drank green tea with a meal felt 51 percent fuller 2 hours afterward than those who sipped on water. Adding another flavor to your meal, without adding significant calories, may promote satiety, as do the catechins found in both hot and cold teas. Try Honest Tea Community

THE SATIETY INDEX

In a landmark 1995 study, Australian researchers measured the "satiating capacity" of 38 different foods. What they found: Foods high in fiber, protein, and water are best at satisfying hunger for the longest period of time. Here's a useful guide of common foods ranked from least satiating to most. The higher the score, the more satisfying the food.

LEAST SATISFYING FOODS

47	Croissants
65	Chocolate cake
68	Doughnuts
70	Candy bars
84	Peanuts
88	Yogurt
96	Ice cream
100	White bread
116	French fries
116	Special K cereal
118	Bananas
118	Cornflakes
120	Cookies
127	Crackers
132	Brown rice
133	Lentils
146	Cheddar cheese
150	Eggs
151	All-Bran cereal
154	Popcorn
154	Rye bread
157	Whole-wheat bread
162	Grapes
168	Baked beans
176	Steak
188	Whole-grain pasta
197	Apples
202	Oranges
209	Oatmeal
225	Fish
323	Boiled potatoes

MOST SATISFYING FOODS

Green Tea, which is higher in antioxidants and lower in sugar than most bottled brews.

■ **START WITH SOUP** Eating a high-fat soup as an appetizer can actually help you lose weight. When your small intestine absorbs fat, it releases hormones that make you feel full. Eat 2 cups of a bisque, chowder, or cream soup with no more than 100 calories per cup, then wait half an hour before diving into your entrée. This gives your appetite time to catch up.

■ **. . . OR SALAD** In a recent Penn State University study, people who ate a salad with their meal consumed 11 percent fewer calories than when they skipped the course. Credit the superfilling but low-calorie fiber in greens.

BONUS BENEFIT!

Romaine lettuce—one of the dark-leaf varieties—is loaded with vision-preserving vitamin A, as well as vitamin C and vitamin K, an essential nutrient for blood clotting.

■ **SAVOR YOUR FOOD** If you wolf down your dinner, you're more likely to go back for round two, since it takes about 20 minutes for your stomach to realize it's full. In fact, slow eaters consume about 67 fewer calories per meal, according to University of Rhode Island research. Need a slowdown strategy? Try holding your fork in your nondominant hand. This gives you the time to recognize fullness.

■ **DIM THE LIGHTS** The glow of the Golden Arches is dangerous in more ways than one. "Bright lights encourage you to eat faster than you otherwise would because they make you feel stressed," says Brian Wansink, PhD, director of the Cornell University Food and Brand Lab. But don't eat by candlelight, either. Mood lighting tends to lower your inhibitions, encouraging you to cap off your meal with a dessert. Medium-wattage incandescent bulbs (60 to 75 watts) are your best bet.

■ **GO BANANAS** If you don't have the self-control to hit slo-mo, opt for foods that are impossible to scarf: produce you have to peel, nuts in the shell, or spicy foods (which may also give your metabolism a boost!).

■ **FILL UP ON FISH** The benefits of seafood keep adding up. In a recent study from Iceland, dieters who ate salmon felt fuller 2 hours later than those who didn't eat seafood or dined on cod, a fish with little fat. The omega-3s found in fatty fish boost your levels of the satiety hormone leptin, the scientists say. Top sources? Spanish mackerel packs 1,140 milligrams (mg) of omega-3s, sockeye salmon offers 766 mg, and pollack contains 484 mg per 3-ounce serving.

■ **SNACK ON RAW CARROTS** Carrots are more filling when they're uncooked, according to researchers in Ireland. Try dipping baby carrots in hummus—both are loaded with belly-filling fiber—or dice the orange veggie up and add it to your salads and slaws.

■ **CHOOSE STARCHES WISELY** If you need a starch fix, opt for yams or white potatoes (with skin) over a fluffy croissant or a yeasty roll. Research shows they're far more filling. Just make sure to bake or roast your spuds instead of frying them.

■ **PUMP UP YOUR SMOOTHIE** Skip the sugary juices and syrups. Instead, build your smoothie around low-fat yogurt and frozen fruit, then add 1 or 2 tablespoons of whey protein powder to your drink. The extra protein punch may trigger the release of the hormones that make you feel full.

■ **AVOID DRIED FRUIT** Think of it this way: For the same amount of calories, you can eat an entire cup of grapes or an unsatisfying 3 tablespoons of raisins. Whole fruit allows you to consume larger portions, plus the water content helps fill you up. Swap your Raisin Bran for shredded wheat topped with fresh blueberries, raspberries, or strawberries (or all three).

■ **TALK AS YOU EAT** Taking breaks while you dine may help you stay fuller longer, according to Dutch scientists. In their study, people who spent 2 hours eating a meal—with a few 20-minute breaks—reported a higher level of satiety afterward than those who took less time to eat. The explanation: A leisurely pace allows your fullness hormones to gradually increase. The perfect duration? Half an hour. If you linger around the table too long, you may be tempted to dish out seconds.

■ **CRANK UP THE HEAT** It's not just internal signals that determine how full you feel. Temperature can also influence your satisfaction—the cooler a room, the more people tend to eat. (This is why restaurants are usually slightly chilly.) At mealtime, turn up the heat a few degrees.

■ **PULL UP A CHAIR** When you sit down to eat for a 20-minute dinner, it tells your brain, "This is a meal." But when you eat in the car or standing over the sink, you tend to speed eat, so your brain doesn't recognize it as a meal. The result? You don't register fullness. Make a point to put your food on a plate and eat at the table for breakfast, lunch, and dinner.

■ **CONTROL YOUR SENSES** Even the smell of a fresh-baked cookie can induce insulin secretion, making you think you're hungry. Likewise, the sight of a tempting treat can trigger your appetite, so avert your eyes (or ask the waiter to remove your plate before you scarf the rest).

■ **FILL UP ON WATER** Don't forget to drink. If you take a sip of water after every bite, you'll not only slow down your shoveling, but you'll also fill up on liquid instead of calorie-dense food. Water helps stretch out your stomach—and once the stomach reaches its max capacity, your brain knows it's time to stop chowing down.

■ **TAKE SMALL BITES** Mind your manners to lose more weight. In a recent Dutch study, people who took large bites of food and chewed for 3 seconds consumed 52 percent more food before feeling full than those who noshed on small bites for 9 seconds. Before you dive in, try cutting your food into bite-size pieces no larger than an inch, and chew at least 20 times before swallowing. Chewing is thought to stimulate nerves in your jaw connected to the brain region that controls satiety.

■ **APPRECIATE YOUR FOOD** Any chef will tell you that taste isn't everything. Presentation—how the food looks on the plate—and other sensory factors play a role in your perception of fullness. If you take the time to smell your food, look at it, and think about each bite, you may find that it's more satisfying.

■ **DRAW YOUR SHADES** Losing sleep can meddle with the hormones that switch your appetite on and off. If you aren't well rested, your food won't satisfy you as much as it would if you'd logged your 8 hours. A simple sleep solution: Close your curtain. You'll block out early-morning light (or street lamps) that can dampen your secretion of melatonin, the sleep hormone.

■ **USE THICKER PLATES AND BOWLS** The container you carry your lunch in could influence your fullness. A 2012 Spanish study review found that the heavier a bowl, the more satisfying people expected its contents to be. They also thought that yogurt in a heavy bowl was denser than the same snack in a lighter bowl. It's what scientists call "sensation transference"—your perception of plateware can influence your perception of its contents. So rather than using flimsy paper plates or plastic containers, use more substantial glass dishes and storage containers.

SELF-TEST: DO YOU REALLY NEED TO EAT?
Rate your hunger to gain control over bingeing

You are more likely to stuff yourself if you eat according to external stimuli—what time it is, how many chips are left in the bag, when you're feeling bored—than what your body is telling you. Use this scale to rate your hunger, and aim to eat when you're in the 3 to 4 range. By the time you hit 5 or 6, you run the risk of overeating or making unhealthy choices since you're so famished, says Dawn Jackson Blatner, RD, a nutrition consultant for the Chicago Cubs.

1. You don't feel hungry.
2. Food sounds good, but you couldn't eat an entire apple.
3. Your stomach feels empty.
4. Your stomach is growling.
5. Your stomach and head hurt.
6. You are irritable and can't focus. Eating feels like an emergency.

■ **RECOGNIZE FULLNESS** Pause as you eat to ask yourself, "Do I feel bloated? Does this still taste as good as it did at first?" Your stomach essentially has three settings: stuffed, full, and starving. Learning to rely on internal cues—that is, how your body feels—can help you stop eating when you reach the "full" stage. If you rely on external cues, such as the end of a TV show or a clean plate, you're more likely to overdo it.

■ **SNACK BEFORE DINNER** If you're eating a late dinner out, a healthy snack can help tide you over and prevent a hunger-induced breadbasket raid. Limit your munching to a 150- to 200-calorie snack, such as yogurt with fruit or 2 tablespoons of natural peanut butter. That way, you'll be comfortably hungry, rather than starving, by dinnertime.

■ **LIVEN UP FOODS WITH VINEGAR** The acidity of vinegar enhances other flavors, whether sweet, salty, savory, or bitter. This may explain why it's been shown to boost the satiety of foods. Add vinegar to a marinade, or splash a little on your leafy greens.

N.E.A.T.

50 strategies to burn more calories all day long

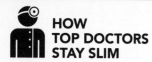

HOW TOP DOCTORS STAY SLIM

"I try to fit in small activities throughout the day. Our campus is pretty big, and I know a lot of shortcuts. But I try to take the longer route, and I take the stairs whenever possible. One year, my assigned parking lot changed, and instead of being a 20-minute walk from my building, it was a 5-minute walk. I gained weight that year, and the only thing that changed was my walk to and from the car—proof that little things add up."

—**DAVID SARWER, PhD,** a psychologist at the University of Pennsylvania's Center for Weight and Eating Disorders

Your metabolism has three components: basal metabolism (the calories you burn to stay alive), the thermic effect of food (the calories you burn digesting food), and finally, physical activity. This includes exercise—lifting weights, playing basketball, going for a jog—but also the little physical actions you perform over the course of your day. This could be walking across the parking lot, typing on your keyboard, cooking dinner, even nervously bouncing your leg as you sit at the computer. The calories you burn during such activities are called "non-exercise-activity thermogenesis." "N.E.A.T. is the amount of energy expended by your muscles during incidental movement," explains Alex Koch, PhD, an exercise scientist at Truman State University.

These everyday small movements can easily add up to 350 calories burned per day. In fact, "a conscious effort to spend more time on your feet might net a greater calorie burn than 30 minutes of daily exercise," says Brandon Alderman, PhD, an assistant professor of exercise science at Rutgers University. However, N.E.A.T. is the most variable metabolic component: In overweight people, it can run as low as 15 percent of total calories burned. In leaner folks, it can exceed 50 percent.

Why the variability? Simple: We've made it easy to engineer activity out of our lives, with everything from remote controls, elevators, leaf blowers, even self-cleaning ovens. (And some of us take more advantage than others.) Research suggests that these seemingly small reductions in daily calorie burn could cause you to pack on an extra 10 pounds per year! If you're already working out frequently and watching what you eat, your only remaining fat-blasting option is to reengineer activity back into your daily life. Think of the time you're at home, your desk, or even the grocery store as untapped weight-loss potential. Need some inspiration? Try these 50 simple strategies:

1. Take the stairs instead of the elevator.

2. Stand up during phone calls at work.

3. Carry each family member's laundry upstairs separately.

4. Hand-wash your dishes rather than using the dishwasher.

5. Straighten up your house during TV commercials.

6. Bathe your dog instead of taking him to a groomer.

7. Turn up the volume on your cell phone ringer, then leave your phone in a far-off corner of the house. That way, you have to stand up and walk to it when it rings.

8. Take a stretch break every half hour you work.

9. Use the restroom that's across the office (or up a floor) from your cubicle.

10. Hide your remote. If you must watch TV, at least walk across the room to change the channel.

11. Chop fresh veggies instead of buying frozen ones.

12. Repaint your kitchen, hang up your family portrait—complete those home-improvement tasks on your to-do list.

13. Rather than yelling for family members in other rooms, walk over to talk.

14. Wash your car in the driveway instead of paying for a car wash.

15. Put essential items on the top shelf of your pantry, so you have to reach for them.

16. Organize your closets.

17. Plant or weed your garden, or tend to your indoor plants.

18. When sitting, tighten your abs and tap your toes.

19. Cook dinner instead of ordering pizza.

(continued on page 44)

HOW ACTIVE ARE YOU?

To help estimate people's calorie burn during physical activity, scientists developed something called the "metabolic equivalent of task," or MET. It's a way to gauge the intensity of your activity—the higher the MET, the more strenuous the activity and the more calories you will burn doing it. How do your daily tasks stack up?

Sedentary

1.0 MET
Sitting in the whirlpool

Meditating

Kissing

Getting your nails done

1.5 MET
Watching sports

Sitting in a meeting

Taking a bath

Eating

Having sex

1.66 MET
Helping your kids with homework

1.8 MET
Typing

Standing and talking on the phone

Checking your e-mail

2.0 MET
Cooking

Making the bed

Brushing your teeth

Putting on makeup

Showering

2.1 MET
Pumping gas

2.18 MET
Doing arts and crafts

2.3 MET
Washing the dishes (standing)

Shopping (without a cart)

Ironing

Styling your hair

2.5 MET
Stretching

Fishing from a boat (sitting)

Dusting

Taking out the trash

Clearing dishes from the table

Putting away groceries

Watering plants

Sitting and playing with children

Playing billiards

Moderate

3.0 MET
Light weight lifting

Washing the car

Cleaning the garage

Carrying small children

Painting a wall

Playing miniature golf

Walking the dog

Yoga

3.3 MET

Sweeping

3.5 MET

Standing on the riverbank fishing

Mopping

Vacuuming

Bathing your dog (standing)

Using the leaf blower

Trimming shrubs (with a power cutter)

3.8 MET

Scrubbing the bathtub or floors

4.0 MET

Bicycling for pleasure (<10 mph)

Water aerobics

Playing with your dog

Gardening

Playing table tennis

4.3 MET

Raking the lawn

4.5 MET

Trimming shrubs (with a manual cutter)

Playing golf

Shooting baskets

5.0 MET

Cleaning gutters

5.5 MET

Ballroom dancing

6.0 MET

Bicycling (10–11.9 mph)

Moving furniture

Chopping wood

Tilling a garden

Shoveling snow

Vigorous

6.5 MET

Aerobics

7.0 MET

Riding the stationary bike

Using the rowing machine

Jogging

Backpacking

Skiing

7.5 MET

Carrying groceries upstairs

8.0 MET

Circuit training

Doing pushups and situps

Playing touch football

Playing singles tennis

8.5 MET

Mountain biking

9.0 MET

Carrying boxes upstairs

9.5 MET

Running (11.5-minute mile)

10.0 MET

Running (10-minute mile)

Kickboxing

20. Ask for your paper to be left at the end of your driveway instead of by your front door.

21. Walk to the mailbox instead of checking the mail from your car.

22. Stand up while you open and read your mail.

23. While stuck in traffic, squeeze your butt muscles, then release and repeat.

24. Swing your arms while you walk.

25. Preset the timer on your TV to switch off after an hour. Then go do something more active.

26. Give your significant other a massage.

27. Pop in a CD and dance while you cook dinner.

28. Paint your nails instead of scheduling a manicure.

29. Stand on the balls of your feet while you pump gas.

30. Make foreplay with your partner last longer.

31. Chew a piece of gum.

32. Drink lots of water at work. You'll have to walk to get refills and take trips to the bathroom.

33. Make it a small water cup, so you require more frequent refills.

34. For 15 seconds every hour, hover over your desk chair in a squatting position.

35. Schedule walking meetings instead of booking a conference room.

36. Dust your office once a week.

37. Stand while waiting for a table at a restaurant.

38. Request a workstation that allows you to stand.

39. Take advantage of casual Friday. When you're dressed comfortably, you move around more often.

40. Make friends with someone on another floor. Visit him or her often.

41. Get rid of your office garbage can. Walk trash to the kitchen bin instead.

42. Park your car at the back of the lot.

43. Bag your own groceries.

44. Walk between stores that are close together.

45. Sit up straight instead of slouching.

46. Take a lap around the grocery store before you start shopping.

47. Stand on one leg while you brush your teeth.

48. Exit the bus or subway a few stops early, then walk the rest of the way.

49. Stand up to style your hair and put on your makeup.

50. When picking up your kids from school, get out of the car and greet them with a hug instead of waiting in the car curbside.

Obesogens

8 ways to protect your body from toxins that cause weight gain

Pepperoni pizza and orange soda are easy-to-spot threats to your weight and health. But there are more insidious and covert causes of weight gain. Recent research has discovered chemicals that interfere with the way hormones work in your body, potentially leading to added pounds. "They're called obesogens, and they hijack the systems that control your body weight," says Frederick vom Saal, PhD, a professor of biological sciences at the University of Missouri–Columbia. There's even evidence that these chemicals can program stem cells to become fat cells. In one study, the adult daughters of women who had the highest blood levels of DDE—a by-product of the pesticide DDT—during their child-bearing years were 20 pounds heavier than the daughters of women who had the lowest levels.

Pesticides, unfortunately, aren't the only chemicals you have to worry about. Obesogens are also found in a range of seemingly benign products, including soy foods, plastics in some food and drink packaging, and processed foods. Fortunately, as knowledge

HOW TOP DOCTORS STAY SLIM

"I chop a cup each of organic carrots, celery, radishes, broccoli, and green beans. Then I put them in a bowl filled with water and place it in my fridge. I eat a cup a day as a snack. I feel like Bugs Bunny, but it's healthy, sweet, and low in carbohydrates."

—JAMES DILLARD, MD, medical director of the complementary and alternative medicine program at Oxford Health Plans of their effects spreads, food manufacturers are responding, and research is revealing new ways to protect yourself.

■ **KNOW WHEN TO GO ORGANIC** Foods that require peeling, such as onions and bananas, aren't highly contaminated with pesticides, so the extra money you fork out for organic produce rarely equals extra protection. The Environmental Working Group recently analyzed the pesticide load of popular fruits and vegetables and found these to be the biggest threats:

1. Apples
2. Celery
3. Strawberries
4. Peaches
5. Spinach
6. Nectarines (imported)
7. Grapes (imported)
8. Sweet bell peppers
9. Potatoes
10. Blueberries (domestic)
11. Lettuce
12. Kale/collard greens

■ **SAY NO TO SOY** A few years back, soy protein began cropping up everywhere—in energy bars, protein shakes, even cookies—and was touted as a weight-loss aid, particularly for women. The problem is, soy contains chemicals that mimic the hormone estrogen,

which can trigger the formation of fat cells. If you're trying to up your protein intake, opt for whey protein (from dairy) instead of soy.

BONUS BENEFIT!

Milk proteins digest more slowly than soy, so you enjoy a steadier stream of nutrients.

■ **AVOID HIGH-FRUCTOSE CORN SYRUP** It can be hard to avoid high-fructose corn syrup, which is, scarily, found in everything from bread to ketchup to cereal. The sweet stuff behaves exactly like sugar in your body—but that isn't the only reason to avoid it. Preliminary research suggests that it disrupts your body's hormonal system, possibly even meddling with your levels of leptin (the fullness hormone). You could, of course, meticulously check every label for high-fructose corn syrup. But there's a better, simpler strategy: Eat whole foods whenever possible. You won't find high-fructose corn syrup in a banana.

■ **KICK THE CANS** Bisphenol-A—better known as BPA—is perhaps the most feared obesogen. It's been shown to mimic estrogen, which can lead to weight gain (or, scarier, prostate cancer and heart disease). "You can cut your risk in half if you take the right precautions and eat more fresh food," says biologist Heather Patisaul, PhD, who studies BPA at North Carolina State University. Start by taking canned goods out of your cart. BPA is embedded in the epoxy resin that lines the cans and can easily leach into your food. Instead, buy fresh, frozen, boxed, or pouched foods, or shop exclusively for canned goods by Eden Foods, Edward & Sons, Wild Planet Foods, EcoFish, and Oregon's Choice. These companies use BPA-free resins in their cans.

BONUS BENEFIT!

Choosing light tuna in a pouch over canned albacore reduces your intake of potentially toxic methylmercury. Try Bumble Bee Premium Light Tuna in Water, which has 25 percent fewer calories than tuna in oil.

■ **BEWARE OF BEVERAGE CONTAINERS** The aluminum soda can you're sipping from is most likely laced with BPA, according to an Environmental Working Group study. Stick to filtered water, and use a stainless-steel bottle (with a BPA-free liner) or one made with copolyester, such as those from Nalgene's Everyday line. BPA may also be lurking in the lids of plastic to-go coffee cups. Pour your coffee into your own mug, or let your java cool down a little and throw the lid away.

■ **CHECK YOUR PLASTICS** Is the bottom of your plasticware emblazoned with the number 7? If so, it may contain BPA-carrying polycarbonate. In a Harvard University study, people who drank from a polycarbonate bottle for 1 week experienced a 70 percent increase in their BPA levels. So toss out containers with the unlucky number 7, and purchase glass or plastic containers with the number 5, a signal that it's BPA free. Try Pyrex's glass storage containers, which have BPA-free lids.

■ **REHEAT WITH CAUTION** Before you microwave your leftovers, make sure they're not in a plastic container with recycling codes 3 or 7, which often indicate BPA or phthalates (another type of chemical that mimics estrogen). Fatty foods absorb chemicals from plastic, and heating speeds the process. Microwave food on a glass plate, and toss plastic containers if they're cracked or scratched—toxins escape more easily from plastic that's damaged.

■ **TRIM THE FAT** Hormone-altering toxins are often fat-soluble. That means they lurk in everything from full-fat dairy products to fatty fish to meat. Consuming reduced-fat dairy products and lean meats may cut your exposure to chemicals.

Plateaus

How to break through them and lose those last stubborn pounds

At first, you were dropping a few pounds a week. Now, that fast weight loss has slowed to a trickle. What's going on? It's likely you've reached your first plateau, which typically occurs when you've lost all of your excess water through a special dietary or exercise effort. When you cut calories, your body is forced to burn up stored carbohydrates as fuel. These carbs, also known as glycogen, retain water. So when you use them as energy, you drop water weight, too. That's why the pounds fly off at first.

Plateaus that occur later in your journey to lose pounds are a reflection of your progress. Since you've already shed inches, your body now requires fewer calories because your resting metabolic rate has declined in proportion to the pounds you've dropped. So following the exact diet and exercise plan that helped you get to where you are will ultimately cause you to plateau. At this point, you're easily able to maintain your weight loss, but the number on the scale isn't budging. What that means: It's time to change your diet and challenge your body with a new exercise plan. Deploy these plateau-busting strategies:

■ **ADJUST YOUR MIND-SET** If you see your plateau as a sign of failure, you're more likely to give up—and blow your diet entirely.

So think of plateaus as a sign of progress. You've lost the initial "easy" pounds, and now you're shedding the weight you never thought you could lose.

■ **REASSESS YOUR PLAN** If you keep a food log, compare your early diet with your current diet. Have your portion sizes gradually increased? Have you introduced brown sugar to your once-plain oatmeal? Make sure you haven't made any subtle changes that could be sabotaging your weight loss. If you have, work on cutting out your newly developed bad habits.

■ **CONTROL YOUR CALORIES** It's simple science: A 150-pound person requires fewer calories than a 200-pound person. Which means you need to trim your portions as you trim your waistline. If you've gone a month without seeing the scale budge, recalculate your daily caloric needs. Here's how: Divide your current weight in pounds by 2.2 (to convert it to kilograms). Then multiply the result by 25. This is roughly how many daily calories you should consume to lose about a pound per week.

■ **RAMP UP YOUR WORKOUTS** As you drop weight, there's often an unfortunate side effect: You lose muscle, too. That can cause your weight loss to slow down, since muscle helps you burn more calories, even when you're at rest. Without that extra burn, a diet that worked at first may no longer do the trick. Rev up your workout: Increase your time exercising or perform your moves at a higher intensity.

■ **SHIFT YOUR FOCUS** Even if the number on the scale isn't moving, that doesn't mean you haven't reaped huge benefits from eating healthier and exercising more. Focus on other gains you're making, like lowering your cholesterol or bringing your blood pressure back into the healthy range. Remember, the benefit of healthy habits isn't limited to weight loss. If you can stop obsessing about your weight, you may find that it falls off naturally, as stress eating subsides.

Blood Pressure: 19 Natural Remedies for Hypertension

You've already taken the first step toward lowering your blood pressure: getting your weight under control. Research shows that keeping your body-fat percentage below 22 lowers your risk of hypertension. However, if you have high blood pressure—that is, the top number is 140 or higher, and the bottom number is 90 or higher—you may need to intensify your efforts. Same goes if you're "prehypertensive," which means the top number is between 120–139 and the bottom number is in the 80–89 range. Here's how to give your heart an extra boost:

1 LAUGH IT UP

If you're going to sit in front of the TV set, pop in a funny movie. In a 2006 University of Maryland study, researchers found that laughing at a comedy flick can cause your blood vessels to dilate by 22 percent. Why? The physical act of laughing causes the inner lining of your blood vessels to expand, allowing for an increase in bloodflow and reducing blood pressure, says Michael Miller, MD, director of the University of Maryland's Center for Preventive Cardiology. To experience the benefit, you should be laughing at least 15 minutes—and little chuckles don't cut it. Go for the belly laughs.

2 PUMP UP YOUR POTASSIUM

A potassium-rich diet helps blunt the blood pressure–raising effects of salt. Scientists aren't entirely sure why, but there's evidence that potassium helps your body excrete salt and keeps your blood vessels from constricting. Despite their reputation, bananas aren't the most potassium-packed food in the supermarket. You'll find the mineral in white beans, raisins, baked potatoes (both sweet and white), grapefruit juice, halibut, and cooked spinach. (For more potassium-packed foods, see the table on page 11.) Aim to take in 4,700 milligrams per day.

3 CRANK THE TUNES

There may be healing power in your iPod. Listening to music with a steady beat for 30 minutes a day while performing breathing exercises can lower your blood pressure, an Italian study suggests. Try it: Switch on slow, steady music, breathe in for a few seconds, then take twice as long to exhale. This can help your blood vessels relax. Just make sure you like the music you're listening to; otherwise, you may not reap the full benefit.

4 INDULGE IN DARK CHOCOLATE

A daily dose of dark chocolate may be enough to tame your blood pressure. In an Italian study, people with prediabetes and high blood pressure lowered their systolic BP (the upper number) by 4.5 points and their diastolic (the lower number) by 4.2 points simply by eating a daily 3.5 ounces of dark chocolate for 15 days. Dark chocolate is rich in flavonoids, a type of antioxidant that boosts bloodflow. You shouldn't have any trouble stopping after a square or two: Dark chocolate is richer than milk chocolate, so its flavor goes a long way. Choose a bar that contains at least 65 percent cacao, such as Ghirardelli's Intense Dark 72% Cacao Twilight Delight Bar.

5 BULK UP YOUR BEAN COUNT

Not only do bean eaters have smaller waists, but they also have lower systolic blood pressure than folks who don't eat beans, according to a 2008 study review in the *Journal of the American College of Nutrition*. Beans are loaded with fiber, potassium, and protein, all of which have been linked to regulation of blood pressure, the scientists explain. One cup of kidney beans, for example, packs 11 grams of fiber, 670 milligrams of potassium, and 17 grams of protein.

6 LOAD UP ON LOW-FAT DAIRY

Milk doesn't just bolster your bones. A Harvard University study of 4,800 people found that those who consumed more than three servings of dairy per day were about 36 percent less likely to have high blood pressure than those who ate less than half a serving. Credit dairy's trifecta of BP-lowering minerals: calcium, magnesium, and potassium. What counts as a serving? A cup of low-fat milk or yogurt, or three domino-size chunks of cheese.

7 DRINK TO YOUR HEALTH

In modest amounts, alcohol expands your arteries and makes them more pliable, which lowers your blood pressure. However, men should stop after two drinks, and women after one. Any more than that, and you may experience a spike in BP. A single serving is a 12-ounce beer, a 5-ounce glass of wine, or $1\frac{1}{2}$ ounces of liquor.

8 HAVE MORE SEX

In a 2006 Scottish study, people who had sex at least once over a 2-week period had lower blood pressure than those who engaged in no sexual activity. The frisky people's blood vessels also responded better to stress. Researchers suspect that arousal causes your brain to release hormones that improve circulatory-system function and boost cardiac performance.

9 CONTROL YOUR CAFFEINE

If you're worried about your BP, eliminate coffee. The jolt of caffeine may send your blood pressure skyrocketing. Can't go decaf? Switch to tea: According to a study in the journal *Psychopharmacology*, the combination of caffeine and theanine, an amino acid in tea, may boost alertness without raising blood pressure as much as caffeine does alone. Consider making your tea of choice hibiscus. It's caffeine free and, according to Tufts University scientists, the flavonoids in hibiscus are thought to dilate your blood vessels, allowing blood to flow through more easily.

10 SNUFF OUT SMOKING

A single cigarette may be enough to narrow your blood vessels and cut off bloodflow to your heart, says Woodrow Corey, MD, a cardiologist at Indiana University Hospital. The nicotine can increase your blood pressure and also raise your risk of atherosclerosis (fatty buildup in your arteries), whether you smoke every once in a while or all the time. Eat to quit: A study in the journal *Nicotine & Tobacco Research* found that fruits, vegetables, water, and dairy products like cheese and milk put a bad taste in smokers' mouths, reducing their desire for cigarettes. Add more produce and low-fat dairy to your diet, and you may avoid the urge the light up, the scientists say.

11 RELAX WITH YOGA

When you feel frazzled, your body pumps out cortisol, a hormone that can lead to high blood pressure and a racing heart (not to mention weight gain). If your cortisol levels are constantly soaring, it can damage the lining of your arteries, so your blood struggles to flow freely. Sign up for a yoga class: Studies show that it can ease stress and lower blood pressure.

12 RELAX WITH ACUPUNCTURE

The newest alternative medicine weapon against high blood pressure is acupuncture. Research suggests that weekly acupuncture sessions can slash your systolic blood pressure by up to 20 points. When the acupuncturist stimulates key areas near your elbows and knees, your body releases neurotransmitters that target areas in the brain that regulate your cardiovascular system, explains John Longhurst, MD, PhD, a cardiologist and director of the Susan Samueli Center for Integrative Medicine at the University of California, Irvine. The blood pressure benefit isn't permanent, however. To maintain the results, you need to continue once-a-week treatments.

13 EMBRACE BERRIES

Blueberries, strawberries, raspberries—they're all loaded with vitamin C, which can help lower your blood pressure, according to a German study. Add a handful to your salad, yogurt, or oatmeal, or try nibbling on frozen berries as a sweet summertime snack.

14 TAKE A BRISK WALK

No time to visit the health club? You can still reap the blood pressure–lowering benefits of exercise. A National Institutes of Health study found that short-but-frequent workouts—10-minute sessions, four times a day—produced the same health benefits, including lower blood pressure, as a daily 40-minute session.

15 FIGHT BACK WITH POTATOES

White potatoes have been unfairly vilified. Not only are they loaded with heart-healthy potassium, but they're also rich in kukoamines. These plant compounds can help lower your blood pressure, according to USDA researchers. The healthiest ways to eat your spuds? Roasted or baked.

16 LOAD UP ON PROTEIN

Dieters who devoted a quarter of their calories to lean protein successfully slashed their blood pressure, a recent Johns Hopkins University study found. Make sure to work protein into every meal and snack—your heart and your waistline will thank you.

17 BOOK A MASSAGE

A study in the *Journal of Alternative and Complementary Medicine* found that after people with normal blood pressure had deep-tissue massages for 45 to 60 minutes, their BPs fell significantly. Even a short session can help: In a recent University of South Florida study, people who enjoyed three 10-minute massages a week experienced an 18-point drop in their systolic blood pressure and a 5-point drop in their diastolic blood pressure after just 10 sessions.

18 CUT THE SALT

The average American consumes 3,400 milligrams of sodium a day—that's at least 1,000 mg more than you need! Trimming your salt intake can help bring your blood pressure back into the reasonable range. Instead of adding salt while you cook, season the final product. That way, you'll require smaller amounts to taste its flavor. (For more ways to reduce your intake, see page 252.)

19 TRY THE SEAWEED SOLUTION

Brown wakame seaweed, found in miso soup, can help lower your blood pressure, say researchers at the University of South Carolina. When people ate a heaping tablespoon of dried wakame every day for a month, their systolic blood pressure dropped 10 points. The seaweed may cling to sodium in your body, so it isn't as readily absorbed into your bloodstream, says study author Jane Teas, PhD.

Thermic Effect of Food

3 ways to eat more and weigh less

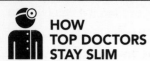

Physical activity isn't the only way to stimulate your metabolism. You actually burn calories simply by eating food. Scientists call this the "thermic effect of food"—the calories you need to digest, use, and store the energy you consume. This generally accounts for 10 to 15 percent of your total calories burned. In other words, for every 1,000 calories you consume, your body is only absorbing 850 to 900.

How it works: Your digestive system breaks down food—whether it's an apple or a cheeseburger—into its most basic building blocks. So, complex carbohydrates, such as whole wheat or oatmeal, are reduced to simple sugars. Fat becomes fatty acids, and proteins are broken down to amino acids. As these molecules circulate through your body, your cells take them in, where they're further broken down into usable energy forms, such as ATP and creatine phosphate. All of these processes require calories.

■ **FUEL UP ON PROTEIN** Your body uses more energy digesting protein than fat or carbohydrates. In fact, studies suggest that you burn up to twice as many calories breaking down protein compared to carbs. To take full advantage of protein's metabolic power, replace half of your typical carbohydrate intake with protein. For most people, this means about a quarter of your calories will come from protein. Aim for at least 10 to 20 grams per meal.

THE THERMIC EFFECT ON MACRONUTRIENTS

NUTRIENT	CALORIES PER GRAM	PERCENT BURNED DURING DIGESTION (APPROXIMATE)
Carbohydrates	4 calories	6%
Fat	9 calories	3%
Protein	4 calories	23%

■ **PICK YOUR POWDER** If you're not a big meat eater, it can be a challenge to consume enough protein every day. That's where powdered protein supplements come in. But before you toss that powder into your smoothie, make sure it contains "whey protein isolate." A recent study in the *American Journal of Clinical Nutrition* found that whey protein has a higher thermic effect than casein and soy proteins.

■ **EAT FISH FOR DINNER** Although fat has a lower thermic effect than both protein and carbs, it still has a place in your diet. Fat is superfilling, plus you need it to absorb fat-soluble vitamins, such as A, E, and K. You just have to choose the right kinds of the nutrient. In a recent Canadian study, men who boosted their intake of fish-derived polyunsaturated fats experienced a 51 percent increase in the number of calories they burned during digestion after 2 weeks. Polyunsaturated fats may actually improve your body's ability to break down fat, the scientists say. You'll find high amounts of the fats in sardines, tuna, sockeye salmon, and rainbow trout.

IS CELERY REALLY A "NEGATIVE-CALORIE" FOOD?

Unfortunately, you won't find a food that requires more calories to digest than it actually contains. Although celery has only 9 calories per stalk (half from sugar, half from fiber), your body simply can't burn all of that during digestion.

Triglycerides

9 ways to lower blood fats

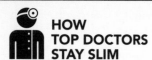

HOW TOP DOCTORS STAY SLIM

"Hummus is the new peanut butter. It's packed with protein and fiber to keep you feeling full and energized. I spread it on everything from pita chips to veggies."

—SUSAN ALBERS, PsyD, a psychologist at the Cleveland Clinic who specializes in weight loss

Cholesterol tends to steal the heart-health spotlight, but triglycerides—another form of fat in your bloodstream—can be just as troublesome. "When your triglycerides are high, your body makes harmful LDL cholesterol particles smaller, which means they can lodge in artery walls more easily," says Patrick McBride, MD, MPH, a cardiologist at the University of Wisconsin. Elevated triglycerides—anything above 150 milligrams per deciliter—have been linked to heart disease and, more recently, to cancer. Losing weight is the first step to taming your triglycerides, but you can accelerate the process with these simple strategies:

■ **PUCKER UP** Tart cherry juice may taste sour, but its benefits are sweet. In an Arizona State University study, people who downed a cup of the stuff per day for 1 month effectively reduced their triglycerides by 10 percent. Other studies have shown similar results for fresh tart cherries. Try stirring tart cherries into yogurt, mixing the dried variety into wild rice pilaf, or adding tart cherry juice to seltzer or tea.

■ **TAME YOUR CARBS** Trimming excess carbs from your diet isn't just about shrinking your belly. "You're reducing the amount of sugar in your bloodstream," says John Elefteriades, MD, chief of cardiothoracic surgery at the Yale School of Medicine. "This makes your body burn an alternative energy source, triglycerides."

■ **CAN THE SODA** In a recent University of California, Davis, study, overweight people who drank a fructose-sweetened beverage with a meal experienced a significant surge in their triglyceride levels. That's because your liver converts fructose to triglycerides, says study author Karen Teff, PhD. Replace soda with unsweetened tea, coffee, or water, and consider diluting your juices with water.

■ **DON'T NEGLECT NUTS** The fats in nuts don't translate to fat in your arteries. In fact, a study in the *Journal of the American College of Nutrition* found that phytosterol, a compound found in pistachios and hazelnuts, can lower your triglycerides by as much as 10 points. Try tossing a few nuts into your yogurt or oatmeal, or bag up a handful as an afternoon snack.

■ **MUSCLE OUT FAT** Muscle helps clear triglycerides from your bloodstream, says Timothy Church, MD, PhD, a preventive medicine expert at Pennington Biomedical Research Center. Start building more. Your goal: at least 15 to 20 minutes of resistance training, two to three times per week.

■ **TAKE A WALK** Brisk walkers may outpace joggers when it comes to taming triglycerides. Duke researchers recently found that people who walked for 50 minutes four times per week experienced a 22 percent drop in triglycerides—nearly twice as much as those who ran for the same amount of time. Lower-intensity workouts may more effectively control triglycerides because they primarily use fats as fuel, whereas high-intensity workouts

rely on glucose, the scientists explain. (See page 335 for walking workouts.)

■ **POP A FISH OIL SUPPLEMENT** The Food and Drug Administration has approved a prescription-only fish oil, Lovaza, to lower triglycerides—but you can reap similar benefits from an over-the-counter supplement. Fish oil is loaded with omega-3 fatty acids, which may help to clear out triglycerides and LDL cholesterol from your blood. Choose a pill that has at least 500 milligrams each of EPA and DHA, the primary omega-3s in fish oil, or add cold-water fish—white tuna, sardines, salmon, Spanish mackerel—to your plate twice a week.

■ **SPICE THINGS UP** What's not to love about cinnamon? It adds a touch of sweetness to your food, and it may also do a solid for your heart. Pakistani researchers recently found that consuming ½ teaspoon of cinnamon per day can reduce your triglycerides by 30 percent. Try sprinkling it over your oatmeal or latte, or use it to coat nuts for a sweet and satisfying afternoon snack.

■ **STRETCH YOUR LEGS** If you're like most Americans, you spend 56 hours every week sitting. It's not just the sedentary quality of sitting that makes it so dangerous. When you sit for an extended period, the enzymes responsible for breaking down triglycerides begin to switch off, says Marc Hamilton, PhD, an associate professor of biomedical sciences at the University of Missouri–Columbia. Interrupt stretches of sitting as often as possible: Take a break and stand every half hour, or try reading e-mails and chatting on the phone while standing.

Burn Notice:
19 More Metabolism Boosters

You can control what you eat and how long you exercise, but it's impossible to know what's going on inside your cells after you eat or exercise. Scientists say your metabolism is the sum of all the bodily processes that keep you alive. But to you, it is simply "fast" or "slow" and determines how quickly you shed weight. And you want to enhance it.

As you age, your metabolism typically slows down. Starting in your thirties, your basal, or resting, rate declines by about 1 percent every 4 years. Plus, for every pound you lose, you burn up to 20 fewer calories a day. But these changes don't have to be inevitable. University of Colorado researchers compared the metabolic rates of older and younger people following the same exercise and eating plan and found no difference. That means your lifestyle may be the most important factor in determining your metabolism. Try these simple tweaks to your diet, workout, and daily routine to accelerate your burn.

1 SPICE THINGS UP

Hot peppers contain a compound called capsaicin that can boost your metabolism while also staving off hunger and increasing post-meal satisfaction. Research shows that eating about 1 tablespoon of chopped red or green chile pepper, which packs about 30 milligrams of capsaicin, can temporarily spike your metabolic rate by 23 percent. Top your food with the hottest sauce you can stand, or sprinkle red-pepper flakes onto pasta dishes and into chili and stews. You can also easily incorporate chile peppers into homemade salsa.

2 GUZZLE A GLASS OF TEA

Green and oolong teas contain catechins, a type of antioxidant that can boost your fat burning. Studies suggest that drinking two to four cups of green or oolong tea daily may result in an extra 50 calories burned every day! Instead of milk or sweetener, add a squeeze of lemon to your tea, which may help your body absorb more of its catechins.

3 GO ORGANIC

Pesticides inundate your body with organochlorines, pollutants that are stored in your fat cells. According to Canadian scientists, these nasty chemicals can lead to a greater-than-normal dip in metabolism as you lose weight. Always opt for organic when buying apples, celery, strawberries, peaches, spinach, imported nectarines, imported grapes, sweet bell peppers, potatoes, domestic blueberries, lettuce, kale, and collard greens. These have the highest pesticide load of any produce, a recent Environmental Working Group analysis found.

4 DRINK COFFEE

The caffeine in coffee (and tea) stimulates your central nervous system, thus increasing your heart rate and breathing. This can rev up your metabolism by 16 percent, according to a study in the journal *Physiology & Behavior*. Just make sure you don't load your drink down with cream and sugar—that will undo any metabolic advantage your joe has to offer.

5 START EVERY DAY WITH BREAKFAST

A study in the *American Journal of Epidemiology* found that people who skip breakfast are 450 percent more likely to be obese. One explanation: Eating in the a.m. jumpstarts your metabolism for the rest of the day. Time is not an excuse: It only takes 60 seconds to heat up a packet of instant oatmeal, an excellent, fiber-rich option.

6 BOOST YOUR WORKOUT INTENSITY

Intense forms of exercise—for example, lifting weights—don't just burn calories while you're doing them. They also activate "afterburn," where you keep burning calories long after you've left the gym. In fact, if you push yourself hard enough, you can expect to burn at least 10 percent of the total calories used during your workout in the hour afterward! That's because your body has to work hard to cool off and repair tiny tears in your muscles caused by exercise. Plus, as you build more muscle, you boost your burn, since muscle uses significantly more calories than fat tissue.

7 SKIP THE LONG RUNS

Your cardio prescription: quick bursts of intense exercise followed by short rest periods. In a Canadian study, women who alternated 4-minute bouts of intense cycling with 2 minutes of easy pedaling burned up to 66 percent more fat during subsequent cardio workouts. Interval training can trigger a boost in metabolism so you burn more fat during exercise and even at rest, says study author Jason Talanian, PhD. You can apply the interval approach to power walking, jogging, or elliptical training. Simply alternate between a pace that leaves you slightly breathless and one that makes speaking more than a few words a challenge.

8 WATCH YOUR IRON INTAKE

Iron helps transport the oxygen your muscles require to burn fat. Men are rarely iron deficient, but women lose iron each month, due to menstruation. The effect: If you don't have enough iron, you may feel sapped and experience a metabolic slump. Top sources of the mineral: fortified cereals, white beans, lentils, cooked spinach, shellfish, and lean meats.

9 BUILD MORE MUSCLE

The weight you may gain from working out isn't a bad thing. For every 3 pounds of muscle you add, you raise your calorie burn by 6 to 8 percent. That can translate to an extra 100 calories torched every day! The best way to gain lean muscle mass is resistance training. For maximum benefit, focus on exercises that use your largest muscles and require two-part movements. That means lots of squats, push-ups, and other exercises that combine upper- and lower-body movements.

10 DO THE RIGHT NUMBER OF REPS

Research shows that completing 8 to 15 repetitions of an exercise produces the biggest boost in fat burning. The caveat: You won't reap the full benefit if you're using too-light weights. You should be struggling by the last repetition.

11 STICK TO TWO TO FOUR SETS

Just one set of a resistance exercise is enough to boost your metabolism, according to Ball State University scientists. But more is better—up to a point. In a recent Greek study, researchers found that there was no metabolic difference between doing four sets and six sets. If you're new to lifting, start with two sets, then gradually go up to four as you make gains in the gym.

12 WORK YOUR ENTIRE BODY

Exercises that activate multiple muscles, rather than isolating one muscle group, result in a greater postexercise metabolic boost. For example, you'll elevate your metabolism much more with squats, which work your legs, butt, and back, than with biceps curls. In fact, in a University of Wisconsin study, exercisers who completed a full-body routine saw an increase in metabolism for 39 hours afterward. Try to work in an intense full-body routine 3 days per week, with a day in between sessions.

13 KEEP REST PERIODS SHORT

Don't rest more than 75 seconds between sets. When you perform 8 to 15 repetitions, a chemical called lactate accumulates in your blood, triggering the release of fat-burning hormones. If you rest too long, you give your body time to clear lactate from your bloodstream. By keeping your recovery time short, you keep levels of lactate—and fat-burning hormones—high.

14 MONITOR YOUR MEDS

Antidepressants boost your mood, but they may depress your metabolism. Although researchers aren't sure why, a German study review pinpointed the meds most likely to produce the effect: Aventyl (nortriptyline), Remeron (mirtazapine), and Paxil (paroxetine). If you've gained weight since you started on an antidepressant, ask your doctor about switching to Wellbutrin (bupropion), which can actually boost your metabolism.

15 DRINK MORE WATER

Every chemical reaction in your body requires water. That includes your metabolism. If you're dehydrated, you may burn up to 2 percent fewer calories than normal, according to researchers at the University of Utah. In their study, people who drank either eight or twelve 8-ounce glasses of water per day had faster metabolisms than those who downed four. How to tell if you're dehydrated? Your urine is dark yellow or amber in color. Make it a habit to drink a full glass of water before each meal and snack.

16 ADD ICE TO YOUR DRINK

Studies have shown that drinking five or six ice-cold glasses of water could help you burn an extra 10 calories per day. That may sound small, but think about this: In a year, that could amount to an extra pound of weight loss. Your body has to heat a cold drink to body temperature, and that process requires calories. Every little bit helps!

17 EAT MORE PROTEIN

Your body burns more calories digesting protein than either carbs or fat. Plus, protein helps your body maintain calorie-torching lean muscle. Shoot for between 10 and 20 grams of protein per meal. Try a cup of Greek yogurt with breakfast, hummus with lunch, and salmon for dinner. Eat a handful of nuts as a snack.

18 ALTERNATE BETWEEN MOVES

This strategy not only saves you time, but it also fires up your metabolism. It's simple: Perform an exercise, rest briefly, then do another exercise that recruits muscles you didn't work with the previous move. For example, you might pair an upper-body exercise with a lower-body move, or an exercise that targets your chest with one that works your back.

19 LOAD UP ON D

Vitamin D is essential for preserving your metabolism-revving muscle tissue. Take in 90 percent of your daily value (400 IU) with a single 3½-ounce serving of salmon. Other D-rich foods: tuna, shrimp, fortified milk and cereal, and eggs.

Part 2

YOUR BRAIN

Think your way thin by tapping into
the power of your mind.

Everybody is gung-ho at the beginning of a weight-loss plan. But how about 6 weeks in? Or even 6 months in? Are you just as devoted to your diet as you were early on? Still exercising every day? Still resolved to ignore those cravings for double chocolate brownies? It's normal that as the newness of your goal wears off, your resolve to move more and eat healthier will wear down—unless you keep your brain engaged. Your brain can be one of your most powerful weight-loss allies—or enemies—since it influences everything from bingeing to willpower, from confidence to happiness. How can you make your brain work *for* your body? This section provides dozens of strategies to employ the power of your mind to control your appetite and keep your weight loss on track.

Binge Eating

12 ways to gain control over a feeding frenzy

Your mother-in-law made you feel inadequate again. Or you just had a blowout with your teenager. You plop down on the couch with a half gallon of ice cream and before you know it, it's gone.

You've just experienced what's known as binge eating or emotional eating—uncontrollable consumption driven most often by stress, anger, anxiety, or depression. After the first bite, you can't stop until the food is gone, you start to feel sick, or worse . . . you realize what you've done and become even more depressed. It becomes a vicious cycle. You binge again.

"Binge eating is a psychological disorder that usually has much deeper roots than a simple food craving," says Mary Ellen Sweeney, MD, an obesity researcher at Emory University School of Medicine in Atlanta. As long as we are eating, we don't have to deal with intense emotional feelings. Doctors say the remedy is to ultimately face those feelings and learn to overcome them. Here are some useful ways to begin that journey as well as tips for avoiding binge eating when your emotions start directing you toward food as relief.

■ **TAKE A BREATHER** Tempted to binge? Just breathe. Try inhaling for 5 seconds, then exhaling for 5 seconds; do this for a full minute. Breathing slowly and deliberately helps your mind calm down, stifling your urge to raid the pantry. "Simply being aware of how your body reacts to stress can lead to decreased cortisol levels in the brain, which lessens the effect of stress," explains Duke University psychologist Jeffrey Greeson, PhD.

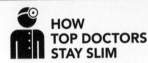

HOW TOP DOCTORS STAY SLIM

"I turn my phone off and sit, focusing on my breath, for 5 minutes twice a day. Thoughts come up and I acknowledge them, and I let them go. Eventually my mind becomes quiet. It may sound flaky, but research shows that mindfulness-based drills not only ease anxiety but also sharpen attention span and lower blood pressure."

—JAMES DILLARD, MD, medical director of the complementary and alternative medicine program at Oxford Health Plans

■ **DISTRACT YOURSELF** "Take your mind away from your forbidden food by focusing on something that takes all your concentration, like the Sunday crossword puzzle," says Dori Winchell, PhD, a psychologist in private practice in Encinitas, California. "Once your mind is engaged in a task that you enjoy and must pay attention to, you're less likely to be fixated on food."

■ **TAKE A TIME OUT** If you feel the urge to binge, set the kitchen timer for 15 minutes, grab a piece of paper and a pencil, and write down how you are feeling. Try to figure out what's making you want to stuff yourself with sugar cookies. Gaining that knowledge and putting it into perspective will start to give you a sense of control over your emotions and the mindless-eating response.

■ **BLOCK NIGHTTIME BINGES** Emotions aren't always the trigger for binge eating. Consuming too few calories can also be the cause, says Jan McBarron, MD, a weight control specialist and director of Georgia Bariatrics in Columbus, Georgia. By depriving yourself physically and psychologically of enough food during the day, your body and mind may take over in a pantry raid at night where your body tries to fill a desperate nutrition gap. The best thing you can do to help yourself is to eat small healthy meals throughout the day. "Eat a sensible breakfast and lunch, and you're less likely to clean out your refrigerator at night," says Susan Zelitch Yanovski, MD, director of the Obesity and Eating Disorders Program at the

National Institute of Diabetes and Digestive and Kidney Diseases at the National Institutes of Health.

■ **EAT SOMETHING SPICY** As anyone who in a moment of bravado ordered the "atomic" buffalo wings knows, it's very difficult to binge on very spicy foods. So, pepper your meal with chiles and Tabasco sauce. In addition to incapacitating your taste buds, spicy foods fill you up faster than bland or sweet foods, and they may help burn calories faster.

■ **RECORD YOUR BINGES** You can even gain a sense of control after bingeing on a box of chocolates—it's not too late to do something about it. Journal about what triggered the binge so you can learn from the experience and plan what to do differently the next time the emotion strikes.

■ **FORGIVE YOURSELF** You didn't start bingeing overnight, and you won't be able to stop that quickly, either, doctors say. Each small step that you take away from bingeing will help you feel better about yourself, but it can take a few years to change your behavior completely. To succeed, the trick is to try and try again.

■ **ASK FOR HELP** Women almost always binge alone. With friends, you'd be able to talk out your feelings instead of eating them away. The key is to recognize when those feelings of anxiety or depression are starting so you can call a friend before raiding the fridge.

■ **SEE A DOCTOR** If you feel you are a binge eater who can't stop, see a doctor or counselor trained in eating disorders. To locate qualified professional help in your area, contact:

National Eating Disorders Association at www .nationaleatingdisorders.org

National Association of Anorexia Nervosa and Associated Disorders at www.anad.org

Center for the Study of Anorexia and Bulimia in New York at www.icpnyc.org/center-for-study .html

American Society of Bariatric Physicians at www.asbp.org

■ **STAY AWAY FROM WINDOWS** Talk about unhappy meals: A recent study in the journal *Public Health Nutrition* found that folks who regularly received food through a drive-up window over a 6-year period were 41 percent more likely to become depressed than those who skipped the greasy grub. (It's a vicious cycle—if you're depressed, you may be more likely to binge eat.) Blame the trans fats in fast food, which are thought to inhibit your brain's production of mood-stabilizing chemicals, scientists say. Determine the times when you're most prone to hitting the drive-thru— say, on the way home from work or after a night out—and pack a healthy snack in your bag to tide you over during your most vulnerable periods.

■ **TAKE PRIDE IN PROGRESS** You don't have to be at your goal weight to be proud of your body. As you drop weight, take note of— and celebrate!—even the subtlest changes, like the slight definition you detect in your arms or abs. In a recent study from Lisbon, Portugal, women who received body-image counseling lost a higher percentage of weight than those who didn't. Why? Because poor body image can lead to emotional eating, which slows down weight loss, says study author Eliana Carraça, PhD.

■ **MEDITATE ON YOUR MASHED POTATOES** Thinking about your food may help you think twice before overdoing it. Take a favorite snack food—say, a piece of dark chocolate—in your hand, and gaze at it as if it's a foreign object. How does it feel between your fingers? What color is it? How does it smell? Allow any thoughts about the food—positive or negative—to freely enter your mind. Bring the morsel to your mouth, noting the movement of your hand and arm, and observe the way your body anticipates eating it. Chew slowly, taking in the taste, and then make a conscious decision to swallow. Yes, this exercise may feel silly. But by forcing you to focus on the objective qualities of food and eating, it can help break any emotional connection you have with food, a recent study from the National Institutes of Health suggests.

Cheating

5 guilt-free strategies for indulging smartly

Nobody wants to go through life without enjoying burgers, pizza, and ice cream. And you shouldn't feel you have to in order to lose weight. In fact, if you feel deprived, you're more likely to opt for the Monster Burger, the gigantic stuffed-crust slice, or an entire carton of ice cream. "Anytime you withhold something enjoyable from somebody, whether it's television or affection or pizza, they'll only resist it for so long," says Brian Wansink, PhD, director of the Cornell University Food and Brand Lab. "Those are deprivation diets. Effective in the short run, but not sustainable." In school, you were taught never to cheat. Well, when it comes to losing weight, stop feeling guilty because cheating on your diet can be one of your most powerful tools for controlling cravings. Just make sure you cheat the right way . . .

■ **DO IT JUST ONCE A WEEK** If you're exercising regularly and adhering to your eating plan, allow yourself a "cheat" meal once a week, says Jennifer McDaniel, RD, an assistant professor of nutrition at Saint Louis University. Any more than that, and it's not cheating. It's a lack of discipline. Indulge in a burger, a piece of chocolate cake, onion rings—whatever it is that you miss the most. The key: Don't let your cheat meal become a cheat weekend. If you overdo it just 2 days in a row, you're eating poorly nearly 30 percent of the time!

■ **MAKE IT SPECIAL** Rather than holing up at home with a bag of Lay's, choose a cheat food that requires you to go out—say, a cup of lobster bisque from your favorite restaurant, or a brownie from the bakery you adore. It's more rewarding to have a night out than to waste calories on everyday junk, right?

SWEET CHEATS

YOU WANT: CHOCOLATE

Skip this: 8 Hershey's Kisses

Eat this: 50 chocolate raisins

The payoff: Protein, calcium, and fiber

YOU WANT: FRUITY

Skip this: 10 Starburst candies

Eat this: 2 packs Welch's Fruit Snacks

The payoff: Vitamins A, C, and E

YOU WANT: NUTTY

Skip this: 3 fun-size Snickers

Eat this: 20 peanut M&M's

The payoff: Twice the calcium

■ **TIME YOUR TREAT** The ideal time to cheat: after a workout. When you've recently exercised, your meal is more likely to be absorbed by your muscles—a good thing—than to be stored as fat, says Alan Aragon, MS, a nutritionist based in Thousand Oaks, California. Even after a low-intensity training session, your muscles can sponge up large amounts of carbs, preventing fat storage. So don't feel guilty about grabbing a slice of pizza after one workout a week.

■ **SAVE ROOM FOR DESSERT** The anticipation of a reward can keep you motivated. So tell yourself: "If I eat sensibly throughout the day, I can have a small dessert after dinner." "Having a strategy for small indulgences is a good idea," says Aragon. "Snack on something clearly defined in size and caloric intake, such as two or three squares of rich, dark chocolate." To avoid overdoing it, portion out what you're going to eat, then put the container away.

■ **SKIP HAPPY HOUR** Once you start drinking, one beer can easily become three. So skip happy hour—it's only asking for trouble—and enjoy an after-dinner drink instead. Think of it as dessert, and limit yourself to a single glass. That's 12 ounces of beer, 5 ounces of wine, or 1½ ounces of hard liquor. Keep it to once or twice a week, and skip dessert on the nights you imbibe.

Cravings

13 ways to kick cravings to the curb

HOW TOP DOCTORS STAY SLIM

"Most days of the workweek, I eat the same breakfast (a banana with about ½ cup of Greek yogurt, mixed with honey and granola) and the same lunch (a whole-wheat tortilla with organic grilled chicken). I realize that's boring, but it gives me the flexibility to eat a wider range of higher-calorie foods if I have a meeting over lunch or I go out on the weekend."

—**DAVID SARWER, PhD,** a psychologist at the University of Pennsylvania's Center for Weight and Eating Disorders

Here's what most people know about cravings: (1) They're nearly impossible to ignore (especially if you want chocolate), and (2) they rarely involve something healthy. Beyond that, cravings are a bit of a mystery to most dieters.

What exactly is a craving? And how is it different from run-of-the-mill hunger? It's a matter of body versus brain. Hunger is that gnawing "I must eat now" sensation in your stomach—a physiological need for food, which means almost anything sounds appetizing. Cravings, on the other hand, are more often psychological, and they have a specificity that hunger lacks. In other words, you have an intense desire for a certain food. You may be dying for, say, chocolate-covered peanuts. Or ice cream. Or ice cream topped with chocolate-covered peanuts. And only that.

Emotions, situations, and even pleasant associations can trigger a craving, says Susan Roberts, PhD, director of the energy metabolism lab at the Jean Mayer USDA Human Nutrition Research Center at Tufts University. A stressful day, or sitting on the couch where you always snack, or even the memory of the Twinkie your mom used to pack in your lunch could be enough to trick your brain into thinking you *need* that food. Once you bite into it, you experience a pleasurable surge of dopamine—the same chemical that's released when people drink or do drugs. That can become habit forming, if not addictive. It can also lead to massive blood sugar spikes and rapid weight gain, especially if your cravings involve high-fat, sugary foods. Luckily, there are scientifically proven strategies to switch off your cravings. Many of them are as simple as they are effective.

■ **TAKE TIME TO SMELL THE CHOCOLATE** Don't dive into your dessert face first. Savor the sweet moment: "When you take the time to slow down and be more mindful of what something really tastes like, you'll feel more satisfied," says Lesley Lutes, PhD, an assistant professor of psychology at East Carolina University. To give in without going crazy, try this simple strategy: Dish out a single serving of your favorite treat and spend a full minute smelling it, looking at it, and thinking about it. Then take a little bite. Chew slowly, moving it around your mouth and observing the texture and taste. After you swallow, ask yourself: Do I want another bite? Or am I satisfied? If you still want more, repeat. Continue this cycle for as long as you want or until you finish the treat (it should take about 10 minutes). You may find that you're content after only a couple of bites, says Lutes.

■ **EAT PROTEIN FOR BREAKFAST** Aim to take in at least 30 grams of protein at breakfast, says Donald Layman, PhD, a professor emeritus of nutrition at the University of Illinois. A protein-rich breakfast can help you feel full for hours and can reduce cravings later in the day. A couple of solid breakfast choices: ham and egg on a whole-grain English muffin or a fruit smoothie made with protein-packed, low-fat yogurt.

BONUS BENEFIT!

Don't go the egg-whites-only route. The yolk houses most of the egg's nutrients, including cancer-fighting choline and antioxidants that help preserve your vision. And don't worry about the cholesterol and saturated fats in the yolks. Two new studies from the University of Connecticut found that eating eggs actually *improved* cholesterol levels and reduced disease-causing inflammation in the body. Lecithin, a substance found in the yolk, helps remove cholesterol from the tissue and transport it to the liver, preventing buildup in your blood vessels, says study author Maria Luz Fernandez, PhD.

■ **SLACK OFF OCCASIONALLY** Super-restrictive diets only fuel your cravings. Think about it: If you're eating rice cakes all day, a heaping slice of chocolate cake becomes tougher and tougher to resist. "When you forbid a food, it only becomes more attractive, and you become likely to overeat," says Janet Polivy, PhD, a professor of psychology at the University of Toronto. So allow yourself a cheat meal once a week. Although flexible dieters experience just as many cravings, they're more likely to get back on track quickly after indulging than rigid dieters are. "If you're doing a good job of sticking to your diet, let the foods you're craving be a reward by scheduling them into a meal," says Joshua Klapow, PhD, a psychologist at the University of Alabama at Birmingham.

■ **FILL UP ON FRUIT** Yes, fruit is high in carbohydrates. But it still has less of an impact on your blood sugar than grains and other starchy foods do, thanks to its payload of fiber. That means eating a couple of servings of fruit per day can help you avoid the cravings that occur when your blood sugar spikes and then crashes. Next time your sweet tooth comes calling, grab a fresh piece of fruit. The best ones for fighting cravings are the richest in fiber: raspberries, apples, strawberries, bananas, and oranges.

■ **BREAK THE SALTY CYCLE** Your salt craving is nothing more than a bad habit. If you can cut your intake of salty foods for a couple of weeks, it'll most likely fade away, says Thomas Moore, MD, of Boston University Medical Center. Besides, it may be the crunch of pretzels and chips, not the salt, that you're actually craving. Swap in carrots and celery, and if that doesn't calm your craving, munch on a few reduced-sodium pretzels.

■ **TAME CRAVINGS WITH TRIDENT** Most cravings pass given half an hour or so. You just need to occupy your mouth in the meantime. So pop in a piece of sugar-free gum—the act of chewing, even if you're not consuming many calories, can help control your urge to binge. In fact, in a 2011 study in the journal *Appetite*, people who chewed gum after lunch were significantly less likely to crave sweet and salty snacks than nonchewers were.

■ **MAKE SMART SWAPS** It's tempting to try to eat around your cravings. But you'll only end up nibbling until you've taken in 500 calories, without feeling the least bit satisfied. So instead of fighting your urges, find healthier ways to quiet them. For example, calm your sweet tooth with fruit—natural sugars can be incredibly satisfying. (Hint: Frozen grapes taste like an ice pop.) Or satisfy a craving for savory foods with a hearty serving of lean meat. When it comes to chocolate, however, research suggests that imitations won't hit the spot. So get your fix in 150-calorie doses. That's about one snack-size chocolate bar.

■ **ACCEPT DEFEAT** You've most likely noticed: The more you try to ignore your cravings, the worse they become. So admit to yourself that you want a gooey slice of cake. Then choose not to act on it. In a recent study, people who resisted gorging themselves on Hershey's Kisses used a similar strategy: Acknowledge the craving, accept it, and move on.

■ **SKIP ARTIFICIAL SWEETENERS** Sugar substitutes don't quash cravings. In fact, they fan your fire of desire even more because they are often sweeter than sugar itself. Aspartame, for example, is 160 to 220 times sweeter than sugar! What that means: Artificial sweeteners can increase your overall preference for sweetness, thus boosting your cravings for sugar, according to a 2010 paper in the *Yale Journal of Biology and Medicine*. These sugar imitators are hiding in everything from diet soda to reduced-fat foods.

■ **TAKE A WALK** A short walk can slash chocolate cravings. In a 2011 study in the journal *Appetite*, people who took a brisk 15-minute walk ate 46 percent less chocolate while performing a mental task than nonexercisers did. Try it: Instead of having dessert immediately after dinner, go for a walk around the block. (If you're dining out, walk to another spot for dessert.) You may find that you no longer want something sweet.

■ **PRACTICE MIND CONTROL** To stop thinking about that burger, start thinking about going for a quiet run in the park. In a recent McGill University study, the intensity of people's food cravings decreased when they imagined themselves engaging in their favorite activities. Cravings are based on mental imagery, so focusing your attention elsewhere reduces your desire to binge. But it doesn't have to be a run—just conjure up something you find pleasant. Your short-term memory has limited storage, so it can't simultaneously obsess over a cheeseburger *and* vacation in Cancún.

■ **EAT DESSERT FOR BREAKFAST** It may sound like a recipe for weight gain to start your day with cake. But new research from Tel Aviv suggests that eating dessert for breakfast may actually diminish your cravings throughout the day, since the sweets trigger a feel-good serotonin surge that can last for hours. In their study, dieters who ate a small treat after a protein-rich breakfast lost an average of 40 pounds more than those who didn't indulge. Try a 150- to 200-calorie piece of dark chocolate.

■ **TWIDDLE YOUR THUMBS** Fighting the urge to indulge doesn't have to be torturous. In fact, it can be fun. A recent study from the United Kingdom found that working with your hands can help curb cravings. The researchers had chocoholics manipulate modeling clay, and found that after 10 minutes, their desire for chocolate waned. What's going on? Playing with clay engages your "visuospatial memory," effectively distracting your brain from food fantasies, explains study author Jackie Andrade, PhD. Making Silly Putty sculptures isn't the only activity that can conquer cravings—tasks like solving a Rubik's Cube may offer a similar benefit.

Journaling

12 ways tracking your progress can boost your motivation

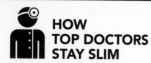

HOW TOP DOCTORS STAY SLIM

"I monitor my weight by tuning in to the difference between 'head hunger' and 'biological hunger.' Chances are, if I ate recently, it's the former and has a psychological cause: Am I bored? Stressed? Tired?"

—**MADELYN FERNSTROM, PhD,** founding director of the University of Pittsburgh Medical Center Weight Management Center

There is power in the pen. Keeping a food log helps you control your calorie intake in two ways: First, it's a reality check, since dieters tend to underestimate what they eat ("I really ate six cookies?"). Second, it builds your awareness *as* you eat, so you avoid the postmeal guilt. The evidence in favor of journaling keeps piling up. In a University of Arkansas study, people who wrote down everything they ate for at least 3 weeks dropped 3½ pounds more than those who didn't. A 6-month study found that people who put pen to paper lost twice as much weight as those who didn't. According to Kaiser Permanente research, food journaling is a better predictor of weight loss than exercise! Here's how to harness the weight-loss power of journaling:

■ **ANALYZE YOUR EATING HABITS** Don't simply record your meals then never look at your log again. Analyze them closely, looking for key patterns, says Lesley Lutes, PhD, an assistant professor of psychology at East Carolina University. Take note of bad habits: Do you skip meals? Do you gorge yourself on the weekends? Are you especially susceptible to sweets after work? "Knowing your routine helps you figure out what changes are right for you," she says.

■ **KEEP IT SIMPLE AT FIRST** In the beginning, don't bother tallying fat, protein, or calories. Rather, focus on establishing the habit of recording everything that makes it into your mouth. Then once you see it all on paper, look for small, painless ways to cut back. For example, switch from a roast beef sandwich on a bun with Cheddar and mayo to roast beef on whole grain bread with light Swiss and mustard. Simple swaps like this one can add up to major weight loss.

■ **DON'T FORGET THE SMALL STUFF** Write *everything* down—not just major meals and snacks. Your journal should include your morning coffee, the french fries you swiped from your child's plate, and the samples you snacked on at the grocery store. Building awareness of your sneakiest sources of calories can help you find simple ways to save.

■ **LOG YOUR PORTIONS** Recording "Cheerios and milk" isn't too painful. But what if you're talking 3 cups of cereal and enough milk to sink half a box of O's? That's a different story. Make sure to estimate the portion size of everything you eat, so you can accurately gauge your intake and problem areas.

■ **RATE YOUR HUNGER** Every time you eat, record whether or not you're hungry. This can help you identify the times you eat for social or emotional reasons, or simply out of boredom. (For a hunger rating chart, see page 434.)

■ **COUNT SWIZZLE STICKS** It's easy to lose track of how much alcohol you imbibe. So grab a cocktail napkin, and throughout the evening, write down the number of alcoholic beverages you drink. The next morning, calculate the number of calories, carbs, and sugars you took in. Prepare for a reality check.

■ **ACKNOWLEDGE YOUR FEELINGS** If you notice consistent trouble spots in your diet— say, bingeing on desserts or overdoing it at lunch—try journaling about your feelings in your food log. This can help you identify the emotional triggers that compel you to eat; once you're consciously aware of your weak spots, it's easier to overcome them.

■ **GO DIGITAL** Do you hate writing everything down? Move your journal to an online platform, such as NutritionData.com or MyFitnessPal.com. (You can even download an iPhone app for on-the-go tracking.) Bonus: These sites offer free nutrient analysis, so you'll know if you're overdoing it in any one area (like sugar or sodium). You can also try e-mailing your daily intake to yourself or keeping track of it in an Excel document.

■ **TRACK YOUR WEIGHT** It's not just food that belongs in your journal. Each morning after you step on the scale, jot down your weight. It's extremely motivating to see your long-term progress ("Wow, I've lost 6 pounds in 3 weeks!") on paper. You can even create a line chart to help you see the magnitude of your progress.

■ **LOG YOUR EXERCISE** Carry a scratch pad with you to the gym. After each exercise, record the number of sets and reps you completed, as well as the weight you used. This not only spurs you to beat your personal record, but it also helps you track how far you've come.

■ **BRAINSTORM FUN WORKOUTS** Jotting down ways to make exercise more fun can help you work out longer, a study in the *Journal of Applied Biobehavioral Research* found. Every week, exercisers wrote down ideas for making activity more pleasurable—for example, "hitting the trails with friends," "listening to music," or "trying a new fitness class." After 2 months, they were exercising twice as long as those who listed reasons to exercise, such as "to lose weight." You may find it more motivating to base your ideas on positive past experiences, like that 10-mile bike ride with your buddies, rather than abstract ideas, says study author Laura Ten Eyck, PhD.

■ **KEEP A "REVERSE" DIARY** Try mapping out your menu ahead of time. Then promise yourself that you're going to stick to it, and build in small rewards for the days that you adhere to your plan. A similar strategy: Write down what you eat *before* you dive in. If you've already recorded your intake, you won't want to amend it.

Motivation

24 simple strategies for sticking to your plan

Motivation may be the weight-loss X factor. It's what keeps you in the gym and helps you resist the drive-thru. And even if you set the loftiest of goals, you won't achieve them if your motivation is lacking. If you're low on enthusiasm, try these strategies to keep your head in the game:

■ **THINK ABOUT YOUR FAMILY** Consider what you'll look and feel like 5 years from now if you don't make a change. Then ask yourself how that will affect your family. You can even write down your answer—putting it on paper may help it seem concrete. Even if personal goals don't motivate you, thinking about loved ones surely will.

■ **TRACK YOUR VICTORIES** Remember those gold stars from kindergarten? It's time to bring them back. When keeping your food log, flag your healthy choices with a gold star. It sounds cheesy, but the positive reinforcement will help motivate you. After you've earned a certain number of gold stars, plan a reward—for example, a fun day trip.

■ **SIGN UP FOR A CHARITY RACE** It's hard to blow off a commitment you've made to lots of people. Plus, if you sign up for a race, you're not only committing to the event (and the money you shell out for the entry free) but also to the training it requires. The motivation may last well after the finish line: A recent Temple University study found that people who participate in a race (especially newbies) often keep exercising afterward if they enjoy the event. Visit

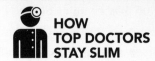

HOW TOP DOCTORS STAY SLIM

"I watch old television series, either on DVD or DVR, while I'm on the treadmill. Once I've gotten into a series, it's much easier to get back on the treadmill each morning and stay on for the entire hour."

—**DAVID SARWER, PhD,** a psychologist at the University of Pennsylvania's Center for Weight and Eating Disorders

Active.com to search for events in your town.

■ **FOCUS ON THE DAY-TO-DAY** Obsessing over your final goal—say, losing 20 pounds—can actually wreck your motivation. The reason: When you've only shed 2 pounds, dropping another 18 can sound daunting, so you may be inclined to give up. University of Iowa scientists found that people are more likely to stick with their belly-off plans when they focus on specific actions instead of the desired result. So make a list of fitness and nutrition goals, such as eating a serving of vegetables with every meal or exercising three times a week. "Setting goals that target specific behaviors helps you see progress, even before it shows up on the scale," says study author Faryle Nothwehr, PhD. "This encourages you to keep at it." Avoid goals that aren't clearly defined, such as "being healthy." These give you too much leeway.

■ **WEIGH YOURSELF ONCE A DAY** If you weigh in every day, you'll be more likely to stick to your plan and maintain your losses. In a study of 3,500 people from the National Weight Control Registry (NWCR) who've maintained 60 or more pounds of weight loss for at least a year, researchers found that 44 percent of them weighed themselves daily. As long as you keep it to once a day, it won't become an unhealthy obsession. Rather, it acts as an early warning system to help you prevent weight regain, says James Hill, PhD, cofounder of NWCR and director of the Center for Human Nutrition at the University of Colo-

rado. "If your goal is to keep your weight at a certain level, you have to have feedback to see whether you're successful."

However, if you step on the scale too often—for example, in the morning and evening—you'll only derail your efforts. Your weight naturally fluctuates throughout the day, and of course, you'll weigh more after a full day of eating (even healthy eating). Seeing that extra pound, even if you know it's not permanent, at the end of the day can be discouraging. Stick to once-a-day weigh-ins, ideally in the morning.

■ **CHART YOUR PROGRESS** Weighing yourself on a daily basis is a start. But you can up the motivation factor by writing down your weight each day. Take it a step further by using your computer to create a line graph that tracks your progress. Whenever you feel discouraged, you can review your long-term progress to help you stay on track.

■ **ELEVATE YOUR EXPECTATIONS** Why settle for 10 pounds when you could lose 20? Setting bigger goals can help you lose more weight, according to University of Minnesota research. Another study in the *International Journal of Obesity* found that women who set big weight-loss goals shed more flab over 2 years than those who set less lofty goals. (And the dieters who failed to reach their goal weight didn't give up, either.) Better yet, set at least two specific goals: one for weight loss ("I want to lose 20 pounds") and one for fitness ("I want to run a 10-K"). That way, if your progress has stalled according to the scale, you can still make headway in the gym.

■ **GIVE YOURSELF A DEADLINE** If you have a time frame, you're less likely to put healthy eating and exercise on the back burner. (Think about it: Brides-to-be are always miraculously able to lose weight.) So choose a specific day—say, your birthday or the first day of summer—and mark your calendar. "Specific goals help focus your attention and increase your effort, which helps you persist longer," says Gary Latham, PhD, a professor of organizational effectiveness at the University of Toronto. A word of caution: Don't select a day when you want to impress others, such as your class reunion, as your endpoint. (See "Lose Weight for Yourself" on page 80.)

■ **LIFT HOW MUCH YOU'VE LOST** At the gym, work out with dumbbells that correspond to the number of pounds you've shed. It will help remind you of how far you've come— and that you don't want to ever carry that excess weight around again!

■ **SCHEDULE A MASSAGE** Research suggests that accepting your body can actually improve your eating habits. One way to improve your self-image: Stretch out on the massage table. Allowing another person to touch you—even if you haven't yet reached your goal weight—can help you feel more comfortable with your body, says Mitch Klein, a licensed massage therapist in New York City. And that's incredibly motivating.

■ **FIGHT THROUGH DISCOMFORT** The first few times you exercise, you *will* feel sore. Don't let that discourage you—see your pain as a sign of progress. If you view it as pushing you one step closer to your goal, you'll suddenly find that you look forward to your postexercise soreness.

■ **REVIEW YOUR DIET** Keeping track of your diet can help you lose twice as much weight, a recent study in the *American Journal of Preventive Medicine* found. Jot down everything you eat for 7 days, look for simple ways to shave calories, then incorporate those changes the following week. When you see your success on paper, it motivates you to keep at it.

Plus, it keeps you from falling into a rut. It can be tempting to stick with the same diet you started with—after all, it helped you lose weight at first. But as you slim down, you need to make subtle adjustments to keep your metabolism in gear and to avoid a plateau. So try to address one problem area each week. For example, if you're still raiding the cookie jar at 3:00 p.m. every day, start swapping in fruit. Then next week, tackle your diet soda addiction.

■ **BUILD A WORKOUT PLAYLIST** You're more likely to stick with an exercise program if you listen to music while working out, suggests a recent study by the North American Association for the Study of Obesity. One reason: Music distracts you from any discomfort you're feeling during exercise, making your workout more enjoyable, says Costas Karageorghis, PhD, of the sports psychology department at Brunel

University in the United Kingdom. Compose a playlist of songs that inspire you, or check out JogTunes.com. The site allows you to select your workout pace, then download playlists that have a tempo to match your target heart rate.

■ **BREAK OUT YOUR SKINNY CLOTHES** Remember that *great* dress you wore in college? Or that expensive shirt you haven't been able to wear in years? Unearth it from the back of your closet. "I tell clients to take out an outfit they love and haven't been able to wear for a long time," says Christopher Warden, CSCS, a personal trainer in New York City. "Just pulling it out of the closet serves as a visual reminder of the goal they're trying to accomplish."

■ **FACE YOUR REFLECTION** When you feel fat, it's tempting to shun mirrors entirely. But you should do just the opposite. Checking out your physique while refusing to give in to your usual critical thoughts can boost your body image, research shows. This, in turn, can motivate you to stay committed to your belly-blasting plan. As you gaze at yourself, avoid negative thoughts. Say things like "I can tell I've been doing lunges," not "I still have a big butt."

■ **LOSE WEIGHT FOR YOURSELF** Research shows that half of the people who start an exercise program slack off within 6 months. That's because many of the reasons people work out—say, shaping up for a significant other or obeying doctor's orders—aren't for themselves. Internal motivation is much more effective. So set a self-serving goal such as "I want to feel more confident," or "I want to be able to walk up steps without feeling winded." If you decide to get fit because you want to feel stronger or healthier, you're more likely to be successful and stay motivated.

■ **FOCUS ON HOW YOU FEEL** It's easy to fixate on the weight or inches you've lost. But that's only one part of your purpose at the gym. You're also there to give yourself a boost, both emotionally and physically. One study found that people who signed up for exercise classes because they wanted to feel good were more likely to attend than those who did it to look good. After your workout, take a moment to enjoy the endorphin rush, while noting positive changes in your body, such as less back pain or tension in your neck.

■ **FIND A WORKOUT YOU LOVE** If Pilates makes you feel powerful, find a studio in your area. Or if running is more your style, sign up for a 5-K or join a local running group. When you feel exhilarated by your workout, it's easier to push yourself and find the motivation to do it again.

■ **ELIMINATE FAILURE AS AN OPTION** Are you going to eat healthy snacks? Yes! Will you make a protein-rich breakfast part of your day? Yes! Will you make it to the gym tomorrow? Yes! Answering positively to a yes-or-no question boosts your likelihood of success, according to a recent Washington State University study. The researchers found that when people said they would visit the health club, they boosted their consumption of healthy snacks and felt more committed to a new healthy lifestyle. Stating your intentions out loud can help, so have a close friend or family member ask you each night, "Are you going to the gym tomorrow?"

■ **BEFRIEND YOUR INSTRUCTOR** Move to the front of your yoga or Zumba class and make an effort to connect with your instructor. Getting to know your group fitness leader can help you feel involved—and may compel you to come to class more often. In fact, Springfield College scientists found that hiding out in the back of the fitness class prevents you from learning and feeling competent. Make friends with class regulars, too. You'll be embarrassed to face them if you play hooky, and the promise of socializing while you exercise can motivate you to attend.

■ **BRIBE YOURSELF** Nothing motivates like money. In a study in the *Journal of Occupational and Environmental Medicine*, researchers offered overweight or obese people either $7, $14, or nothing for every 1 percent drop in weight. After 3 months, those who were offered the most had lost the most weight. For every pound you lose, stash away $10. Once you reach your goal, treat yourself to a manicure, tickets to a sporting event, or a new pair of shoes.

■ **FIND A WORKOUT ALTERNATIVE** If you have a busy schedule, you probably won't be able to make it to the gym every day. But that doesn't mean you can't be active every day. Come up with a plan B: "If I miss the gym, I'll run around the block or do lunges and squats in my living room." This will help you maintain your fitness momentum, even when life makes it tough to stick with it.

■ **DON'T OVERDO IT** Compulsively exercising sucks the fun out of it, draining you of all motivation to continue hitting the gym. Don't think of your workout as a chore you *have* to do. Think of it as a way to decompress after a long day or as a midday break from the office. Diversifying your workouts can help: Play tennis one day, take a Spin class the next, and then lift weights a couple of times per week. Trying new activities will bust any boredom that threatens your resolve. And, remember, not every workout has to be an hour-long session. You can keep it short and sweet a couple of times per week.

■ **ENLIST YOUR DOG** If you can't get your butt off the couch, your dog will! Research shows that dog owners are more devoted to exercise, since they don't want to deprive their pooch of a walk. Make a walk around the block a nightly commitment for you and your dog. Note: This doesn't work for cat owners.

Social Influences

10 ways to make friends and family your weight-loss allies

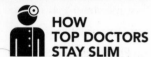

HOW TOP DOCTORS STAY SLIM

"My wife and I do not keep sweets in the house. When our kids go to birthday parties, they scrape the frosting off the cake because it tastes too sweet to them. People think the problem with sugar is that it makes you fat. But it's not just inches around your waist. Sugar is a potential toxin. The liver becomes fatty, and it starts to release small, dense particles of LDL, which are the most damaging kind for blood vessels. Ice cream is my weakness. But I've got to walk to get it—the store is more than a mile away. I'll walk there with the girls once a month."

—SANJAY GUPTA, MD, an assistant professor of neurosurgery at Emory University and CNN's chief medical correspondent

You've dutifully stuck to your diet plan all week. Then comes Friday night, when you find yourself face-to-face with a cheesy fried appetizer intended to be shared among friends. Or you go out for after-work drinks and are tempted by the supersweet martinis, since all of your girlfriends are drinking them. "Women tend to match each other's behavior at the table," says Marisa Moore, RD, a nutritionist based in Atlanta. Men, on the other hand, feel a social pressure to eat up, having been raised to equate manhood with a ravenous appetite.

Neither are conducive to weight loss. In fact, people who dine with one other person take in about 35 percent more calories than when they dine alone. Join a party of eight, and you'll nearly double your intake! You don't have to ditch your friends and family to lose weight. Simply equip yourself with these strategies—which can even help you use your social network as a motivating force.

■ **PREPARE A COMEBACK** If you refuse to eat those chili-cheese fries, your friends are undoubtedly going to ask, "Why aren't you eating?" You may even feel pressure to eat because others think you're not enjoying yourself, says psychologist Martin Binks, PhD, the former director of behavioral health at the Duke Diet and Fitness Center. To avoid being met with groans, say something as simple as "I had a late lunch." Or if you don't have a viable excuse, come armed with stories. If you're carrying the conversation, you can't stuff yourself, too!

■ **TAKE IT SLOW** Nibble on appetizers like you'd nurse a cocktail. Your friends will see that you're munching, so they won't start quizzing you. Plus, eating slowly helps you feel fuller. Another strategy: Dive into the appetizer last and you'll keep your calories down. That plate will be empty well before you can grab seconds.

■ **BUILD A WEIGHT-LOSS TEAM** In a study of people who lost weight and kept it off, 70 percent said they had strong social support, compared to only 38 percent of those who regained lost weight. Another study found that socializing with others who have successfully shed weight improves your odds of maintaining your weight loss. "You can improve your self-control by being strategic with your social network," says Michelle vanDellen, PhD, a social psychology researcher at Duke University. Ask a friend who's also trying to slim down to hold you accountable, or find a dieting partner at WeightLossBuddy.com.

■ **KEEP GATHERINGS SMALL** If it feels like a party, you may feel free to eat like it's a party. A recent study in the journal *Appetite* found that women who lunched with four friends took in 150 calories more than those who dined with three. Until you feel strong enough to resist that Bloomin' Onion, limit the size of your lunch-date crowd.

■ **CHOOSE YOUR DINNER PARTNER WISELY** Your thin friends could be thwarting your weight-loss efforts. If you watch a fit person order a lot of food, you may be more inclined to eat heartily, too, according to researchers at the University of British Columbia. In their study, people who watched a skinny person dish out 5 tablespoons of M&M's ate three times as much candy as when they indulged alone. "You assume you can also stay thin by eating the same amount," says study author Brent McFerran, PhD. His advice: Dine with health-conscious friends. A separate study found that you may order less when dining with people who watch what they eat.

■ **FIND A LIKE-MINDED WORKOUT PARTNER** Are you looking to lose 20 pounds? Shed your cellulite? Tone up your stomach? Find a friend who has similar goals and ask him or her to join you at the gym. (Or make it your significant other. A recent Duke study found that people were 50 percent more likely to start exercising if their partner joined them.) "When people do something together, they're more likely to stick with it," says Karen Miller-Kovach, RD, author of *He Loses, She Loses*. Instead of a competition, establish a friendly camaraderie, which is more encouraging, say Canadian researchers. Make a pact to push each other toward your mutual goals, and schedule a standing gym date at least three times per week.

■ **DROP WEIGHT TOGETHER** Falling in love can make you fall off the wagon. It's suddenly easier to skip your workout or have pizza for dinner instead of eating your normal grilled chicken and roasted veggies. "When we get comfortable in a relationship, we establish new habits together that aren't always the best for our weight," says Amy Gorin, PhD, an assistant professor of psychology at Brown University. Of course, your mate can act as an accountability partner in your quest to lose those love handles.

In fact, couples who diet together are more likely to succeed, according to recent Israeli research. "Sharing dishes and eating together helps the dieters stick to a diet—there won't be temptations on their plates," says study author Rachel Golan, RD, MPH. Map out a weekly meal plan you can both agree to, then cook together at least 5 nights a week. Dining at home could save you about 290 calories per day!

■ **COUPLE UP AT THE GYM** A study in the journal *Obesity* found that couples who live together for at least 2 years are less likely to be active. But you can also be each other's biggest ally at the gym, says Gorin. Women who work out with a partner tend to lose more weight than those who sweat solo, according to research in the *Archives of Internal Medicine*. So join the gym together and meet up a few times a week after work. If one (or both) of you hates the gym, train together for a 5-K, or make your Saturday dates something active, like riding bikes or hiking.

■ **AVOID EATING LIKE A KID** Parents, beware: People with kids at home are significantly more likely to scarf pizza, cheese, ice cream, bacon, and salty snacks, according to a study in the *Journal of the American Board of Family Medicine*. Parents averaged an extra 5 grams of fat every day—nearly 2 of which were saturated. That's the saturated-fat equivalent of a slice of pepperoni pizza! When you're feeding a family, it's easy to settle for grab-and-go foods you know your kids will eat, the scientists say. Try preparing a week's worth of meals every Sunday night, then freezing them to eat throughout the week. That way, you won't fall into the convenience-food trap.

■ **RECRUIT YOUR COWORKERS** Ask your workplace to launch an official fitness incentive program. A study in *Eating Behaviors* found that when female coworkers teamed up to lose weight, they were more likely to exercise and shed weight faster. It also benefits your employer: Research suggests that workplace fitness programs increase productivity!

HOW YOUR DOG CAN HELP YOU LOSE WEIGHT

Walking your pooch can help shrink your paunch. People who logged 20 minutes of leash time five times a week dropped an average of 14 pounds in a year, University of Missouri-Columbia research found. Dog owners have also been shown to be better at overcoming exercise barriers, such as a busy work schedule. One reason: Pets are enthusiastic exercise partners—they're always game, regardless of the weather or what's on TV. To maximize your workout, throw in some high-energy games like chase, tug-of-war, and Frisbee.

If you're ready to start running, don't ditch your dog. Once he establishes a routine—say, a morning jog—he'll be sure to remind you (cue the wet nose). Plus, his steady pace will help you stick to a more strenuous training plan. Even if you don't have a dog, you can still reap the benefits. Find an animal shelter at www.aspca.org, and volunteer to run or walk a pound pup.

Stress

10 stress-busting tips to help you lose weight faster

There's a reason you want to munch on a brownie instead of Brussels sprouts after having a tough day at the office. Your body releases a flood of the hormone cortisol when you're stressed. You usually don't feel its effects for about an hour, but when it hits, you know it: Cortisol essentially turns your body into a carb- and fat-seeking missile. (There's a reason fried foods and desserts are considered "comfort" foods.) In fact, a recent British study linked high levels of the hormone to increased munching on junk food.

"Cortisol is one of the most potent appetite signals we have," says nutritional biochemist Shawn Talbott, PhD. Research suggests that it may meddle with the hormones that control your appetite (ghrelin) and help you feel full and satisfied (leptin). So when your cortisol levels skyrocket, you're more likely to crave a decadent dessert—and lack the willpower to resist.

But the bigger danger doesn't necessarily involve the pathway from your couch to your kitchen. Chronically elevated cortisol levels encourage your body to store excess fat, particularly in your belly. "Abdominal fat is rich in cortisol receptors, which facilitate the process of turning the unburned fat you eat into visceral fat,"

HOW TOP DOCTORS STAY SLIM

"I think stress reduction is important for weight control, so I try to find time to take a bubble bath, get an occasional massage, and practice mindfulness and prayer. And I spend time outdoors with my kids at Golden Gate Park and our neighborhood playgrounds."

—NAOMI STOTLAND, MD, a doctor at the Center for Obesity Assessment, Study, and Treatment at the University of California, San Francisco

says George Blackburn, MD, PhD, associate director of nutrition at Harvard Medical School. Cortisol may also slow your production of testosterone (women have it, too), a hormone essential to building muscle. And low muscle mass ultimately translates to a slower metabolism.

Unless you quit your job and move to Fiji, you can't always avoid stress or stop your body's automatic response to it. But you *can* help control it. Try these easy stress-stamping strategies:

■ **HIT THE SACK EARLIER** A healthy diet and regular exercise can help ward off stress and belly fat—but only if you're getting enough sleep. Skimping on shut-eye causes your cortisol levels to rise, while also triggering an increase in deep abdominal fat—the most dangerous kind. In a Canadian study, scientists found that people who averaged 5 to 6 hours of sleep per night were nearly 60 percent thicker around the middle than those who logged 7 to 8 hours. You may not even need as much snooze time as you think: A study in the journal *Sleep* showed that more than 8 hours of shut-eye could lead to weight gain.

■ **BOOK A MASSAGE** Stop thinking of a massage as an indulgence. Think of it as an important stress-fighting, fat-blasting tool, since massage can help lower your cortisol levels. In one study, one 15-minute chair massage lowered people's cortisol levels by 24 percent. Not only did they feel less stressed, anxious, and depressed, they solved math problems faster

and more accurately after the massage! That may translate to higher productivity at work. If you can't break away from your desk during the day, keep a handheld back massager in your office and take periodic massage breaks.

■ **CHEW GUM** Chewing gum can dampen your cortisol response to stress, helping you feel less anxious and more alert, according to a 2009 article in *Physiology & Behavior*. The scientists aren't sure why it works, but they speculate that the act of chewing boosts blood-flow to your brain. Or a simpler explanation: Chomping on Extra distracts you from your feelings of mental overload.

■ **EAT BEFORE AND AFTER EXERCISE** Fueling up on protein before and after you hit the gym can dampen the effects of cortisol, which is released in response to exercise. Eat a snack rich in both carbs and protein, such as an apple and peanut butter, about half an hour before your workout. Then have a protein-rich meal immediately after.

■ **LAUGH OUT LOUD** Laughter can help lessen the toll cortisol takes on your body. That's because it signals your body to release relaxing endorphins, also known as "happy chemicals." It can be as easy as watching a funny 3-minute video on YouTube. You have time for that, right?

■ **DISTRACT YOURSELF** Cortisol doesn't linger in your bloodstream forever. So if you can resist the call of those Twinkies for 2 or 3 hours, you'll be in the clear. Buy your favorite magazine and cozy up on the couch for a couple of hours. Or hit the gym for an intense sweat session. You'll forget all about the "feed me now!" call of cortisol.

■ **GET MOVING** Yoga isn't the only stress-relieving exercise. Any form of physical activity performed 30 minutes a day can combat cortisol. Instead of "steady-state" cardio, where you work at a consistent pace the entire time, try interval training, where you exercise in short, intense bursts. This type of exercise is thought to influence your hormones faster than regular cardio, thus enhancing the stress-squashing benefit of exercise. Try it: After warming up, sprint for 1 minute, then walk for 1 minute. Repeat 10 to 12 times.

■ **LOAD UP ON VITAMIN D** Vitamin D, found in fortified milk and fatty fish, is thought to partner with calcium to slow your body's production of cortisol. This not only helps control your stress levels but may also help burn up belly fat!

■ **CRANK UP THE DOPAMINE** A 2011 study in *Nature Neuroscience* found that listening to favorite tunes or anticipating a certain point in a song can cause a pleasurable flood of dopamine. Your music Rx: Slip in your earbuds and listen to a few songs at a time, several times per day. "These doses of dopamine can lower your stress," says Edward Roth, MT-BC, a professor of music therapy at Western Michigan University.

■ **ADOPT A NEW HOBBY** Learn to play badminton. (Just kidding.) Practice the guitar. Master the art of grilling. Any activity that gives you a sense of mastery can activate your brain's mesocorticolimbic system, a key reward region, which causes the release of stress-fighting dopamine. Plus, as you practice your new hobby, you'll enter a psychological state called "flow." "You lose track of time and are completely immersed in what you're doing," says Michael Addis, PhD, a psychology professor at Clark University. "It's incredibly relaxing to the mind."

Willpower

6 exercises to strengthen your resolve

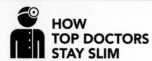

HOW TOP DOCTORS STAY SLIM

"I try to look at most meals as energy rather than fun, so I choose foods that will give me the nutrients I need. Meals that are packed with protein are filling enough that I'm not starving and keep me from being tempted by unhealthy treats at the coffee shop."

—**DAVID SARWER, PHD,** a psychologist at the University of Pennsylvania's Center for Weight and Eating Disorders

Willpower is like gas in your car: Once your tank is empty, you're not going anywhere (except, perhaps, the ice-cream aisle). Studies suggest that people have only a limited reserve of willpower. And it's not just fighting temptation that taps into your supply. Controlling your emotions, paying attention during meetings, performing your best at work—all of these things are thought to deplete the same supply of mental energy you need to resist that doughnut. Unfortunately, it's often when your willpower is sapped that you're most tempted to cave to the Krispy Kreme diet.

Your self-control, however, doesn't rest on mental strength alone. Physiological factors, such as blood sugar, brain chemistry, and hormones, also influence—and can undermine—your ability to say no. Here's how to reclaim your willpower:

■ **GO EASY ON THE COCKTAILS** Alcohol is more than a source of empty calories. It may also weaken your willpower, so you find yourself impulsively ordering a platter of wings or a 600-calorie cocktail. That's because booze slows the flow of glucose—your fuel for mental tasks—to the parts of your brain responsible for self-control, according to a 2007 Florida State University review of studies. You don't have to abandon it all together. You simply need to pace yourself. Try holding your drink in your nondominant hand, so you don't raise your glass to your lips as automatically.

■ **FUEL YOUR RESOLVE** When you're eager to shed weight, it's tempting to eat like a rabbit. But depriving yourself of a healthy meal or snack also drains your body of glucose, so your brain lacks the energy to resist a pig-out. (Plus, starving yourself curtails production of leptin, a hormone that helps regulate appetite.) Your move: Spread your calories out—three meals of about 500 calories and two snacks of 100 to 200 calories, ideally with both complex carbs and protein. This helps keep you satisfied, so you never feel an overwhelming need to raid the pantry.

■ **ADJUST YOUR MIND-SET** If you tell yourself, "I can never eat potato chips again," you're going to obsess over the Lay's in your office vending machine. So switch your weight-loss mind-set by mentally repeating, "I'm starting a new, healthy routine." Then focus on what you *can* have.

■ **INDULGE ON OCCASION** If you're constantly telling yourself no, you may eventually lose all willpower and dive into that tub of ice cream. Rather than always choosing the healthy option, allow yourself one indulgence a week. This can actually boost your resolve in the long term. In a recent study in the journal *Obesity*, eating chocolate mousse decreased people's desire for bread and desserts more effectively than a cottage cheese snack did. When following a healthy-eating plan, it may be better to consume a real dessert than a "healthy" substitute, says study author Sofie Lemmens, PhD. The occasional indulgence satisfies your cravings—and helps control your intake of other foods.

■ **BEAT HUNGER PANGS WITH FULLNESS** Fiber-rich foods help you feel fuller longer, which means hunger pangs won't override your willpower. Aim for at least 25 grams (women) or 38 grams (men) per day—whole grains (especially bulgur), beans and peas, artichokes, and raspberries are all great sources.

■ **DON'T SKIMP ON SLEEP** Logging too little sleep can weaken your self-control, especially as the day drags on. One reason: A lack of shut-eye has been linked with elevated levels of ghrelin, a hormone that triggers hunger, possibly making you more prone to bingeing when you're sleep deprived. One study found that when people slept only 4 hours for 2 nights in a row, their appetites increased by 23 percent, particularly for salty snacks and sweets. Shoot for 7 to 8 hours per night.

Part 3
YOUR DIET

The most critical element
of weight loss

A recent analysis of 33 weight-loss studies concluded that diet—the food you put into your body—controls about 75 percent of your ability to lose weight. While exercise is important for overall good health, your eating habits wield the greatest influence over whether you are heavy or lean. But successful weight loss is not just about cutting calories out of your diet. That rarely works over the long term because when you give your body fewer calories, it responds by reducing the amount of energy it uses, says Keith Berkowitz, MD, medical director of the Center for Balanced Health in New York City. Your body senses the change and compensates by slowing down your metabolism to conserve energy.

How do you overcome that natural tendency of the body to be frugal? You feed it metabolism-revving foods while cutting out "empty calories," calorie-dense foods that have very little nutritional value, such as breakfast muffins, cheese curls, and supersize sodas. (These are the foods that also tend to raise blood sugar and trigger cravings for more.) This section of the book shows you how to cut calories the smart way, not simply by eliminating junk foods but by adding good foods that turn your body into a highly efficient fat-burning machine.

Alcohol

15 ways to drink up and slim down

You're at the bar with your friends, and you order a Chardonnay or maybe a gin and tonic. You promise yourself—and your waistline—that's all you're going to have. But then your friend buys a round, and you can't say no. Down goes drink number 2. Did we mention the wings with blue cheese and the plate of nachos he ordered for the group? You can't be rude, so you partake. "Between the drinks and the bar food, you could put away 1,000 calories at happy hour," says Susan Bowerman, MS, RD, assistant director of the UCLA Center for Human Nutrition.

A single serving of alcohol won't trigger weight gain. In fact, it can help you lose: Recent research shows that people who have one drink a couple of times a week are less likely to become obese than teetotalers. However, regularly drinking any more than one drink (or two for men) may be the fastest route to larger Levi's. In fact, folks who consume more than four drinks daily boost their odds of obesity by 46 percent.

Unlike fat, carbs, and protein, the calories in alcohol can't be stored in your body (it's essentially a toxin), so they have to be used immediately. That sounds like a smart way to enjoy free calories, until you consider the side effect: Your body is

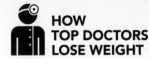

HOW TOP DOCTORS LOSE WEIGHT

"My wife wasn't happy about it, but we got rid of all the red wine glasses that we received for our wedding."

–BRIAN WANSINK, PhD, director of the Cornell University Food and Brand Lab (His research shows that oversized wine glasses can trick you into pouring more than one serving.)

forced to use alcohol as fuel instead of fat, so the fat stays right where it's at. The average drink contains 12 to 14 grams of alcohol—that's 84 to 98 calories your body has to burn before it can break down anything else. Research shows that downing the alcohol equivalent of just two drinks can decrease your fat burning by 73 percent! Sorry to throw a wet blanket on your happy hour, but alcohol is a major factor in weight gain and belly fat.

And it's not just the calories in your glass that you have to worry about. British researchers found that people who drank alcohol-spiked juice half an hour before lunch ate 15 percent more at a buffet than juice-only drinkers. Alcohol is thought to whet your appetite and make food tastier. There may also be a psychological component: Cocktails can undermine your willpower. "Alcohol breaks down inhibitions, so it's harder to make healthy food choices," says Gary Foster, PhD, director of the Center for Obesity Research and Education at Temple University. After a couple of beers, you may suddenly find it easier to ditch your diet and order a basket of fries. Tame your intake with these strategies:

■ **HAVE A DRINK FOR DESSERT** When you slide onto the stool for happy hour, you're in the state of mind to indulge. So you do. And when you have a cocktail *before* dinner, you risk depleting your healthy-eating resolve as you become a little tipsy. So save your wine or

beer for after dinner. Since you're already full from your meal, you're less likely to face alcohol-induced munchies. Think of your drink as your dessert—you wouldn't have more than one slice of cheesecake, right? Limit your imbibing to a single serving one to three times a week. That's 12 ounces of beer, 5 ounces of wine, or 1½ ounces of hard liquor.

■ **SAVOR THE FLAVOR** It's easy to chug supersweet drinks—margaritas, martinis, sangria—since they taste less like alcohol and more like dessert. So opt for high-quality drinks that you'll want to savor, like vintage wine or single malt scotch, instead. These beverages will also have a less-pronounced effect on your blood sugar.

■ **LIGHTEN UP YOUR COCKTAILS** What you need to know about cocktails: sugar + alcohol = lots of calories. If it tastes sweet or has a salty rim, it's probably bad news. Most cocktails have 2 to 5 ounces of alcohol—significantly more than a serving—plus sugary mixers, like grenadine or Midori. Skip the martinis and instead mix a little white wine, seltzer water, cranberry juice, and lime juice as a healthier alternative, suggests dietitian Kristin Kirkpatrick, RD, of the Cleveland Clinic Wellness Institute. (Just make sure your cranberry juice is 100 percent juice rather than a sugar-laden "cocktail" blend.) Another reasonable choice: tequila and club soda.

■ **SKIP SLUSHY DRINKS** If you *do* decide to indulge in a cocktail, order it on the rocks instead of frozen. The slushy drinks are more likely to be made with supersugary mixers than those served on ice.

■ **COUNT BOTTLES** Give yourself a reality check: Jot down how much beer, wine, or other alcoholic beverages you drink in a week. Then calculate the calories. Surprised? A "reasonable" two beers per night can add up to more than 2,000 calories a week—a day's worth of calories! Researchers at the Alcohol Research Group in Emeryville, California, found that people who record every drink consume less alcohol than those who don't keep track of their intake.

■ **GO ON AN ALCOHOL FAST** Try to stop drinking, but just for a week. Over those 7 days, monitor your weight and how your pants fit. You'll undoubtedly notice a difference if you're a regular drinker. Once you realize that you can indeed survive without it, you can go back to having one daily drink—which you may find you no longer desire.

■ **DRINK BOOZE WITH BENEFITS** Choose a beverage that's good for more than getting drunk. Pinot Noir, for example, packs more disease-fighting antioxidants than any other alcoholic drink. And when whipping up cocktails, replace sugar-packed mixers with juices, such as 100 percent pomegranate juice, which is loaded with heart-healthy antioxidants. But remember, even good calories are still calories, so be sure to practice moderation.

■ **STOCK YOUR BAR WITH HIGHBALLS** The type of glass you use can influence how much you pour. In a Cornell University study, researchers asked bartenders to pour a standard 1½-ounce shot of whiskey or rum into either a tall, skinny highball glass or a short, fat tumbler of equal volume. They were right on target with the highballs, but they overpoured by 37 percent into the tumblers. It's a trick of the eye: We perceive tall glasses as larger than short, squat ones. As a result, you're more likely to fill a short glass to the brim, but you stop halfway with a highball. Similarly, balloonlike red wine glasses can trick you into overdoing it. Use a Champagne flute instead.

■ **DOWNSIZE YOUR GLASSES** America has even supersized its barware. Glasses now range from 7 to 13 ounces, even though traditional drink recipes call for no more than 5 ounces of liquid. Shop for 2½-ounce shot glasses, 4½-ounce cocktail glasses, and 10-ounce highball glasses.

■ **SAVE IT FOR THE WEEKEND** Even a bottle of ultra-low-carb beer has 95 calories. Which means if you abstain on weeknights, you could save nearly 500 calories per week! If you can't wait until the weekend, choose one night a week to unwind with a single glass.

■ **OFFSET THE NEGATIVE EFFECTS** If you plan to party tonight, cut back during the day. Eat a low-calorie but filling lunch, like soup or salad. Then, before heading out for a drink, tell yourself you can only go if you hit the gym first. Finally, grab a healthy snack beforehand—try veggies and hummus, turkey with whole-grain crackers, or half a cup of oatmeal

(continued on page 98)

WHAT'S ON TAP?

Calorie counts per serving of popular beers and other alcoholic beverages

BEER

Ales: 150–350 calories

Blue Moon: 171 calories

Brooklyn Brown Ale: 205 calories

Budweiser American Ale: 182 calories

Coopers Sparkling Ale: 180 calories

Newcastle Brown Ale: 180 calories

Redhook ESB Original Ale: 179 calories

Samuel Adams Irish Red: 190 calories

Sierra Nevada Bigfoot: 330 calories

Sierra Nevada Draft Ale: 157 calories

IPAs: 180–240 calories

Samuel Adams Latitude 48 IPA: 206 calories

Sierra Nevada Ruthless Rye IPA: 205 calories

Sierra Nevada Torpedo Extra IPA: 236 calories

Lagers: 130–180 calories

Budweiser: 144 calories

Coopers Premium Lager: 180 calories

Coors: 142 calories

Corona Extra: 148 calories

Foster's Lager: 150 calories

Heineken: 166 calories

Michelob: 155 calories

Michelob Honey Lager: 178 calories

Miller Genuine Draft: 143 calories

Molson Canadian: 143 calories

Pabst Blue Ribbon: 144 calories

Rolling Rock Extra Pale: 132 calories

Samuel Adams Boston Lager: 175 calories

Yuengling Traditional Lager: 135 calories

Light lagers: 55–140 calories

Amstel Light: 95 calories

Beck's Premier Light: 64 calories

Bud Light: 110 calories

Bud Light Lime: 116 calories

Bud Light Platinum: 137 calories

Budweiser Select: 99 calories

Coors Light: 100 calories

Corona Light: 99 calories

Heineken Premium Light: 99 calories

Labatt Blue Light: 108 calories

MGD 64: 64 calories

Michelob Light: 123 calories

Michelob ULTRA: 95 calories

Miller Chill: 100 calories

Miller Lite: 96 calories

Molson Canadian Light: 113 calories

Natural Light: 95 calories

Pabst Blue Ribbon Light: 113 calories

Sam Adams Light: 119 calories

Pale ales: 130–200 calories

Bass Pale Ale: 156 calories

Moosehead Pale Ale: 135 calories

Sierra Nevada Pale Ale:
175 calories

Pilsners: 120–170 calories

Bitburger: 146 calories

Pilsner Urquell: 156 calories

Porters: 140–220 calories

Samuel Adams Honey Porter:
194 calories

Sierra Nevada Porter:
194 calories

Stouts: 125–320 calories

Beamish Irish Cream Stout:
146 calories

Guinness Draught: 125 calories

Guinness Extra Stout:
176 calories

Rogue Brewery Shakespeare
Oatmeal Stout: 201 calories

Samuel Adams Cream Stout:
189 calories

Sierra Nevada Stout:
225 calories

Wheat beers: 150–176 calories

Blue Moon Belgian White:
164 calories

Bud Light Golden Wheat:
118 calories

Samuel Adams Cherry Wheat:
176 calories

HARD LIQUOR (per 1½ ounces)

Rum: 100 calories

Vodka: 64–128 calories (depending on proof)

Whiskey: 100 calories

MIXED DRINKS

Black Russian: 192 calories

Bloody Mary: 118 calories

Cosmopolitan: 300 calories

Eggnog: 591 calories

Gin and tonic: 146 calories

Gin rickey: 114 calories

Hot toddy: 164 calories

Irish coffee: 147 calories

Margarita: 450 calories

Mojito: 180 calories

Piña colada: 245 calories

Presbyterian: 123 calories

Screwdriver: 146 calories

Vodka soda: 120 calories

Whiskey sour: 184 calories

WINE: ~120 calories

Chardonnay: 120 calories

Merlot: 123 calories

Pinot Noir: 121 calories

Red Zinfandel: 129 calories

Riesling: 120 calories

Sauvignon Blanc: 119 calories

**CHAMPAGNE: 110–130 calories
(per 5 ounces)**

with almonds. Food slows the rise of alcohol in your blood, and snacking beforehand reduces the chance that you'll order the deep-fried mozzarella sticks.

■ **DRINK PLENTY OF WATER** You've heard it before, and we'll say it again: "After one alcoholic drink, order something nonalcoholic," says Charla Schultz, RD, a dietitian at the Mayo Clinic. Ideally, your between-beer beverage will be water. This helps you pace yourself (although we don't recommend more than one or two drinks) and can help you cut back by a glass or more.

■ **LIMIT YOUR SUPPLY** Keep only one bottle or can of beer in the refrigerator at a time. If you bought a six-pack, store the other five in the pantry. "The more you can hamper raw convenience, the more likely you are to curb mindless drinking," says Brian Wansink, PhD, director of the Cornell University Food and Brand Lab. And no one wants to crack open a warm beer, right?

■ **COUNT AS YOU POUR** It can be tough to estimate serving size for vino—especially if you're pouring into a giant-size glass. Your trick: Count to five Mississippi, then stop pouring. That should give you about 5 ounces of wine, which is one serving.

■ **TRACK YOUR INTAKE** If you're planning to imbibe in alcoholic beverages, decide ahead of time how many drinks you'll have (ideally one or two). Then set aside a bottle cap or swizzle stick from each drink you have. If you have a physical reminder of how much you've already consumed, you may be inclined to down fewer drinks, studies suggest.

Artificial Sweeteners

Keep these imposters out of your life

Although artificial sweeteners will save you calories, recent research has linked foods sweetened with them to weight gain. In a study at the University of North Carolina at Chapel Hill, people who drank diet soft drinks instead of regular soft drinks ate more desserts and bread than those who drank water instead of soda. A separate study at the University of Texas found that drinking just three diet sodas per week could raise your risk of obesity by more than 40 percent.

Although *you* know the difference between diet and nondiet foods, your body doesn't. When you consume artificial sweeteners, your brain simply registers "sweet," which triggers a feedback loop that may increase your drive for sugar, says Barry Popkin, PhD, author of the University of North Carolina study. Artificial sweeteners like Splenda, stevia, Sweet'N Low, and Equal are hundreds of times sweeter than sugar. That means regularly consuming the sugar substitutes may actually increase your overall preference for sweetness. And they're not limited to diet drinks. These days, artificial sweeteners are lurking in everything from reduced-calorie yogurts to canned fruit to sugar-free pancake syrups. Here are some ways to keep artificial sweeteners from sneaking into your daily diet:

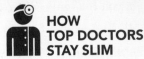

HOW TOP DOCTORS STAY SLIM

"Lunch is often bean salad—chickpeas and black beans are my favorites, with some fresh salsa and olive oil—or when I regress a bit, a sandwich of toasted rye bread with Koeze's all-natural chunky peanut butter and a bit of fig preserve."

—**JOHN BUSE, MD, PhD,** a professor in the division of endocrinology and metabolism at the University of North Carolina at Chapel Hill

■ **ELIMINATE SODA ENTIRELY** Whenever you see a can of soda, conjure a mental picture of yourself opening the can and pouring it into a glass and watching 10 to 12 teaspoons of granular white sugar settle at the bottom of the glass. Maybe that image will help you to avoid reaching for the can—even if it's diet soda. If you want a fizzy drink, guzzle a glass of seltzer flavored with a slice of lemon or lime. Seltzer has zero calories and is blissfully free of artificial sweeteners. Just don't be fooled by clear sparkling beverages that look like seltzer but contain sugar substitutes—they're just as dangerous as diet soda. (For more soda alternatives, see "Liquid Gold.")

■ **WEAN YOURSELF OFF OF SUGAR . . . WITH SUGAR** Satisfying sugar cravings with an artificially sweetened treat isn't as smart as food manufacturers would have you believe. "Substitutes may not signal the same satiety hormones as sugar, making it easier to overeat," says Lona Sandon, RD, an assistant professor of nutrition at the University of Texas Southwestern Medical Center in Dallas. That may be because real sugar triggers a more prolonged release of satisfying dopamine than artificial sweeteners do.

Instead of trading sugar for chemicals, replace your normal indulgences with portion-controlled desserts that have nutritional benefit. For example, instead of high-calorie chocolate cake, break off a few squares of antioxidant-rich dark chocolate.

Or instead of a sugary Popsicle, munch on frozen berries or grapes.

■ **OPT FOR NATURAL SUGARS** The healthiest way to satisfy your sweet tooth is to grab a piece of fruit. Artificial sweeteners are generally reserved for unhealthy processed foods, which add zero nutritional benefit to your diet. By swapping in fruit, you're folding in better-for-you natural sugars. Grapes, mangoes, and sweet cherries are some of the sweetest fruits on the shelf.

■ **SWEETEN WISELY** The best sweeteners

HOW SWEETS IMPACT YOUR BRAIN

There's a reason you equate sweets with serenity. When you consume dessert, your prefrontal cortex, a part of your brain that helps control emotions, lights up, says James Herman, PhD, a professor of psychiatry and behavioral neuroscience at the University of Cincinnati. Sugar also triggers the release of feel-good endorphins that make you want more and more. What's the purpose of your craving for cake? Simple: In the caveman era, sugar carbs were an important source of fuel, since they help keep us alert (and aware of danger).

The wooly mammoth is no longer a threat, but your brain doesn't know that—we're still wired to desire the foods we needed for thousands of years. Here's the thing: It's not calories alone that determine the reward value of food; the actual act of eating can have a calming, pleasurable effect. So instead of switching to low-calorie, artificially sweetened desserts, buy a single-serve treat made with real sugar, and take half an hour to eat it. The more you savor the flavor, the more rewarding it will be.

are those that offer extra health benefits. Honey, for example, is loaded with antioxidants and is thought to have antibacterial properties. And University of Rhode Island researchers found that real maple syrup packs 54 different antioxidants. But keep in mind: Unlike artificial sweeteners, both honey and maple syrup have roughly the same number of calories per teaspoon as sugar, so drizzle them sparingly.

LIQUID GOLD

Sometimes you just want flavor—*not* another glass of water. But before you reach for a soda, diet or otherwise, grab one of these delicious, health-boosting drinks.

Iced green tea

Who knew a little leaf could rev your metabolism—and help you live longer? In a recent study in the *Journal of the American Medical Association,* women who downed about 3 ounces of green tea per day were 31 percent less likely to die from heart disease than those who drank less. Credit the tea's high levels of EGCG, an antioxidant known to be both life extending and metabolism boosting. Brew your own: Steep four bags of green tea per cup of boiling water, then chill it in your refrigerator. If you need a shot of sweetness, stir a little antioxidant-rich honey into your glass.

Low-fat chocolate milk

Add chocolate to that milk mustache. University of Barcelona scientists recently found that people who drank chocolate milk (made with cocoa powder) every day for a month had lower levels of the inflammation that causes heart disease than those who drank regular milk. The polyphenols found in cocoa may suppress inflammation, explains study author Ramon Estruch, MD, PhD. Sip on low-fat chocolate milk, such as Horizon Organic Lowfat Chocolate Milk, or stir a tablespoon of unsweetened cocoa and sugar to taste (just a little!) into low-fat plain milk. You'll silence your sweet tooth without breaking the calorie bank.

Ruby red grapefruit juice

Juice is generally something to avoid, since it's often dense in calories and high in sugar. But ruby red grapefruit juice is the healthy exception. It's packed with flavor, and its acidity may help slow your rate of digestion, so you feel fuller longer. The key is portion control: Stick to an 8-ounce serving to avoid adding too many liquid calories to your day.

THE SKINNY ON SWEETENERS

Nonnutritive (zero calorie)

Acesulfame K (Sweet One, Sunett)

Origin: Combination of potassium, sulfur, nitrogen, carbon, and hydrogen

Taste: Slightly bitter-metallic aftertaste; 180 to 200 times sweeter than sugar

Danger: It's FDA approved, even though a few animal studies suggest a link to lung and breast tumors.

Stevia (Stevia in the Raw, PureVia, Truvia, SweetLeaf)

Origin: Dried leaves of a South American shrub

Taste: Ultrasweet, sometimes with a licorice-like aftertaste; 200 to 300 times sweeter than sugar

Danger: After some concerns about toxicity, the stevia production method was refined and designated "generally recognized as safe" by the FDA. In 2008, the government agency approved it as a food ingredient. Studies have shown that it doesn't affect blood sugar and doesn't increase the risk of cancer.

Sucralose (Splenda)

Origin: Chlorine atoms are substituted for hydrogen-oxygen groups in ordinary sugar

Taste: The closest to sugar, with virtually no aftertaste; 600 times sweeter than sugar

Danger: Since it's derived from real sugar, rather than chemicals, it's among the safest of sugar substitutes.

Aspartame (Equal, NutraSweet)

Origin: Two amino acids combined with methyl ester

Taste: Sugarlike, but with a faint bitter aftertaste; about 200 times sweeter than sugar

Danger: Once thought to be linked to cancer, but the FDA says it's not a health risk. It was approved for use in all foods and beverages in 1996.

Saccharin (Sweet'N Low)

Origin: Sulfur and other components combined in a chemically complex stew

Taste: Cloyingly sweet, with a metallic aftertaste; 200 to 700 times sweeter than sugar

Danger: In the 1970s, animal studies prompted the National Toxicology Program to indicate it as a probable carcinogen. No such link was found in human studies, so it was eventually declared safe. Your body can't digest it, so more than four packets a day can lead to stomach issues.

Nutritive (contains carbs and calories)

Agave

Origin: Nectar from the same Mexican cactus that yields tequila, cooked to 140 degrees

Taste: Light versions have a floral taste, while dark agave is more like molasses; 25 to 40 percent sweeter than sugar

Nutrition: 20 calories, 16 grams carbs, 1 gram fiber per teaspoon

Danger: Can be up to 90 percent fructose, more than you'll find in high-fructose corn syrup. Fructose overload can trigger weight gain and high blood pressure.

Honey

Origin: A fructose-glucose mix regurgitated by bees

Taste: Varies depending on where it's harvested, but no aftertaste; 100 to 150 percent sweeter than sugar

Nutrition: 64 calories, 17 grams carbs per tablespoon

Danger: None.

Sugar alcohols (sorbitol, mannitol, xylitol, lactitol, isomalt, erythritol)

Origin: Sugar combined with hydrogen

Taste: Convincingly sugarlike; only about 30 to 70 percent as sweet as sugar

Nutrition: 1.5 to 3 calories, 2.6 carbs per gram (A piece of sugar-free gum contains about 1 gram.)

Danger: Just 10 grams of sorbitol is enough to make you gassy or to cause diarrhea since your body can't digest sugar alcohols. Plus, they can spike your blood sugar since they contain carbs.

Breakfast

20 secrets for starting your day right

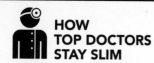

The world's worst breakfast isn't last night's leftovers. It's eating no breakfast at all. After 8 hours of sleep, your body is essentially in starvation mode, which means your levels of insulin and leptin (the fullness hormone) have dropped and your metabolism has slowed to a crawl. If you don't wake up your body with food, your metabolism will stay sluggish all day long, even though you may feel hungrier than normal! That's a dangerous combination—and one that could show up on your waistline. A University of Massachusetts study found that people who regularly skip breakfast are 450 percent more likely to be obese.

If you load up on the right foods in the morning, you can enhance your weight loss. "Eating helps rev your metabolism, which starts your calorie burn," says Susan Bowerman, MS, RD, assistant director of the UCLA Center for Human Nutrition. In a Virginia Commonwealth University study, dieters who started their day with a protein-rich, high-calorie breakfast lost more weight over 8 months than those who only consumed 290 calories and a quarter of the protein. The big-breakfast eaters found it easier to adhere to their diet, even though both groups ate similar amounts of calories each day. So what makes the ideal morning meal? Heartiness—it should include protein, whole grains, whole fruit, and a little dairy. Follow these rules to pull off the perfect breakfast:

■ **EAT BREAKFAST EVERY DAY** A study of successful dieters found that 78 percent of them eat breakfast every single day! Commit to grabbing breakfast—even if it's something small—every day. This is one habit that you don't want to break.

■ **ELIMINATE EXCUSES** The biggest reason people skip breakfast: "I don't have time." So prove to yourself that you do. This weekend, time how long it takes you to zap a bowl of instant oatmeal and eat it. It's most likely *not* long enough to make you late for work. Then remind yourself why it's so important. "Not eating breakfast may reduce your metabolic rate by 10 percent," says Leslie Bonci, RD, MPH, director of sports nutrition at the University of Pittsburgh Medical Center. If even instant oatmeal is pushing it, keep a protein-rich breakfast bar in your car, or prepare a yogurt-and-berries parfait the night before.

■ **EASE YOUR WAY IN** If you're a recent breakfast convert, you don't have to dive in with a 500-calorie meal. But you do need a little something. So try drinking your calories: Start with a glass of milk, which gives you 8 grams of protein plus fat-burning calcium, or sip on a latte made with low-fat milk. If you can stomach solid foods, grab a piece of whole-wheat toast topped with a slice of melted cheese. As your body becomes accustomed to morning feeding, you can increase the size of your meal.

■ **DIVIDE AND CONQUER** Don't have the stomach for a big breakfast? Try eating half of it when you first wake up, then eat the other half once you settle in at the office. Zap a packet of instant oatmeal with low-fat milk at home, then bring an apple or banana to eat at work while you check your e-mails. This helps you frontload your calories—which can boost your satiety all day long—without giving you a bellyache.

■ **HURRY TO THE TABLE** Sure, you've heard this advice before. But for good reason: If you sleep for 8 hours then delay breakfast, your body is essentially running on fumes by the time you make it to work. And that sends you desperately seeking sugar. Aim to eat breakfast within an hour of waking. The instant shot of energy—at least 300 calories' worth—awakens your metabolism for the coming day. Plus, it keeps ghrelin, your appetite hormone, from kicking into gear.

■ **FIND YOUR CALORIE RANGE** Ideally, you'll consume at least a quarter of your day's calories at breakfast. For most people, this falls somewhere in the 350- to 500-calorie range. In fact, breakfast should be your largest meal of the day. Think about it: Your morning meal is fuel for the entire day, so packing in calories in the a.m. is the only strategy that makes sense.

■ **RISE AND SHINE WITH PROTEIN** Protein makes an appearance in almost every chapter of this book—and for good reason: It fills you up more effectively than other nutrients and takes your body more time to digest and absorb. Problem is, people consume 65 percent of their protein after 6:00 p.m., according to a University of Illinois study. That's a big mistake: The researchers found that to preserve your muscle as you lose weight, you need to consume protein with every meal. "The most important diet upgrade for people who want to lose weight is to eat protein for breakfast," says Louis Aronne, MD, director of the Comprehensive Weight Control Program at New York–Presbyterian Hospital/Weill Cornell Medical Center.

Not only will you feel more satisfied, but you'll also burn more calories and eat less throughout the day if you load up on protein. Studies show that people who pack in protein burn about 71 more calories per day, and those who eat a protein-rich breakfast consume 200 fewer calories a day than carb-heavy breakfast eaters. Fortunately, several classic breakfast foods are packed with the superfilling nutrient—eggs, Greek yogurt, ham, Canadian bacon, and peanut butter on whole-grain bread are all great sources. Ideally, you'll consume 30 grams of protein at breakfast.

■ **DON'T FORGET VEGETABLES IN THE MORNING** It can be a challenge to eat the recommended five servings of vegetables every day. That makes working them into your morning meal essential. The perfect vessel for veggies? Eggs. Try folding chopped bell peppers, spinach, or broccoli—all high-fiber, low-carb options—into your omelet or scrambled eggs.

■ **PICK YOUR MORNING MEAT** A common dieter's mistake: buying turkey bacon instead of classic pork cuts. Although turkey is relatively lean, turkey bacon can contain up to twice as many additives as regular bacon and significantly more sodium. Besides, the difference in calories between the two is negligible. Stick to a couple slices of the classic pork stuff, which is also a smarter pick than sausage. Ham and Canadian bacon are worthy choices, too.

■ **EMPHASIZE EGGS** Eggs may very well be the perfect breakfast food. Dieters who started their day with two eggs and toast dropped 65 percent more weight than those who ate a bagel with cream cheese, a study in the *International Journal of Obesity* reports. Another study found that eating eggs for breakfast effectively staves off hunger for the rest of the day. For the 143 calories in two large eggs, you net nearly 13 grams of belly-filling, hunger-fighting, muscle-building protein. Just don't ditch the yolk. This is where most of the nutrients are housed, including brain-boosting choline; vision-preserving vitamin A, lutein, and zeaxanthin; and vitamin D and calcium. Australian scientists found that loading up on vitamin D and calcium in the a.m. can blunt your appetite.

■ **CUT EMPTY CARBS** Carbohydrates from processed grains elevate your insulin levels. And the more insulin circulating through your body, the more fat your body produces! Plus, these fast-burning carbs won't keep you satisfied for long. Bagels are the primary offender, but you'll also find the dangerous carbs in white toast, pancakes, muffins, waffles, and sugary cereals. If you're eating a grain for breakfast, make sure it's 100 percent whole grain or whole wheat.

■ **SHOP FOR THE RIGHT CEREAL** If you choose the right box, you can add a hefty load of fiber to your meal. Ignore the claims on the front of the cereal box—even Cookie Crisp boasts about its whole grains—and focus on the nutrition panel on the side. Look for at least 3 grams of fiber, fewer than 200 calories per serving, and no more than 8 grams of sugars per serving. Then check the ingredients: Every grain should include the word "whole," not "refined." A few cereals that fit the bill: Post Shredded Wheat, Fiber One Honey Clusters, and Cheerios.

■ **PRACTICE PORTION CONTROL** Don't just fill your bowl to the brim. Cereal serving sizes vary, so make sure to check the nutrition panel. Then use a measuring cup to dish out the appropriate amount, says Roberta Anding, RD, a dietitian and director of sports nutrition at Baylor College of Medicine. (You can even keep a measuring cup in the box as a reminder to portion it out.) If your bowl of cereal looks measly (and unsatisfying), try pouring it into a coffee mug—you'll trick your mind into thinking you're eating more. Whatever you do, don't eat cereal straight out of the box. You'll end up overdoing it.

■ **DRINK WATER WHILE YOU WAIT** Is your oatmeal in the microwave? Your omelet in the pan? Grab a glass of water! Researchers from the Virginia Polytechnic Institute found that overweight people consumed fewer calories at breakfast when they drank water beforehand. Even if you're carefully controlling your calories, water is still an easy way to boost fullness and satisfaction.

■ **PLAN YOUR GRAB-AND-GO STRATEGY** If your only breakfast option involves a drive-thru, don't panic—you can find healthy meals if you know what to look for. Surprisingly, one of your safest fast-food options comes from McDonald's. The Egg McMuffin contains a reasonable 300 calories, with 12 grams of fat and 18 grams of protein. If you prefer breakfast wraps, choose one that contains eggs and veggies—and doesn't include the words "loaded," "meaty," or "cheesy" in its name or description. As for grab-and-go oatmeal, here's the restaurant breakdown:

RESTAURANT	CALORIES	FAT	SUGAR	FIBER	PROTEIN
Starbucks Perfect Oatmeal	140	2.5 g	*	4 g	5 g
Jamba Juice Steel-Cut Plain Oatmeal with Brown Sugar	220	3.5 g (1 g saturated)	12 g	5 g	8 g
Au Bon Pain Apple Cinnamon Oatmeal (medium)	280	4.0 g (1 g saturated)	14 g	7 g	8 g
Jamba Juice Steel-Cut Fresh Banana Oatmeal	280	4.0 g (1 g saturated)	23 g	6 g	9 g
McDonald's Fruit & Maple Oatmeal	290	4.5 g (2 g saturated)	32 g	5 g	5 g

* Not stated

■ **CHOOSE THE RIGHT BEVERAGE** A hot cup of coffee? Go for it. It's chock-full of antioxidants, plus the caffeine can give your metabolism a jolt. A cold glass of milk? Absolutely. The protein and fat will help you stay full throughout the morning while also promoting muscle building and fat burning. Juice? Not so fast. The juice in your fridge may be nothing more than sugar water. Even if it's 100 percent juice, it should contain no more than 120 calories per serving. You're better off sticking to whole fruit. A cup of orange juice has 110 calories. But a whole orange contains just 60 calories. Plus, unlike juice, whole fruit is loaded with fiber, which helps counteract its natural sugars.

■ **LOAD UP ON OATMEAL** Oatmeal contains a type of fiber called beta-glucan, which can help control appetite for up to 4 hours, according to a study in the journal *Nutrition Research*. Your perfect pick: steel-cut oats. They're made from chopped oat grains (aka groats), whereas instant oatmeal consists of chopped and flattened groats. "The enzymes in your gastrointestinal tract take a longer time to penetrate the unrolled groats in steel-cut oatmeal," says David Jenkins, MD, PhD, a nutrition and metabolism researcher at the University of Toronto. "This results in a slower uptake of glucose, and that makes steel-cut oatmeal better." Plus, steel-cut oats pack 8 grams of soluble fiber per cup—twice the amount in instant oats. Try Arrowhead Mills Organic Steel Cut Oats. (See "10 Ways to Upgrade Your Oatmeal.")

■ **. . . OR EXPLORE OATMEAL ALTERNATIVES** Tired of the Quaker man? Try Ralston, which is essentially a whole-grain, fiber-rich version of cream of wheat. For a shot of flavor, drizzle it with a small amount of honey or real maple syrup. Another option: hulled buckwheat, which packs nearly 6 grams of protein per serving. The downside is that it takes a while to prepare, so make a big batch that you can reheat throughout the week.

■ **BUILD A HEALTHY SMOOTHIE** If you need a 60-second breakfast, homemade smoothies are one of your healthiest choices—but only if you choose the right mix-ins.

EASY HEALTHY BREAKFASTS!

1. Spread natural peanut butter and a drizzle of honey on a piece of whole-grain bread. You can even add a few almonds.
2. Stir ¼ cup almonds, ½ cup berries, and ⅓ cup high-fiber cereal into low-fat Greek yogurt.
3. Prepare your oatmeal with ½ cup 1% milk and cinnamon to taste. Eat ¾ cup reduced-fat cottage cheese with 3 tablespoons almonds on the side.
4. Top two frozen whole-wheat waffles with ½ cup part-skim ricotta, ½ cup berries, 1 tablespoon slivered almonds, and a sprinkling of cinnamon.
5. If you're a bagel addict, opt for a whole-grain version, then scoop out the doughy part. Spread on 2 tablespoons of low-fat cream cheese.
6. Whip up a two-egg omelet and add ½ cup mixed peppers and onion. Pair that with ¼ cup steel-cut oats mixed with ¼ cup berries.

10 WAYS TO UPGRADE YOUR OATMEAL

Prepare your oats with 1% milk, then stir in one of these deliciously healthy combinations.*

Brain Booster

2 Tbsp fresh blueberries + 1 Tbsp chopped walnuts + ½ Tbsp ground flaxseed

Per serving: 73 calories, 5 g fat (0 g saturated), 6 g carbs, 2 g fiber, 0 mg sodium, 2 g protein

Trail Mix

1 Tbsp raisins + 1 tsp cinnamon + ½ tsp vanilla extract + 2 Tbsp roasted pumpkin seeds (unsalted), chopped

Per serving: 130 calories, 7 g fat (1 g saturated), 12 g carbs, 3 g fiber, 6 mg sodium, 5 g protein

Juicy Pear

¼ cup diced pears + 2 tsp real maple syrup + 1 Tbsp chopped walnuts

Per serving: 106 calories, 5 g fat (0 g saturated), 16 g carbs, 2 g fiber, 2 mg sodium, 1 g protein

Asian Fusion

1 Tbsp sliced almonds + ½ tsp ground ginger + 1 tsp honey + 1 Tbsp ground flaxseed

Per serving: 90 calories, 4 g fat (0 g saturated), 12 g carbs, 4 g fiber, 0 mg sodium, 3 g protein

Banana Nut Bread

1 sliced banana (large) + 1 Tbsp pecan pieces + 1 tsp cinnamon

Per serving: 175 calories, 5 g fat (1 g saturated), 34 g carbs, 6 g fiber, 2 mg sodium, 2 g protein

Nutrition information is for the toppings only.

Peanut Butter Banana

1 Tbsp natural peanut butter + ½ sliced banana (large)

Per serving: 161 calories, 8 g fat (1 g saturated), 19 g carbs, 3 g fiber, 61 mg sodium, 4 g protein

Apple Pie

½ cup apple slices + 1 Tbsp sliced almonds + ½ tsp apple pie spice

Per serving: 64 calories, 3 g fat (0 g saturated), 9 g carbs, 2 g fiber, 1 mg sodium, 1 g protein

Banana Split

¼ cup sliced strawberries + ¼ cup banana slices + 1 Tbsp dark chocolate chips + 1 Tbsp dry-roasted peanuts (unsalted)

Per serving: 167 calories, 9 g fat (3 g saturated), 23 g carbs, 1 g fiber, 2 mg sodium, 3 g protein

Tropical Breeze

½ cup pineapple cubes + 1 Tbsp macadamia halves (unsalted)

Per serving: 100 calories, 6 g fat (1 g saturated), 12 g carbs, 2 g fiber, 1 mg sodium, 1 g protein

Tin Roof

1 Tbsp unsweetened cocoa powder + 1 Tbsp dry-roasted peanuts (unsalted) + 1 Tbsp ground flaxseed

Per serving: 121 calories, 9 g fat (2 g saturated), 10.5 g carbs, 6.5 g fiber, 5 mg sodium, 6 g protein

Drinking a protein-rich smoothie for breakfast, compared to a carb-heavy or fat-laden one, can help you consume fewer calories at lunch, according to a study in the *European Journal of Clinical Nutrition*. Try using 1% milk as your base (a little fat helps you absorb milk's nutrients), or add low-fat Greek yogurt as your thickening agent. A cup of 1% milk contains 8 grams of protein, while a 6-ounce cup of low-fat Greek yogurt packs in 17 grams.

■ **BRING ON THE DAIRY** Morning dairy isn't confined to milk drinkers. Try stirring berries into Greek yogurt, or melt Swiss cheese on your English muffin sandwich. They all contain calcium, a nutrient shown to boost fat burning. Always opt for low-fat dairy—it has just enough fat to help you absorb key nutrients, such as vitamins D and E, but not enough to send your calorie count through the roof.

Calcium

How boosting your bone strength can help you lose weight

Growing up, you most likely heard your mother say, "If you don't drink your milk, you won't build strong bones!" She was right—but preventing osteoporosis isn't the only reason that calcium is important. The mineral is also critical for muscle function, and it may even speed up your fat loss. The reverse is also true: There's evidence that calcium deficiency can slow down your metabolism, says nutritionist Tammy Lakatos Shames, RD.

In an *American Journal of Clinical Nutrition* study, dieters who had the highest intake of calcium from dairy lost 60 percent more weight than those with the lowest. Obese women who raised their daily intake from 600 milligrams to 1,200 lost an average of 11 pounds more than those who didn't boost their calcium consumption, a study in the *British Journal of Nutrition* found. If you're not currently getting your daily dose of calcium, you may notice an even more pronounced fat-blasting effect once you increase your intake.

Your body can't make its own calcium, so it's essential that you take in 1,200 milligrams a day through your diet. In fact, if you don't take in enough of the mineral, your body may begin to release calcitriol, a hormone that promotes fat storage. To meet your calcium needs, look for foods that have at least 200

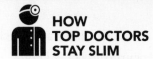

HOW TOP DOCTORS STAY SLIM

"When I need to wake up sleepy taste buds, fresh chopped cilantro does it. The nutritional powerhouse is high in iron and disease-fighting flavonoids, and it tastes great in wraps, salsa, and yogurt."

—**CHRISTINE GERBSTADT, MD, RD,** a spokesperson for the Academy of Nutrition and Dietetics milligrams listed on the label; work them into your diet every day.

TOP SOURCES OF CALCIUM

Part-skim ricotta cheese (1 cup): 668 mg calcium

Low-fat plain yogurt (8 ounces): 452 mg calcium

Collards (1 cup cooked): 357 mg calcium

1% milk (1 cup): 305 mg calcium

Spinach (1 cup cooked): 291 mg calcium

Swiss cheese (1 ounce): 224 mg calcium

Provolone cheese (1 ounce): 214 mg calcium

Black-eyed peas (1 cup cooked): 211 mg calcium

Part-skim mozzarella (1 ounce): 207 mg calcium

Low-fat cottage cheese (1 cup): 206 mg calcium

Cheddar cheese (1 ounce): 204 mg calcium

Muenster cheese (1 ounce): 203 mg calcium

BONUS BENEFIT!

Ramping up your calcium intake may help lower your cholesterol while you're dieting. In a Canadian study, dieters who added 1,200 milligrams of calcium to their daily diet saw a 200 percent greater decrease in cholesterol than those who didn't up their quota. It's the same reason calcium helps you lose weight: It seems to prevent the absorption of fat, especially the saturated kind.

Calories

9 ways to calculate your calories— and make the most of every one

You eat them. You count them. You loathe them. You burn them. But do you really know what calories are? And are they all created equal?

The short answer: Calories are a measure of heat, or energy, in food, and not all calories are created equal. Chances are, that flies in the face of everything you think you know about calories. But the truth is, your body burns and stores the 500 calories in a slice of cheesecake differently than the 500 calories in a giant pile of celery.

Your diet consists of three basic types of energy: carbohydrates, protein, and fat. And your body processes each of them differently. For every 100 calories of carbs you consume, you burn about 6 of those calories during digestion. You burn roughly half that many digesting an equivalent amount of fat. The big winner is protein: You use around 23 calories digesting 100 calories' worth of protein. All of this is to say that the classic "calories in, calories out" formula can be misleading. Which most likely leaves you wondering: How can I properly calculate the calories I consume? And how can I make sure that I burn them all off?

■ **DON'T TRUST THE TREADMILL** It's certainly motivating to see the calories add up with every stride. But don't count on the "calories burned" display on the cardio machine being accurate. The number includes the calories you'd burn even if you were doing absolutely nothing. (By some estimations, cardio machines inflate your energy expenditure by 30 percent.) "Depending on your size,

HOW TOP DOCTORS STAY SLIM

"I eat a diet of foods that score highly on the NuVal rating system, which I helped create. That includes plant foods high in fiber, like vegetables, fruits, beans, lentils, whole grains, nuts, and seeds. It also means high-quality protein like fish and seafood; low-fat organic dairy products; dark chocolate; and, in moderation, good beer and wine. By eating well, you fill up with fewer calories."

—David Katz, MD, MPH, director of the Yale-Griffin Prevention Research Center you burn about 1.2 calories a minute while you're sleeping," says Alex Koch, PhD, an exercise scientist at Truman State University. "So to know how many extra calories you're burning with exercise, you have to subtract that number from your total."

■ **LEAN ON PROTEIN** As previously mentioned, your body burns more calories digesting protein than it does breaking down carbs or fat. So take advantage: Make sure to include at least 10 to 20 grams of protein from lean sources like eggs, chicken breast, and sirloin steak at every meal. Ideally, your snacks will also be high in the belly-filling stuff. Think about it this way: If you consume 200 calories from protein instead of fat, you'll burn an extra 40 calories simply digesting your food.

■ **FILL UP WITH FIBER** Your body processes different types of carbs at different rates. Glucose and starch, both simple sugars, are rapidly absorbed. But fiber lingers in your digestive tract. A particular type of fiber, called insoluble fiber, may even block the absorption of other calories. The daily fiber recommendation is 25 grams for women and 38 grams for men, but this is one situation when overdoing it is okay.

■ **SPEND MORE TIME ON YOUR FEET** Despite what most people think, you don't burn the majority of your calories at the gym. Most of your calories go toward bodily functions (which you can't do much about), but there's a certain percentage that you burn through everyday movements, like walking to the bathroom or shivering in the cold. It's what scien-

tists call non-exercise-activity thermogenesis, or N.E.A.T. Raising your N.E.A.T. can be as simple as taking the steps to the third-floor bathroom every day instead of using the one down the hall. Or parking in the back of the lot rather than scouting out a prime spot. For 50 easy ways to boost your N.E.A.T. and burn more calories, see page 40.

■ **DON'T BE FOOLED BY DIET FOODS** If you judge foods by calories alone, "diet" foods will seem like worthy choices. Healthy Choice Roasted Sesame Chicken, for example, contains 440 calories. Reasonable enough for a dinner, right? But upon closer inspection, you'll find that it also packs 27 grams of sugars! If you want to make sure you're burning the calories you take in as efficiently as possible, you need to know where they're coming from. Consume no more than 20 grams of sugars per day if you're a woman and 36 grams if you're a man, and try to buy foods that have fewer milligrams of sodium than calories (sodium doesn't contain calories, but a high amount is a sign of a poor-quality food). Finally, shelve any foods that contain heart-clogging trans fats—or sneaky sources of them, such as hydrogenated or partially hydrogenated oils.

■ **STOP OBSESSING** You should have a rough idea of how many calories you consume in a day. However, if you fret over every bite you take, it can actually be counterproductive. A study in the journal *Psychosomatic Medicine* found that dieters who counted calories experienced an increase in cortisol, a stress

9 EASY WAYS TO CUT CALORIES

Trim the fat

Next time you're baking, replace the oil in the recipe with unsweetened applesauce or pureed pumpkin. You can also use Sunsweet Lighter Bake prune-and-apple blend.

Reconsider your chowder

Instead of creamy New England clam chowder, heat up a bowl of tomato-based Manhattan clam chowder. You'll save about 80 calories per cup!

Stay away from coffee syrup

A few pumps of Starbucks syrup could easily cost you 100 calories. Rather than flavoring your coffee with syrup, sprinkle it with cinnamon and nutmeg. While you're at it, skip the whip.

Change your spaghetti ratio

If you eat more pasta than sauce, turn that around. Fill your plate with one serving of pasta and two servings of red sauce. Don't do this if your sauce is named Alfredo.

Tune up your tuna

Instead of buying canned tuna that's packed in oil, purchase water-packed tuna to save about 30 calories per serving.

Tweak your sweets

Rather than eating a cup of ice cream, savor ½ cup ice cream (or even better, sorbet) topped with ½ cup sliced strawberries.

Swap your dippers

Use fresh vegetables, such as sliced bell peppers, celery, or carrots, as vessels for your salsa or guacamole instead of chips.

Switch your spread

Substitute 2 tablespoons hummus for the mayo you normally spread on your sandwich. You can also try mustard.

Stop at the crust

Leave the ruffled edge of your pie on the plate. The edges and bottoms of baked goods can be especially caloric, since they absorb the butter used to grease the pan.

hormone that has been linked to weight gain (especially in the belly). "Too many people are counting calories instead of focusing on the content of food," says Brandon Alderman, PhD, an assistant professsor of exercise science at Rutgers University. Concentrate on making smart food choices—vegetables, fruits, lean protein, whole grains, low-fat dairy—rather than spending unnecessary hours comparing nutrition panels on processed foods.

■ **AVOID CRASH DIETING** When you take calorie cutting to an extreme, you accomplish one thing: slowing down your metabolism. You'll see the pounds fall off at first. But once you shed that initial weight, your progress will most likely slow to a crawl, just like your metabolism. The reason: Drastically cutting calories causes you to lose muscle, your primary calorie-burning tissue. You're better off trimming a moderate number of calories and exercising regularly. Your weight-loss target should be 1 to 2 pounds per week.

■ **LOAD UP IN THE MORNING** Here's the eating plan most dieters follow: a small breakfast, a medium-size lunch, and a big dinner. That's not a smart move. Saving the heft of your calories for the evening may cause your hunger hormones to go haywire, compelling you to eat more. Plus, when you pack in calories before bed, you're only fueling your body for sleep, when you require the least number of calories. To lose weight, frontload your calories with a big breakfast of about 350 to 500 calories. You'll stay satisfied throughout the day, making you less likely to binge or make unhealthy food choices.

■ **WATCH YOUR PORTIONS** You know you should control the number of Doritos you eat when you're cheating. But do you practice moderation when eating healthy foods? A recent study found that people tend to underestimate the number of calories in nutritious items, such as yogurt, fish, and baked chicken. Just because a food is healthy doesn't mean you can eat big portions. Take nuts, for example: One handful can easily contain 200 calories. Although those are healthy calories, you still don't want to down 600 calories of nuts in a single sitting. Make sure to control your portion sizes, regardless of what you're eating. (For easy ways to monitor your portions, see page 220.)

7 Dangerous Eating Habits— And How to Overcome Them

1 OVEREATING DURING THE HOLIDAYS

Holiday meals aren't inherently evil. Your dining room table is, of course, piled with food, but the occasional cheat meal is good for you. The real issue is the idea of a holiday *season*— that month between Thanksgiving and Christmas when you let loose, or the weeks before and after Halloween when you treat candy like an essential food group.

Change Your Outlook

Think of holidays as isolated days: Thanksgiving Day, Christmas Day, Halloween. Then splurge on those individual days—not for a week before and after. Try to limit yourself to a couple of small indulgences per holiday; it's okay to cheat, but you should still practice self-control when doing so.

Pace Yourself

It's tempting to stuff your face at a rapid-fire pace during Thanksgiving dinner. But are you really enjoying that turkey and gravy when you down it in 30 seconds? A recent study in the *Journal of the American Dietetic Association* found that women who wolfed down their food ate nearly 70 calories more but felt less satisfied than those who took their time. Take advantage of talk time during holiday dinners—catching up with your family members will slow down your shoveling. You can also try taking smaller bites, chewing thoroughly, and setting your fork down in between bites.

Go Easy on the Alcohol

Celebrations warrant a couple of drinks. But they don't warrant an entire bottle of Champagne. It's not just the calories that are dangerous. Being tipsy lowers your inhibitions, so you're more inclined to take a second (or third) trip to the buffet. Limit your celebratory sipping to one or two drinks. A single serving is 12 ounces of beer (the amount in one bottle), 5 ounces of wine/Champagne, or $1\frac{1}{2}$ ounces of liquor (a shot glass–full). On New Year's, make it ultra brüt Champagne, which is significantly less sugary than other varieties.

Offer to Host

If you're hosting, you can control the menu. Which means instead of offering the standard fried, cheese-laden finger foods, you can serve up figure-friendly appetizers. Try melon wrapped in proscuitto (great with Pinot

Grigio), raw oysters (pair with Sauvingon Blanc), veggies and black bean dip (perfect for Pinot Noir), or dark chocolate (ideal for Merlot).

Snack in Advance

Before you sit down to a holiday dinner, eat a protein-rich snack, like a small bite of cheese or an apple with natural peanut butter. Snacking before a meal sounds counterintuitive if you're trying to save calories. But by filling up on protein beforehand, you'll reduce the temptation to overdo it on high-calorie foods at dinner.

Buy One Kind of Candy

There's nothing fun about fun-size candy bars. Consider this: If you eat a fun-size Butterfinger, Snickers, and Baby Ruth, you've just taken in more than 250 calories! Keep your candy-bowl choices to a minimum, since variety can compel you to eat more. As for brightly hued candies, like M&M's, buy the holiday versions, which usually contain only two or three colors.

2 FREQUENTING CONVENIENCE STORES

Perhaps you're on the go constantly, or you have only 15 minutes to eat lunch every day. Or maybe you're a working mom, trying to prepare a spread for a family of four. So what do you do? You grab a bite from the gas station, cruise through the drive-thru, or stock up on frozen meals. The problem: These convenience foods are usually loaded with unhealthy fats, unnecessary calories, and undesirable additives. Over time, you wreak havoc not only on your waistline but also on your heart and every other part of your body.

Keep Healthy Snacks on Hand

Rather than relying on gas station granola bars—or worse, Little Debbies—store good-for-you snacks in your glove box or purse. That way, when hunger strikes, you're not tempted to fill your belly with junk. Try to cap each snack at 150 to 200 calories, and only choose items that contain belly-filling protein. A few smart picks: low-fat string cheese, a handful of unshelled pistachios, or Jack Link's Beef Jerky.

Plan Your Fast-Food Strategy

Sometimes fast food is unavoidable. If you regularly find yourself in a mealtime pinch, review the nutrition facts on the Web site of your most frequent fast-food stop. Determine your healthiest options and stick to those when you're forced to hit the drive-thru. (Believe it or not, there are a few bright spots on most fast-food menus.) By planning your meals, you reduce the chance that you'll cave to the call of the Monster Burger combo.

Say No to Takeout

A recent University of Minnesota study found that parents and kids who ate takeout for dinner were more likely to be obese than those who ate at a sit-down or fast-food restaurant or had dinner delivered. Your best option: none of the above. Sit down once a week, plan your menu, then cook in bulk. You can freeze dinner-size portions and reheat them throughout the week.

Shop the Perimeter

Make it a personal policy to steer clear of the supermarket's center aisles, since this is where processed, nutritionally empty foods generally hide. If you work the perimeter of the store, you're much more likely to fill your cart with produce, low-fat dairy, and lean meats—the makings of healthy meals. The exception: Venture into the frozen aisle for unseasoned vegetables. Just avert your eyes as you pass those frozen pizzas!

3 RESTRICTIVE EATING

The harder you try, the harder you may find it to lose weight. Over the long term, severe calorie restriction can cause you to pump out more ghrelin, the hunger hormone, and less leptin, the fullness hormone. And the more you restrict your diet, the more attractive "forbidden" foods become. Give it a few weeks and you may find yourself elbow deep in that bag of Doritos.

The effects of extreme calorie cutting can also show up *inside* your body, too. By sending your body into starvation mode, you face a metabolic slowdown and begin to burn up muscle tissue, which is your body's calorie-burning engine. It's no wonder people who follow a very low-calorie diet regain significantly more weight than those on a more forgiving plan, according to a recent study in the journal *Obesity*. If you lose weight on a 1,000-calorie diet, you'll start gaining the weight the second you start eating a 1,300-calorie diet.

Swap Smart

If you repeatedly deny yourself certain foods, you may just strengthen your cravings until you give in and binge. Dying for a brownie? Eat it, but forgo the cream in your coffee this afternoon. Or if you *must* have a slice of cake, eat a smaller dinner. Instead of viewing foods as "off-limits," think of them as things you can have occasionally. Smart dieters know when to indulge!

Practice Carb Control

Don't cut out carbs altogether. Rather, limit your intake of the kinds that cause your blood sugar to spike—that is, the "enriched" or "refined" carbs you'll find in candy, soda, and junk food. Focus on the healthy carbs found in vegetables and whole grains.

Spread Your Calories Out

It's true: You have to trim your calories to lose weight. But you can do so without feeling deprived. If three meals won't cut it, divide your calories among three small meals and two snacks. By eating consistently throughout the day, you'll never have that "feed me now" impulse that drives you to overeat.

Never Restrict Your Produce Intake

You simply cannot eat too many fruits and vegetables. Potatoes are the exception: They contain few calories, little starch, and lots of fiber. Otherwise, eat produce with abandon.

Strive for Slow and Steady

To avoid losing muscle mass, aim to lose no more than 1 to 2 pounds per week. To meet this goal, most people need to scale back by 500 calories per day through a combination of diet and exercise.

4 EATING LATE AT NIGHT

Your metabolism doesn't suddenly slow down at 9:00 p.m. And your body processes calories no differently at night than at 3:00 in the afternoon. So why does late-night snacking have such a bad reputation? Simple: People tend to munch at night out of boredom or routine—for example, they've always eaten a bowl of ice cream before bed, so they keep up the habit.

After a full day of eating, nighttime eating only tacks on unnecessary calories right before you enter a sedentary state for the next 8 hours. Plus, if you load up on calories at night, you might not be hungry for breakfast. That's bad news: A University of Massachusetts study found that breakfast skippers are 4.5 times more likely to be obese than those who eat a morning meal.

Fuel Up Around 3:00 P.M.

Starving yourself during the lunch-to-dinner stretch can predispose you to late-night bingeing. So in the late afternoon, grab a protein-rich snack, such as a handful of almonds or a hard-cooked egg. Make sure you don't skip meals, either. This can also trigger a 10:00 p.m. pantry raid.

Eat an Early Dinner

A recent Northwestern University study concluded that regularly eating after 8:00 p.m. may increase your risk of obesity. The shocking part: Late-night munching was related to BMI, independent of sleep timing and duration. What that means: It's not simply because people who eat late have more hours to chow down. Try to sit down for dinner between 5:30 and 7:30 p.m.

Snack on Cereal

Going to bed with a growling stomach is bound to disrupt your sleep. So if you're truly hungry (not just bored), have a small but satisfying after-dinner snack of about 150 calories. Your go-to bite: ½ cup of whole-grain cereal, topped off with 1% milk. A Wayne State University study found that people who ate cereal at least 90 minutes after dinner lost more weight in a month and ate a smaller percentage of their calories at night than noncereal eaters. Plus, the healthy carbs create tryptophan, which helps your brain make serotonin.

This feel-good chemical then triggers the production of melatonin, the sleep hormone.

5 EATING WHILE YOU WATCH TV

As if the sedentary nature of tube time isn't bad enough, Americans have a particular passion for adding a bowl of potato chips to the experience. It's a double whammy: You ingest a load of calories while burning next to none. (You burn only about 0.2 calorie more per minute watching TV than you do sleeping.) One study found that people who watch TV while eating consume 300 calories more per sitting than those who don't. Plus, the more TV you watch, the less active you tend to be.

Keep Dinner at the Table

When you don't eat at the table, you think of your dinner as more a snack than a meal. Not only that: "When you're distracted by the TV, you rely on external cues, like the end of the show, to tell you when to stop eating, instead of stopping when you feel full," says Brian Wansink, PhD, director of the Cornell University Food and Brand Lab. So fold up that TV tray and take your plate to the kitchen table. As you eat, pay attention to how your body feels—not how much food is left on your plate.

Snack Cautiously

If you *must* have a snack while you watch your show, make it popcorn—it's a high-volume food, so it will fill you up fast. But don't pop just any pack. Although popcorn is a fiber-rich snack, it's too often adulterated by ungodly amounts of fake butter. So opt for a plain, lightly salted popcorn, such as Orville Redenbacher's Natural Simply Salted, which has just 60 calories per 2 cups (popped). Or if you need a little flavor, try Orville's Spicy Nacho popcorn. It sounds like a nutritional disaster, but the flavoring actually comes from real jalapeño chile peppers, which contain metabolism-boosting capsaicin.

Don't Let Ads Suck You In

The BK King may be creepy, but he can still entice you to eat. In a 2009 Yale University study, people (especially men and restrained eaters) tended to eat more after watching television advertisements for fast food, soda, or candy bars. If you feel the urge to eat during a commercial break, distract yourself: Take your dog out or sort your mail. Even better, do some jumping jacks, run in place, dance around your living room—anything that makes you feel somewhat out of breath. Keep this up during every commercial break, and you could burn 100 to 135 calories after an hour of TV. Plus, you'll stamp out your urge to eat.

6 CUTTING LOOSE ON WEEKENDS

It's a good idea to schedule a cheat meal once a week. If that meal happens to be Saturday night's dinner, so be it. It's only when you allow that cheat meal to become a cheat *weekend* that you enter dangerous territory. A 2008 study in the journal *Obesity* found that people eat an average of 111 calories more on Saturday than on weekdays. That doesn't sound significant, until you consider what weekend eaters are piling onto their plates. The researchers found that people's protein consumption *declines* on weekends, whereas their fat intake spikes. The effect: Study participants gained an average of 0.17 pound every weekend—which, over a year, adds up to nearly 9 pounds.

Take Advantage of Breakfast

You're not in a hurry on Saturday morning, so why not enjoy a leisurely breakfast? It's the perfect time to appreciate breakfast the way it's supposed to be: an omelet mixed with diced veggies, a cold glass of 1% milk, a banana on the side. Once you realize the merit of a proper morning meal, you may just find the time to whip one up on weekdays.

Plan Activities, Not Meals

If your weekend plans sound something like this: "dinner and drinks Friday night, ice cream on Saturday night, and brunch on Sunday," you may need to rethink your day planner. When you dine out with friends, you consume 50 percent more than you do when you're alone, according to Penn State research. It's not necessarily the food that's the problem, but rather a tendency to prolong the meal to keep the good times going. So instead of suggesting dinner or dessert, plan nonfood activities with your friends, such as visiting an art museum or going hiking. If you do want to grab a bite, suggest lunch—it's easier to keep your meal light, and you're less inclined to order cocktails.

Anticipate Your Hunger

You're at the mall and hunger strikes. So what do you do? Head to the food court, naturally. What you find there: Chinese buffets, fast food, and giant cookies. All bad ideas. On the weekend, you should never leave the house without a healthy option on hand. Stow a low-calorie protein bar in your glove box or purse so you're not tempted by mall food or the drive-thru.

Skip Drinks Before Dinner

Even the most diligent of dieters can fall victim to the call of alcohol on the weekends. It helps you unwind and is an easy way to socialize. So have a drink, just not before dinner. Alcohol lowers your inhibitions, so when you imbibe before a meal, you may feel less guilty ordering the bacon double cheeseburger with curly fries. Have wine with your meal, or better yet, designate it as dessert.

Drop the "Last Supper" Mind-Set

Sunday night can be a particularly vulnerable time. It's the end of the weekend, which means you have to resume your diet in approximately 12 hours. So you overdo it. Big mistake. Making healthy choices shouldn't have an on/off switch—it should be a way of life, says Dave Grotto, RD, a Chicago-based nutrition consultant. In fact, research has shown that people who eat consistently day after day are 150 percent more likely to maintain their weight loss than those who diet only on weekdays.

Ironically, the best way to prevent a Saturday free-for-all is to cut yourself a little slack during the week. Have a light beer one night, or indulge in a small cup of fro-yo. That way, you don't feel so deprived during the week that you go wild on the weekends. Besides, if you abandon all nutritional standards over the weekend, you may find it tough to get back on track come Monday.

Stock Up on Healthy Snacks

When you feel famished after a night out, that leftover cake on your counter can be irresistible. Keep junk (if you have any) out of sight and, instead, place a bowl of fruit on your kitchen table. That way, when you come in late and want to grab the first thing you see, it will be fruit, not dessert.

7 EATING DURING TIMES OF HIGH EMOTION

You easily bypass the vending machines at work. You breeze through cocktail party buffets without a hitch. So why do you find yourself housing a tub of ice cream after a rough day, or raiding the pantry when you feel stressed? You're engaging in what's called "emotional eating"—in other words, self-medicating with food. Unfortunately, emotional eating often leads to bingeing, where you eat not one but three scoops of ice cream in an attempt to calm whatever negative emotions you're feeling. You can surely see how this leads to weight gain.

And it's usually not carrots and celery that you turn to. When you're feeling grumpy or emotional, your brain is probably pumping out less mood-regulating serotonin. This deficiency can cause you to crave carbohydrates, which contain an amino acid that's necessary for production of serotonin.

Boost Your Mood Every Hour

Once an hour, take a minute to watch a funny video on YouTube or surf a blog you enjoy. By adding small doses of positive emotions to your day, you make yourself less susceptible to the negative ones that can lead to an after-work binge.

Cast Off Negativity

Visualize your negative thoughts riding by on a conveyor belt. Label each one ("Project due tomorrow!" or "Fight with my spouse!"), then picture it chugging off into oblivion. Research subjects at Temple University's Center for Obesity Research and Education report that this visualization method helps them avoid emotional eating.

Love Your Body

Poor body image can lead to emotional eating. So look in the mirror, and instead of focusing on perceived flaws, check out the areas you love, like the muscles in your calves or the beginnings of your abs. In a study at the Technical University of Lisbon, in Portugal, women who were counseled to improve their body image lost a higher percentage of their body weight than those who weren't.

Identify Your Triggers

Do you overeat after logging extra hours at work? Or before first dates? Keep a food diary and jot down how you're feeling every time you eat. Eventually, you'll notice trends that can help you identify which emotional triggers cause you to overeat. Then plan what you'll do instead of raiding the pantry—for example, taking a walk or calling a friend.

Breathe Slowly

If you're on the brink of a bad-mood binge, pause for 60 seconds: Focus on the center of your chest and inhale for 5 seconds, then exhale for 5 seconds. Keep repeating this slow-breathing cycle to force your mind to calm down. It sounds simple, but it actually can help—it gives you a window of time to realize what you're about to do. That's often enough to stop you from overeating. If that doesn't work, imagine an attractive celebrity sitting next to you. You most likely won't want to eat that box of Twinkies anymore.

Carbohydrates

19 smart strategies for low-carb eating

Carbohydrates have a nasty reputation. Over the past decade, they've been vilified as one of the primary reasons for American obesity. But really, you shouldn't fear carbs. They're your body's go-to source of instant energy, and they help replenish your glycogen, a type of stored energy that fuels exercise. Carbohydrates are also essential for the production of serotonin, a brain chemical that helps you feel calm and content.

So why do so many people cut them out entirely? For one, your body burns significantly fewer calories digesting carbohydrates than it does breaking down protein. Not only that, but carbs can elevate your blood sugar, says Barbara Gower, PhD, an obesity researcher at the University of Alabama at Birmingham. This triggers a flood of insulin, a hormone that tells your body to stop burning and start storing fat. Then comes the inevitable crash—which triggers another cycle of carb and starch cravings, says Valerie Berkowitz, MS, RD, director of nutrition at the Center for Balanced Health in New York City.

That sounds like plenty of reasons to eliminate carbs. But here's the thing: You only experience these unwanted effects when you (1) overdo it or (2) consume the wrong kind of carbohydrates. Unfortunately, most of us are doing both. The average American takes in about twice the recommended daily servings of grains, generally in

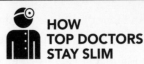

HOW TOP DOCTORS STAY SLIM

"I love substituting spaghetti squash for the noodles in pastalike dishes. I certainly don't miss the carbs, and 1 cup of spaghetti squash has only 42 calories! Plus, it's packed with carotenoids, which may actually help prevent UV damage to the skin."

—MEGHAN O'BRIEN, MD, a dermatologist based in New York City

the form of white bread, pasta, and sweets.

The simple carbs lurking in that bagel or cupcake send your blood sugar soaring almost immediately. And if you're downing them all day, you'll be in constant fat-storing mode. On the other hand, complex carbohydrates—the kind found in whole grains—are broken down slowly, so you avoid a body-stressing blood sugar spike. These are the carbs you want.

■ **SKIP REFINED CARBS** Refined carbohydrates are rarely satisfying, plus they boost your appetite and send your blood sugar through the roof. Translation: You'll need to eat more of them to feel full, but you will quickly be hungry again, all while directing fat to your midsection. These hunger-stimulating carbs are lurking in sweets, white bread, white pasta, crackers, cookies, and other baked goods, and sugary cereal, which you should banish from your diet. In fact, refuse to eat grains that are not whole grains. Just don't rely on food labels to tell you what's inside. Even "whole wheat bread" may not be 100 percent whole grain. So flip over every box or bag and check the ingredient list. Every grain should include the word "whole" in its name. If not, you're eating refined carbs.

BONUS BENEFIT!

Cutting refined carbs may help slash your cancer risk. Eating too many calories can boost your levels of insulin-like growth factor, a hormone that has been shown to increase growth of tumors. The best way to control your levels? You guessed it: consuming less sugar and refined carbs.

■ **MAXIMIZE GRAINS** Whole grains are always preferable to refined. But some whole grains are better than others. Actual whole grains—bulgur, millet, amaranth, quinoa, brown rice, and oats, for example—are healthier than foods made from flour (even whole-grain flour), such as breakfast cereals. (For a primer on true whole grains, see "8 Simple Carb Substitutions" on page 130.)

■ **SWITCH TO LOW-CARB ALCOHOL** Unless you're an endurance athlete, you don't gain much benefit by loading up on carbohydrates, as you do with adding protein. That means cutting back on filler carbs—those that aren't necessary but that you regularly consume—can be the simplest way to trim calories from your diet. Start with alcohol: Drink no more than one (or two, for men) alcoholic beverages per sitting, and opt for red wine, which has fewer carbs than white, or a low-carb beer. You can expect to see the effects: Even modestly reducing your carb intake can help you burn more belly fat, compared to cutting back on fat, according to University of Alabama researchers.

■ **SET LIMITS** If you're not banishing carbs entirely, it can be tough to find your sweet spot. Luckily, science has shed light on the ideal carbohydrate zone. In a University of Florida study, dieters who ate less than 100 grams of carbohydrates per day dropped an average of 4 pounds more fat every month than those who consumed more. The explanation is simple: As your carb intake decreases, so does your level of insulin, says study author James Krieger, MS. Rather than cutting back on fruits and colorful vegetables, place limits on the most carb-dense foods, such as grains and potatoes—try to eat no more than one fist-size serving per meal. To gain a little carb perspective, check out the chart below:

FOOD	CARBOHYDRATES
1 slice whole-grain bread	11–18 g (depending on size)
½ cup cooked brown rice	23 g
1 cup cooked broccoli	11 g
Apple (medium)	25 g
Russet potato (medium)	38 g

■ **SIP ON TEA** Why don't tea bags have nutrition labels? Simple: Unsweetened varieties typically contain less than 1 gram of carbohydrates per serving and thus have virtually no calories. That makes them the ideal drink for carb-conscious dieters—especially if you have a sweet tooth. You can find teas in dessertlike fruit, vanilla, and berry blends that will satisfy your sugar cravings without impacting your blood glucose levels. Just don't make the mistake of adding a glut of sugar to your brew.

■ **CHOOSE THE RIGHT FRUIT** Fruit may be the ultimate dessert: It contains carbs and natural sugars, which are healthier than the sweet stuff you'll find in cookies or cake. Plus, the carbohydrates in fruit act as fuel for your muscles, without spiking your blood sugar as

significantly as starchy foods. This helps you avoid the cravings and binges that you experience when your blood sugar skyrockets then crashes.

Keep in mind: Not all fruits are created equal. Pears, bananas, and dried fruits aren't unhealthy per se, but for the amount of carbs they contain, they offer relatively few nutrients. You don't have to banish them entirely, though. (If you do have the occasional handful of dried fruit, make sure it contains no more than 19 grams of sugars.) Just make blackberries, raspberries, and papaya your priority. These fruits contain far fewer carbs, plus they offer a load of fiber and powerful nutrients. Aim to eat at least two servings of carb-friendly fruit per day.

■ **REPLACE SOME CARBS WITH PROTEIN** You don't have to follow a no-carb diet in order to lose weight. But you *should* emphasize protein over carbohydrates. A USDA study found that substituting 55 grams of carbohydrates with an equivalent amount of whey protein for 23 weeks can help you lose weight. One reason: Eating protein boosts your satiety and results in less of a blood sugar spike than eating carbs alone. Try making simple swaps first: Instead of a second piece of toast, add an egg to your plate. Or instead of spreading your bread with jelly, swap in peanut butter.

■ **DON'T FEAR CARROTS** Dieters have long shunned carrots, assuming they're packed with sugar. Wrong: A cup of chopped raw carrots contains 12 grams of carbs, only half of which are from natural sugars. (The rest are from fiber and slow-digesting complex carbs.) That's fewer carbohydrates than you'll find in a cup of milk or a medium piece of fruit. Plus, vitamins, minerals, and fiber accompany the sugar in the orange veggie (something you won't find in sugary desserts). Reintroduce them to your diet: Top your salad with shredded carrots or dip baby carrots in hummus for a fiber-filled snack.

■ **DON'T FEAR CORN, EITHER** Yes, high-fructose corn syrup comes from corn. But beyond the name, the two have little in common. Corn does contain carbs, but they're the high-quality, complex kind—similar to what you'll find in whole grains. And while high-fructose corn syrup has had all of the nutrition and fiber sucked out of it, a large ear of corn packs 15 percent of your daily fiber plus a quarter of your thiamin, a mineral that helps your body convert carbs into usable energy. The key: Think of corn as more of a grain than a vegetable—which means you should eat it in controlled portions. Try stirring fresh kernels into salads or homemade salsa.

■ **ADD COLOR TO YOUR PASTA OR RICE** If you've quit eating pasta in the name of carb cutting, you can put it safely back on your plate with this strategy: more sauce, less pasta. Flip the traditional ratio of noodles to sauce so the pasta's still integral to the meal, just not the focus. To bulk up your meal, heat up a cup or two of chopped onions, peppers, broccoli florets, or spinach and mix them into your cooked grains. Although whole-grain pasta and brown rice are full of healthy carbs, vegetables contain fiber-rich, less-starchy carbs. (Ideally, you'll consume no more than two daily servings of whole grains, beans, and high-starch veggies, and you'll take in the rest of your carbs from fruits and low-starch vegetables.)

■ **REPLACE CARBS WITH FATS** The healthy fats in an avocado, olive oil, and peanut butter aren't to be feared. They won't make you fat—in fact, when swapped in for carbs, healthy fats may help you lose weight, according to researchers from the University of Alabama at Birmingham. While carbs can trigger blood sugar fluctuations that prime you to overeat, fat has no such effect and also keeps you fuller longer. Try these simple swaps: Spread a small pat of butter on your toast instead of jam, or sip on 1% milk instead of a sports drink after exercise.

■ **LEARN TO NAVIGATE THE BREAD AISLE** The bread aisle can be intimidating. There are dozens of choices, and if you're not knowledgeable, it can be tough to find the right loaf. Here's what you need to know: The only bread that belongs in your cart is 100 percent whole grain. This will eliminate more loaves than you think—even breads that claim to be "whole wheat" may not be 100 percent whole grain. So flip the package over and make sure that every grain in the ingredient list includes the word "whole." You can also look for the Whole Grain Council's "100% Whole Grain" stamp.

Compare calories and fiber. The ideal slice has no more than 100 calories and contains at least 3 grams of fiber per slice. (Hint: If you're having trouble finding lower-calorie options, look for thin-sliced bread.) Martin's 100% Whole Wheat Potato Bread, Vermont Bread Company Soft Whole Wheat, and Oroweat Double Fiber are all smart picks.

■ **AVOID THE WRAP TRAP** No one thinks burritos are healthy. So it's a mystery as to why people consider wraps a diet food. If not chosen carefully, a single tortilla can cost you more calories and carbs than two slices of bread. In fact, we found that one popular commercially made 12-inch wrap contains 290 calories and 50 grams of carbohydrates! As with bread, limit your search to 100 percent whole-grain products (that means no enriched wheat in the ingredient list), including brown rice or corn tortillas, and choose a wrap with around 100 calories and a few grams of fiber. And don't be sucked in by spinach or veggie wraps—they don't count as vegetables. You're much better off piling a plain whole-grain wrap with actual vegetables.

■ **RECONSIDER YOUR SALTY SNACKS** Pretzels have an air of innocence—they're light, crunchy, and low in calories. The perfect diet food, right? Far from it. Chomping on pretzels is essentially the same as eating sugar, since they're full of empty carbs and have no redeeming qualities, like protein or healthy fats. Likewise, most crackers are vessels for refined carbs and added sugars. If you love salty snacks, stick to 100 percent whole grain varieties that have at least 2 grams of belly-filling fiber per serving. (White flour is often listed as wheat flour, so make sure "whole-grain flour" or "whole-wheat flour" is the first and only flour on the ingredients list.) Unique Essential Eating Sprouted 100% Whole Grain Pretzel Puffs are a reasonable option. As for crackers, try Wasa Crackers or Kashi Snack Crackers Original 7 Grain, which are packed with whole grains and fiber.

■ **MAKE UP FOR MISTAKES** It's not always easy to control your carb intake. When you're dining out, for example, the bad guys seem to be hiding in everything from salad dressing to marinara sauce. If you eat refined carbs, munch on another food that has protein or healthy fat, such as hummus. This will help you avoid the blood sugar spike-and-crash, says Cathy Nonas, RD, director of the New York City health department's nutrition program. And whenever

ARE YOU GLUTEN INTOLERANT?

If you can't lose weight, despite eating a healthy diet, you may have gluten intolerance. In a recent study from New Zealand, men who were unable to shed excess pounds stopped eating gluten—a protein found in wheat, rye, oats, and barley—and they immediately began losing weight. In some people, gluten chronically elevates insulin levels, thus signaling fat storage, the study authors explain.

Medical tests for gluten intolerance are often inconclusive. The easiest way to find out if you're intolerant: Eliminate gluten from your diet for 4 to 6 weeks and monitor your weight and general health. If you can tolerate gluten, there is no evidence of a benefit to cutting it out. (Eliminating gluten may actually lead to weight gain.)

you do eat a higher-carb food, make it a policy to eat at least three lower-carb meals or snacks before resuming your normal intake.

■ **FOCUS ON FIBER** Believe it or not, fiber *is* a carbohydrate. That may sound crazy—considering the evil reputation of carbs and the fat-burning reputation of fiber. The belly-filling nutrient is one of the primary reasons that eliminating carbs is a bad idea. You need fiber to slow down digestion so you stay satisfied and keep your bowels moving. In fact, unlike other types of carbohydrates, such as starch, fiber doesn't spike your blood sugar. "The more carbohydrates you eat, the more fiber becomes important to help minimize the wide fluctuations in blood sugar levels," says Jeff Volek, PhD, RD, a nutrition researcher at the University of Connecticut.

8 SIMPLE CARB SUBSTITUTIONS

You want: chips
Eat this: baked cheese Before you say, "It's okay. I eat veggie chips," consider this: These "healthy" chips are usually made from starchy root vegetables, so their carb count is similar to that of potato chips. Baked cheese has the same crunch you crave, without the carbohydrate cost. Place thin slices of cheese on a baking sheet, pop them into a 350°F oven, and bake for 5 to 6 minutes, or until light brown. Let them cool before eating.

You want: hash browns
Eat this: summer squash When cooked, summer squash tastes similar to potatoes but has just a fraction of the carbs. Grate the squash, mix in an egg, form patties, and pan-fry them in olive oil.

You want: a wrap
Eat this: romaine lettuce You can jam everything from turkey to chicken salad into a leaf, roll it up, and eat it just as you would a wrap.

You want: spaghetti
Eat this: spaghetti squash Once cooked, the flesh of spaghetti squash turns into noodle-like strands. Simply cut the squash in half, seed it, then place each half (cut side down) in a dish with ¼ cup water. Zap it in the microwave for 10 minutes, or until it's soft. After it's cooled, scrape out the flesh and top with pasta sauce.

Work more fiber-rich foods that are mixed with water—think brown rice, oatmeal, and whole grain pasta—into your diet. A study by the British Nutrition Foundation found that fluid-rich foods keep you fuller longer than dry foods. Another ideal way to eat more roughage: Stock up on produce, particularly nonstarchy vegetables, such as broccoli, spinach, Brussels sprouts, and peppers. These veg-gies are low in calories, so you can fill up your plate without a second thought. Stir 'em into ½ cup cooked whole grain pasta or brown rice to make your meal more substantial.

■ **EAT POTATOES THE RIGHT WAY** The no-carb craze framed spuds as nutritional villains. Even though nonstarchy veggies are best, pota-toes still have a place—albeit a small one—on your plate. When boiled or baked, their starch

You want: salad dressing

Eat this: tuna mixed with olive oil mayo Tuna blended with a small amount of olive oil mayonnaise—which has about half the calories and fat of the normal spread—is the perfect stand-in for bottled dressing. Plus, you gain a satisfying load of protein.

You want: mashed potatoes

Eat this: mashed cauliflower Steam fresh or frozen cauliflower in the microwave, then spritz it with olive oil. Add a little half-and-half and puree the mixture in a food processor. Season with salt and pepper to taste, then fold in roasted garlic, curry powder, or even chopped pistachios for a flavor boost.

You want: breading

Eat this: flaxseed Breading serves only to add a little flavor and texture—but at a hefty carbohydrate cost. Sprinkle 2 tablespoons of flaxseed over cooked salmon or chicken breast instead.

You want: dessert

Eat this: melons Cantaloupe and honeydew are rich in slow-digesting carbs that calm your cravings. Plus, the sweetness of a fresh scoop of the fruit is not too far off from ice cream.

absorbs water and swells, and once chilled, some of it may crystallize into "resistant starch," meaning it resists digestion. In your large intestines, this resistant starch ferments and produces fatty acids that may block your body's ability to burn carbs. The effect: You burn fat instead. (If you reheat the potatoes, resistant starch levels plummet.) The positives of potatoes are, of course, negated if you fry them or soak them in sour cream or butter. So stick to boiled or baked potatoes (skin on), and make your potato salad with vinegar instead of mayo. Keep your potato portions to fist size.

■ **EAT CARBS BEFORE EXERCISE** Exercising on an empty stomach won't prime you for increased fat burning. The opposite, in fact. When you don't fuel up beforehand, your blood sugar drops during your workout, which can enhance your appetite. Snacking on simple, fast-digesting carbs an hour before you hit the gym will give you a quick surge of energy to fuel your sweat session.

Rather than tangling with Twinkies, munch on the healthiest source of simple carbs: fruit, paired with a little protein, such as peanut butter or cheese. This carb/protein combination raises your insulin levels just enough to expand your blood vessels, permitting increased bloodflow during your workout. The nutritional duo may also help you burn fat. In a Syracuse University study, people who downed a carb/protein shake before exercise had higher metabolic rates the following day than when they consumed carbs alone. If you

don't have a full hour before your workout, sip on a preformulated shake, such as EAS Myoplex Lite, that contains a blend of protein and carbs. Liquid food is digested much more quickly than solids, so you won't feel sick.

■ **REFUEL AFTER A WORKOUT** The first 15 minutes after exercise are an essential time for consuming carbs. During your workout, your body burns up carbs, which allows it to attack your fat stores after you leave the gym. One problem: The longer you wait to eat afterward, when your carb reserves are sapped, the more you'll break down muscle. If you replace lost carbs, you'll slow down your protein loss, encourage muscle growth, and boost your bloodflow so nutrients can be distributed through your body. Pair your carbs with a little protein to provide the amino acids necessary to repair and build muscle. (No need to prioritize fat, since the timing of your fat intake isn't as critical as it is for protein and carbs.)

Keep your snack between 100 and 150 calories—say, an apple and a tablespoon of peanut butter or a glass of chocolate milk (shown to be a perfect postworkout beverage). And don't worry about negating your workout. As long as you keep your calories under control, a postworkout snack can actually help you lose weight. In one study, exercisers who ate a small snack afterward shed more than twice as much flab as those who ate nothing. If you're concerned, you can always save part of a meal for after your workout or schedule gym sessions before meals.

Coffee

5 healthier ways to have a java

Why do so many eating plans ban coffee? Simple: People rarely drink it black anymore. Rather, they load it up with sugar, cream, flavored syrups, whipped cream—all of which overshadow any nutritional value that your morning joe has to offer. On average, gourmet-coffee drinkers—those who prefer coffee from a drive-thru rather than a coffeepot—guzzle 206 more calories a day than regular coffee drinkers.

On the other hand, plain coffee is a perfectly sensible beverage; smart, even. Sipping on the brewed beans has been linked to a lower risk of developing type 2 diabetes, Parkinson's disease, and Alzheimer's disease. And it can also be a major weight-loss ally. The caffeine in coffee excites your central nervous system, kicking your metabolism into high gear. A study published in the journal *Physiology & Behavior* found that the average metabolic rate of people who drank caffeinated coffee increased 16 percent over that of those who drank decaf. That little jolt can amount to an extra 100 calories (at least) burned per day!

■ **DRINK COFFEE ON THE ROCKS** Make your own iced coffee at home. Simply pour black coffee on ice—you can stir in a little 1% milk if you can't stand it black. Research shows that you burn more calories when you add ice to your drink, since it takes a little

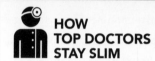

HOW TOP DOCTORS STAY SLIM

"My favorite breakfast: I combine a cup of plain Greek yogurt, a cup of blueberries, 2 tablespoons of flaxseed, and a handful of almonds. I have that almost every day with an 8-ounce glass of Mott's Garden Blend, a double espresso, and a big glass of water."

—**JOHN BUSE, MD, PhD,** a professor in the division of endocrinology and metabolism at the University of North Carolina at Chapel Hill extra energy to bring the cubes up to body temperature.

■ **STOP DRINKING AFTER 4:00 P.M.** It's okay to down more than one cup of coffee a day—as long as you schedule your caffeine hits *before* 4:00 p.m. (Some people may find that 2:00 p.m. is a better cutoff point.) Late-afternoon caffeine can lead to insomnia come bedtime, and sleeplessness can trigger mindless midnight snacking. If you need something flavorful to sip on, switch to noncaffeinated tea, such as hibiscus or chamomile tea, in the evening. (Decaf coffee still contains a small amount of caffeine.)

BONUS BENEFIT!

Coffee is the number-one source of antioxidants in the American diet, according to a study from the University of Scranton. But before you down half a pot, make sure you're sipping the right roast. A 2011 Portuguese study found that light-roast blends offer significantly more antioxidants than dark roasts. Try Starbucks Blonde Roast whole bean coffees, now sold in supermarkets.

■ **ADD JAVA TO YOUR PREWORKOUT SMOOTHIE** If you exercise in the a.m., take advantage of the energy jolt a cup of coffee can provide. Instead of juice, add cool coffee to your preworkout smoothie. Choose a really strong, concentrated blend, like espresso, so it doesn't dilute your drink. Then sip on it at least half an hour before you hit the gym and enjoy a burst of energy on the treadmill.

BREW THE PERFECT CUP

Buy fresh whole beans in small batches every 2 weeks, and invest in your own coffee grinder, since grinding just before you brew yields the best cup. For every 6 ounces, use 1 or 2 tablespoons of ground beans, and only use filtered water. Keep unused beans out of the freezer—the frigid temps will destroy the essential oils that make coffee delicious. Store them on a dark shelf in your pantry in an airtight container.

■ **RECONSIDER SWEETENERS** A packet of sugar contains 16 calories. A packet of Splenda contains zero. Which is preferable? Sugar. That's because artificial sweeteners are often hundreds of times sweeter than sugar, so they can increase your overall preference for sweetness. What that means: If you stir artificial sweeteners into your daily cup, you may actually enhance your drive for desserts. (Or be increasingly tempted by that Frappuccino.) That said, loading up your coffee with sugar isn't exactly conducive to weight loss. If you add sugar to your coffee, scale it back: Stir in a single packet of real sugar, and use a little less of it each week until you can drink it black (or with a little low-fat milk and cinnamon). You'll be surprised at how quickly your taste buds adjust.

BONUS BENEFIT!

If you forgo the sugar in your coffee, you'll reduce your risk of diabetes. In fact, in a Harvard University study, researchers found that guzzling five cups of coffee a day slashed people's risk of diabetes in half, most likely due to the drink's high levels of antioxidants. Headed to Starbucks? Order a Caffè Americano—it's strong, flavorful, and sugar free.

■ **CHOOSE THE RIGHT MIX-INS** Sugar aside, you still face a whole host of other coffee add-ins: creamer, whip, syrup. The list goes on—and not many of these coffee companions are worth messing with. But cinnamon and nutmeg—the spices you'll find in the little shakers at some coffee shops—are different. They add both flavor and health benefits to your mug: Cinnamon can help tame your blood sugar, according to USDA research, and small amounts of nutmeg can calm your stomach. As for dairy, steer clear of anything with the word *cream* in its name. Your safest bet is 1% milk.

BUZZ KILL: HOW COFFEE CALORIES ADD UP

The fancier your cup of coffee, the unhealthier it probably is. Here's what happens to an innocent 16-ounce cup of coffee once the barista starts pumping in those extra ingredients:

Caffè Americano
Ingredients: espresso, water
Nutrition: 15 calories, 0 g fat, 0 g sugar

Caffè Latte
Ingredients: espresso, 2% milk
Nutrition: 190 calories, 7 g fat, 17 g sugars

Caffè Mocha, No Whip
Ingredients: espresso, 2% milk, mocha sauce
Nutrition: 260 calories, 8 g fat, 34 g sugars

Caffè Mocha with Whip
Ingredients: espresso, 2% milk, mocha sauce, whipped cream
Nutrition: 330 calories, 15 g fat, 35 g sugars

Iced Peppermint Mocha
Ingredients: espresso, 2% milk, mocha sauce, whipped cream, peppermint syrup, chocolate curls
Nutrition: 390 calories, 17 g fat, 49 g sugars

Cooking

17 ways to lose pounds in your kitchen

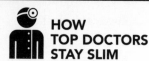

**HOW
TOP DOCTORS
STAY SLIM**

"Before I started my career and met my wife, I had the eating behaviors of your typical single guy in his twenties—big portions of high-calorie and high-fat foods. Now, I try hard to 'practice what I preach.' My wife, Miranda, does much of the cooking at home, and her favorite recipes combine protein and vegetables in one dish. One of our favorites is a chicken and spinach dish that's so tasty you forget the calorie content is very reasonable."

DAVID SARWER, PhD, a psychologist at the University of Pennsylvania's Center for Weight and Eating Disorders

If the recycling bin in your kitchen is full, you may need to overhaul your diet. Why? Because that bin is most likely full of boxes and cans—an indication that you're not eating fresh, whole foods. "One of the biggest signs of unhealthy eating habits is an unused kitchen," says dietitian Amy Baertschi, MS, RD. "It means we're resorting to convenience foods loaded with fat, salt, and preservatives. Get back to cooking and you'll have more control over what you're putting in your mouth." As your number of home-cooked meals increases, your frozen-dinner and fast-food intake inevitably decreases. Not sure where to start? Follow the guidelines below.

■ **PLAN YOUR MENU** When are you most vulnerable to the drive-thru? The minute you ask yourself, "What's for dinner?" If you're both hungry and pressed for time, you're likely to ignore all nutritional red flags and cruise through the McDonald's drive-thru for a quick hit. Don't allow that to happen. One night a week, sit down and plan your home-cooked meals for the week, then devote an hour or two to grocery shopping for necessary items. That way, your answer will be automatic: "Tonight is grilled chicken and asparagus." Suddenly, a greasy burger doesn't sound so appealing. A Centers for Disease Control and Prevention survey found that nearly 40 percent of people who were able to lose weight and keep it off planned their weekly meals.

■ **COOK IN BULK** It can be tough to find time to cook every day. Even so, you don't have to resort to the frozen concoctions at the supermarket. Instead, make it a Sunday-afternoon ritual to cook in bulk, freezing extra portions to eat throughout the week. That way, even after a crazy day, you know you have a healthy meal waiting for you, which makes it infinitely easier to bypass the drive-thru.

A good place to start: chicken breast. It's one of the leanest sources of protein, plus it won't put a major dent in your wallet. Try this: Rub 2 pounds of chicken breasts with pepper and olive oil and place them on a broiler pan. Cook under the broiler at 500°F for 5 minutes, then flip them over and cook for another 5 minutes. Once they cool, seal them in a freezer bag and store them in your refrigerator (or freezer). Season your portion with salt or spices once you're ready to eat.

■ **BANISH PROCESSED FOOD FROM YOUR FREEZER** Frozen, unseasoned fruits and veggies are ideal for your homemade meals. In fact, since they're frozen shortly after picking, they can be even more nutrient-dense than fresh options. But frozen *meals* are another story entirely. Even if they're low in calories, they're most likely laden with sodium and unpronounceable preservatives. If your freezer is currently stocked with Lean Cuisines, allow yourself a month to gradually ease them out of your diet. Then start shopping the perimeter of your supermarket, where you'll find healthy produce, lean meats, and low-fat dairy.

■ **GO EASY ON THE SALT** If you're like most people trying to lose weight, you've prioritized trimming bad fats, cutting calories, and adding protein to your plate. Those are all sound weight-loss strategies. But have you considered sodium? In an attempt to add flavor to reduced-calorie or low-fat foods, dieters have a tendency to sprinkle salt a little too liberally. That's dangerous, since excess sodium can cause you to retain water and may even spike your blood pressure. Rather than salting food as you cook, add just a dash to your meal at the table, using your fingers instead of a saltshaker.

■ **SKIP THE DEEP FRYER** You can enjoy crispy chicken or fish without all the fat of deep-frying it. Simply coat a skillet with 1 tablespoon of extra-virgin olive oil and pan-fry the meat for 10 minutes per side. Use paper towels to blot away extra grease, then transfer your chicken or fish to a 250°F oven and bake it for 15 to 20 minutes.

■ **BRING ON THE BROTH** Even better, instead of stir-frying your veggies or meat in oil, pour ½ cup of chicken, beef, or vegetable broth into your wok. This adds a welcome punch of flavor to your produce without tacking on 1,000 calories in oil.

■ **REPLACE THE OIL IN BAKED GOODS**
Fried foods aren't the only oil-coated crimes in your diet. Even though baked goods don't *taste* oily, most recipes call for a significant amount of the stuff. Try replacing the vegetable oil in baked goods with applesauce, canned pumpkin, or Sunsweet Lighter Bake prune-and-apple blend. You won't miss the calories or fat, since these substitutes maintain the moisture in your cakes and muffins.

■ **PACK IN THE PROTEIN AND FIBER** If you don't make protein and fiber part of every home-cooked dinner, you're more likely to raid the pantry before bed. When planning your menu, focus on lean meats—such as chicken breast, fish, or sirloin steak—for your entrée, and work fiber-rich vegetables and legumes (also a protein source) into your side dishes. To further boost your fiber intake, incorporate one serving of whole grains into your meal.

■ **PLAN FOR DESSERT** Always crave something sweet after dinner? Then make sure to keep whole fruit on hand—it's high in super-satisfying fiber, a nutrient that can help calm your sweet tooth. Or treat yourself to a caffeine-free dessert tea, such as Mighty Leaf Chocolate Mint Truffle, which is blissfully low in calories but rich in flavor. If you prefer wine, sip on a dry white wine or a full-bodied red. The full flavor will keep you from chugging it, so you'll be satisfied with a single glass.

■ **BURN CALORIES WHILE YOU COOK** Ditch the hand mixer and use a wooden spoon instead. Stirring is a more vigorous activity than operating a plug-in mixer, so you'll burn a few extra calories before you sit down for dinner. Another calorie-burning strategy: Crank up the tunes and dance while you cook.

■ **PRACTICE PORTION CONTROL** Even when cooking at home, you're still susceptible to inflated portions, especially if you have no concept of "half a cup" or "8 ounces." Use measuring cups and spoons to portion out things like pasta, sauces, and nuts, or consider investing in a food scale. This handy tool can help you gauge proper portion sizes for tough-to-measure foods like meat and fish. (A serving of beef, poultry, or fish weighs 3 ounces.)

■ **SHRINK YOUR MENU** A simple diet may be the key to weight loss. A study in the *Journal of Consumer Research* found that people eat up to 40 percent more when given a variety of foods than when given a single dish. Your senses are overwhelmed by the array of colors and smells, which can distract you from noticing you're full. In fact, according to Randy Seeley, PhD, an obesity researcher at the University of Cincinnati, sensory cues can heighten your appetite, even when you don't need the calories. Your move: When you're cooking for a small group (or yourself), limit your meal to an entrée and one side dish.

■ **RETHINK YOUR OILS** Corn, soybean, and other vegetable oils are certainly cheap—but you're not doing yourself any favors by adding them to your cart. They're high in omega-6 fatty acids, which can cause inflammation if not counterbalanced by healthy omega-3s. Make heart-healthy olive oil, which is rich in omega-3s, a pantry staple. Even then, use it only when absolutely necessary, since it is still high in calories. (See "Bring on the Broth" on page 137 and "Replace the Oil in Baked Goods," opposite page).

■ **MAKE IT A FAMILY AFFAIR** Where do families most often enjoy a night out? You guessed it: fast-food joints, according to a recent Mintel report. That's far from a "happy meal." People consume far more calories when dining out than when they cook their own meals, research shows. To make dinners at home more fun, invite your kids to participate in the prep work. Set a fixed time for dinner every night, and stick to it.

■ **DON'T BUY THE VALUE SIZE** It's a good idea to cook in bulk. The same can't be said about buying in bulk. In a recent Cornell University study, people who were given large boxes of pasta cooked and ate more of it than those given smaller boxes. You miss out on a savings of a few cents by buying smaller packages, but you could save hundreds of calories.

■ **SERVE FROM THE STOVE** Rather than setting food on the dinner table, leave it on the stovetop. Simply seeing food can tempt you to eat it, even when you're already full. One study found that people who said they didn't want pizza were more inclined to eat a slice anyway when the pie was in front of them. So dish out a single serving of each item, sit down, and eat slowly. Chances are, you won't want to go back for seconds—especially if you can't see it! The exception: If you're serving a tray of fresh fruits and vegetables, keep it on the table. That's the kind of food you *want* to load up on!

■ **TAKE A COOKING CLASS** Food fatigue can tempt you to overeat. ("Oatmeal . . . again?") If you're not sure how to incorporate flavorful ethnic ingredients, such as sriracha sauce or ginger, into foods, look for a cooking class at a local community college. You can learn creative, authentic ways to add new, healthy ingredients to your meals.

Dairy

How a milk mustache can help you lose more weight

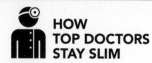
No diet worth following will ban dairy from your plate. It's rich in high-quality protein, healthy fats, and calcium and often fortified with vitamin D, a nutrient found in few foods. "Most people don't get enough dairy products in their diet," says nutritionist Cheryl Forberg, RD. You probably associate protein with meat, but dairy products are also rich in animal proteins. Unlike the protein found in plant foods—nuts, veggies, whole grains—animal proteins are considered "complete," meaning they contain all nine essential amino acids necessary for building muscle. Plus, if you're filling up on low-fat dairy, you have less room for carbohydrates in your diet.

Want proof that dairy won't derail your diet? Check your waistline. In a University of Tennessee study, people who ate three daily servings of dairy lost more belly fat than those who ate significantly less of the stuff. Another study found that dieters who consumed high amounts of dairy lost 70 percent more weight than those who ate the same number of calories but less vitamin D and calcium—the main nutrients you gain by eating dairy (fortified, for vitamin D).

"There's some evidence that calcium deficiency, which is common in women, may slow metabolism," says Tammy Lakatos Shames, RD, a nutritionist based in New York City. The calcium in dairy may block absorption of fat, saturated included, while vitamin D has been linked to greater fat loss, an effect that's enhanced by proteins in dairy. Calcium and vitamin D may also work together to reduce your output of cortisol, a stress hormone that causes you to store belly fat, says Michael B. Zemel, PhD, director of the Nutrition Institute at the University of Tennessee. Of course, covering every entrée with shredded Cheddar won't help you lose weight. Here's how to add dairy to your diet—the right way:

■ **OPT FOR LOW-FAT DAIRY** You know that full-fat dairy can be a recipe for weight gain. But beyond that, the question of fat in your cheese, milk, and yogurt becomes a little murky. Your first instinct is probably to pick up the skim milk or fat-free yogurt, but don't do it: A little fat in your dairy actually helps your body absorb important fat-soluble vitamins, such as D and E. Besides, the caloric difference between skim and low-fat dairy is minimal—maybe 20 or 30 calories, max—and a small amount of fat makes food more satiating. So go ahead, grab the 1% milk.

■ **CHOOSE YOUR CHEESE WISELY** It's not difficult to find delicious 1% milk. But hunting down tasty, diet-friendly cheese can be tough—most low-calorie options you find in the supermarket are mass-produced, flavorless fare. In other words, anything but appetizing. The key is cutting out some, but not all, of the fat. This helps maintain the creamy texture and savory flavor of cheese that you crave while keeping the calories at a reasonable level. You can count on Cabot brand for delicious low-fat cheeses. They make 50 percent reduced-fat sharp Cheddar, jalapeño, and pepper Jack varieties. To keep your portions under control, cut off a chunk no larger than your thumb.

■ **EAT DAIRY WITH EVERY MEAL** To reach your daily goal of three servings, incorporate low-fat dairy at every meal. Try these simple strategies: Eat low-fat Greek yogurt for breakfast, have a slice of cheese on your sandwich at lunch, and drink a glass of milk with your dinner. You can also fold dairy into your snacks. Stir berries into Greek yogurt, or grab a string cheese with a piece of fruit, suggests Forberg.

BONUS BENEFIT!

A Harvard University study found that people who consumed at least three daily servings of dairy were about 36 percent less likely to have high blood pressure than those who ate less than half a serving. Credit the calcium, which may have a BP-lowering effect, as well as the heart-healthy minerals magnesium and potassium.

■ **DRINK CHOCOLATE MILK AFTER A WORKOUT** Your favorite childhood drink may be the ideal postworkout recovery drink. In a 2010 James Madison University study, athletes who drank low-fat chocolate milk after exercise had lower levels of creatine kinase, a marker of muscle damage, than those who downed a high-carb drink. One reason: The whey protein in milk is quickly broken down, while the casein protein in high-carb drinks is slowly released over a longer period of time. Just don't be fooled by "chocolate drink" impostors, like Yoo-hoo. Make sure to choose

HELP! I'M LACTOSE INTOLERANT!

You're not alone—more than 30 million Americans are lactose intolerant. As a result, manufacturers are constantly introducing new nondairy alternatives to milk. (You probably don't have to worry about yogurt and cheese, since they're relatively low in lactose.) Here are the best of the bunch:

Almond milk

Sip this: Almond Breeze Original

Nutrition: 60 calories, 2.5 g fat (0 g saturated), 8 g carbs (7 g sugars), 1 g protein*

This creamy, slightly sweet drink is the least caloric of the milk alternatives and is fortified with calcium and vitamins E, A, and D. You'd think that a nut-based drink would be high in protein, but since the milk consists of ground-up nuts and water, the protein is diluted. Try it in smoothies, cereal, and coffee.

Hemp milk

Sip this: Living Harvest Tempt Original

Nutrition: 100 calories, 6 g fat (0.5 g saturated), 9 g carbs (6 g sugars), 2 g protein

Earthy-tasting hemp milk is naturally high in heart-healthy omega-3 fatty acids, but it's unfortunately low in protein and calcium. It's best mixed into mashed potatoes, muffins, and quick breads. (And don't worry, it doesn't contain the compounds in marijuana that make you high.)

Coconut milk

Sip this: So Delicious Coconut Milk Beverage Original

Nutrition: 80 calories, 5 g fat (5 g saturated), 7 g carbs (6 g sugars), 1 g protein

Coconut milk is lower in sodium than most milk alternatives, plus it's relatively low in calories. The downside: It's high in saturated fat. Use it strictly as a thickening agent for smoothies and oatmeal.

Skip these: soy milk, rice milk

*Nutrition information is per cup.

high-quality chocolate milk, such as Organic Valley low-fat chocolate milk.

■ **AVOID SUGAR-PACKED YOGURT** In a University of Tennessee study, dieters who cut 500 calories and ate three servings of yogurt per day shed 81 percent more belly fat over 3 months than those who didn't dip into yogurt. The caveat: Not just any yogurt will do—even if it's low fat. Yogurt manufacturers have a nasty habit of adding unnecessary sugars to those little cups, some of which pack as much as 30 grams of the sweet stuff! You should be especially leery of fruit-on-the-bottom yogurt, which often contains more sugar than fruit. Your best bet: Stick with plain, low-fat yogurt, then stir in fresh, sliced fruit or whole-grain cereal (as long as it's not granola, a notoriously sugary food).

If only fruit-flavored yogurt will do, follow these criteria in making your selection: A 6-ounce serving should contain no more than 150 calories, 3 grams of fat (any more probably means it contains whole milk or cream), and 22 grams of sugars, and should offer at least 4.5 grams of protein and 15 percent of your daily calcium. Check the ingredient list, too: If high-fructose corn syrup makes an appearance, leave it behind.

■ **SWAP LOW-FAT MILK FOR JUICE** When given the choice between OJ and milk, which do you choose? If you're smart, you go for the milk. Even fruity drinks that boast "100 percent juice" on the label can be high in sugar without having a single gram of fiber to balance out the sugar load. Make low-fat milk your go-to morning beverage, and get your fruit fix in the form of whole fruit.

■ **DON'T BUY INTO DAIRY IMPOSTORS** Avoid the temptation to lump ice cream and queso dip into the same category as yogurt and cheese. Although these foods contain calcium and protein, they also contain a heavy load of preservatives, sweeteners, and unhealthy fats.

6 DAIRY SWAPS FOR WEIGHT LOSS

You eat: ricotta cheese

Try this: cottage cheese Instead of layering whole-milk ricotta into your lasagna, use low-fat cottage cheese. If texture is an issue, you can whip cottage cheese in a food processor or blender until smooth. Try Friendship 1% cottage cheese, also a great sour cream substitute.

You eat: cream cheese

Try this: whipped cream cheese Cream cheese is one of the most caloric spreads in the supermarket. If you consider it a staple, opt for a whipped version, such as Philadelphia whipped cream cheese. The whipping process incorporates air, effectively reducing the number of calories per smear.

You eat: butter

Try this: whipped butter Butter, in moderation, isn't bad for you. In fact, it's healthier than margarine, a source of heart-clogging trans fats. As with cream cheese, choosing a whipped variety, such as Land O' Lakes unsalted whipped butter, can save you significant calories over the stick stuff.

You eat: full-fat Cheddar cheese

Try this: part-skim mozzarella cheese Full-fat Cheddar cheese packs 6 grams of saturated fat per ounce. Switch to part-skim mozzarella and you can cut that in half while saving about 40 calories.

You eat: egg whites

Try this: whole eggs with added omega-3s If you eliminate the yolks, you lose the heft of eggs' nutrients. Instead of removing the yellow stuff, add omegas. Choose a variety high in heart-healthy omega-3s, such as Eggland's Best.

You eat: cheese and crackers

Try this: plain popcorn sprinkled with Parmesan cheese Both cheese and crackers are low-volume foods, meaning they contain very little air, so you have to eat a significant stack in order to feel full. By switching to air-filled popcorn, you fill your belly faster for far fewer calories.

Dessert

21 ways to indulge without harming your health

Dessert is a particularly vulnerable course for a dieter. It's supposed to be indulgent, therefore you may feel justified in ordering the largest milkshake, with extra Oreos and whipped cream to top it all off. But this is the wrong approach to dessert. It's not so much the sugar and calories that satisfy you as it is the *act* of eating—of savoring that milkshake, whether it consists of one scoop of ice cream or three. High-calorie foods certainly taste good, but enjoying those foods is what makes you feel that familiar rush of pleasure afterward. See the difference? The bottom line is that losing weight shouldn't make you feel deprived. So if you absolutely can't live without dessert, then by all means, eat that cake. Just stop after one small slice.

■ **KEEP SWEETS PETITE** If you're baking at home, make your cupcakes in a mini-muffin pan. Roll cookie dough into ½-inch balls instead of golf-ball-size mounds. Or whip up cake lollipops in lieu of your standard double-decker creation. The smaller the

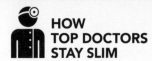

HOW TOP DOCTORS STAY SLIM

"I love dessert. So I allow myself to eat it daily—I don't deprive myself. I just enjoy it in moderation. I try to eat homemade treats. That way, I know the ingredients are all natural. When possible, I revise recipes to make them lower in fat and higher in fiber and protein. I also love dark chocolate, so I always have some with me to snack on. My favorite treat is frozen yogurt with home-baked toppings, such as my mom's cookies and dark chocolate. I even put protein bars on top."

—**REED BERGER, MD,** a weight-management specialist at the University of Illinois Hospital serving size, the less likely you are to overdo it. No single indulgence should cost you more than 200 calories.

■ **DITCH THE DIET SODA** The artificial sweeteners in that Diet Coke could be riling up your sweet tooth. In a University of North Carolina at Chapel Hill study, people who drank diet soda instead of the regular variety ate more dessert and bread than those who sipped on water instead of soda. The reason? Since sugar substitutes are significantly sweeter than the real deal, they may increase your cravings for dessert. Cut out soda—diet or regular—entirely, and sip on water or tea instead. If you need a hint of sweetness, sip on a low-calorie dessert tea, such as Mighty Leaf Chocolate Mint Truffle.

■ **CUT EXCESS SUGAR ELSEWHERE** To make room for dessert, you need to cut back on added sugars in your meals and snacks. Even processed foods that don't seem sweet— pasta sauce, salad dressing, bread, crackers— can be loaded down with sugar. So check the labels and avoid any items that contain unreasonable amounts of added sugar or high-fructose corn syrup. By reducing your intake, you'll naturally slash your cravings for sugar, so smaller portions of dessert will satisfy you.

■ **EAT DESSERT WITH BREAKFAST** It's every kid's dream come true: Scientists now say you should eat dessert first. In a recent Israeli study, researchers found that dieters who ate chocolate, cookies, cake, ice cream, or doughnuts with a protein- and carb-rich breakfast lost 23 percent of their body weight over 32 weeks, compared to 4 percent among those who ate a low-carb, sweets-free breakfast. (They had the same daily calorie intake.) One reason: The dessert-eating dieters experienced greater reductions in cravings for sweets, fats, carbs, and fast food and felt less deprived, making them less tempted to stray from their plan.

■ **REARRANGE YOUR PANTRY** Look inside your pantry: What do you see first? If the answer is cookies or candy, you need to rethink your arrangement. Move indulgent items from eye level to the top shelf—if they're out of sight, you're less likely to grab them. Same goes for your fridge. Take healthy foods out of the crisper and place them on the most visible shelves. Then push the fattening stuff to the back. You'll be more likely to reach for the front-and-center berries than the leftover cheesecake in the back of the fridge.

■ **SIP ON WINE FOR DESSERT** Restaurant desserts can be deceiving. Take, for example, Uno Chicago Grill's Kid's Sundae—you'd think a kiddy portion would be a safe, but this behemoth packs 430 calories and 46 grams of sugars! Unless you've checked the nutrition facts beforehand, play it safe and order a small glass of wine for dessert when you're dining out. And tell the waiter you only want 5 ounces. That way, you avoid imbibing several servings in one sitting. For extra insurance, choose a high-quality vintage wine that you'll want to savor.

■ **PLAN FOR DESSERT** If you do want to eat dessert out, review the nutritional facts ahead of time on the restaurant Web site. Then consider the extra calories when making your entrée selection. For example, if you want to end your meal with a slice of cake, order a healthy appetizer as your entrée. Or if you must order a high-calorie dessert, split it with your dining partner and stop after a few spoonfuls.

■ **INDULGE IN AN AFTER-DINNER FRUIT** Before you scoff, realize that this doesn't necessarily mean eating a plain apple or orange. You can cleverly disguise your favorite fruit as an indulgent dessert. Try garnishing strawberries, banana slices, or melon chunks with a conservative amount of dark chocolate. Or top $\frac{1}{2}$ cup of frozen yogurt with a generous helping of fresh berries or sliced fruit. Cantaloupe and honeydew melon can hold their own alone—a fresh, chilled scoop is just as tasty as dessert.

■ **STOCK UP ON HEALTHY ICE POPS** You don't have to forfeit frozen treats altogether to lose weight, says Marisa Moore, RD, a spokesperson for the Academy of Nutrition and Dietetics. You just need to upgrade your sweets. Buy whole-fruit, low-sugar popsicles, such as Edy's No Sugar Added Fruit Bars, or make your own. Blend fresh or frozen fruit with low-fat vanilla yogurt and freeze the mixture in ice-pop molds.

■ **STEER CLEAR OF 100-CALORIE PACKS** Those little bags of Oreo Thin Crisps seem like a stroke of genius. But really, they're just an invitation to overdo it. Research suggests that dieters register small bites in portion-controlled packs as "diet" food, so they tend to eat more than they might otherwise. (When you finish one bag and still aren't satisfied, you dig in to another—and then another.) Skip the mini cookies and buy regular-size treats in individual portions instead. You can even find your favorite ice creams in small cups.

■ **CHOOSE THE RIGHT CHOCOLATE** Chocolate is the most common and intensely craved food among women, research shows. So don't banish it entirely (you'll eventually cave). Just make sure you choose wisely. The darker the chocolate, the richer it is in heart-healthy antioxidants. That means white chocolate is the ultimate no-no—it doesn't contain a speck of cocoa, the source of the sweet stuff's beneficial antioxidants. Classic milk chocolate is only marginally better. Look for dark chocolate that is at least 70 percent cocoa, such as Green & Black's Organic Dark 70% bar. You'll quickly find that a few squares of high-quality dark chocolate seem more indulgent than a giant bag of M&M's. In fact, in a study from Denmark, people who ate dark chocolate ate 15 percent fewer calories' worth of pizza 2 hours later than milk chocolate eaters did.

■ **DRESS UP YOUR YOGURT** If you haven't worked at least three servings of dairy into your day, consider eating low-fat Greek yogurt for dessert. Rather than eating a fruit-flavored variety, stir fresh fruit into $\frac{1}{2}$ cup of plain

Greek yogurt, or mix in a tablespoon of dark chocolate chips if you need a chocolate fix. When only ice cream will do, choose an additive-free variety, such as Breyers, that has as few ingredients as possible. (Classic flavors, like vanilla or chocolate, are your best bet.) Measure ½ cup into a bowl, then top it with ½ cup fresh fruit.

■ **SAVOR YOUR SWEETS** Don't give yourself a brain freeze: In a study in the *Journal of Clinical Endocrinology & Metabolism*, people who took 30 minutes to eat a bowl of ice cream had higher levels of fullness hormones than those who inhaled it in 5 minutes. "Eating slowly lets food interact longer with the intestinal cells that produce these hormones," says lead study author Alexander Kokkinos, MD, PhD. Stretch out your dessert session as long as possible, making sure to consider the taste and texture of every bite. And banish any dining distractions, like your TV or smartphone, so you fully appreciate the experience.

■ **SPLURGE THE RIGHT WAY** You're enjoying you're weekly cheat meal—so why are you wasting it on Oreos? When it's your day to indulge, choose a sweet that's something special. For example, swing by your favorite bakery for that supersoft sugar cookie you love. Or splurge on the Cold Stone concoction that you've been craving for weeks. "It's more rewarding to have a nice treat than to waste calories on regular things you can have anytime, like potato chips or cookies," says Stephen Gullo, PhD, former chair of the National Obe-

sity and Weight Control Education Program at Columbia-Presbyterian Medical Center.

■ **FIND YOUR WEAK SPOTS** Do you eat a full box of Reese's Pieces every time you see a movie? Or are you always tempted to order the massive cheesecake on date night? You may be more influenced by where you are, what you're doing, and who you're with than by the taste of the food in front of you. Pinpoint your most troublesome times and plan ahead—"I'm going to bring my own bag of trail mix"—or banish your cravings by sipping on water with appetite-suppressing lemon or by chewing gum.

■ **LIMIT YOUR CHOICES** When your pantry is stocked with Chips Ahoy!, M&M's, *and* Nutter Butters, it's harder to say no, since one of them will likely satisfy whatever craving you're wrestling with. In fact, research shows that when presented with a variety of foods, people tend to consume more calories. Keep only one kind of treat on hand, then fill the rest of your shelf space with healthier options, such as whole-grain cereal or nuts (try the cocoa-dusted kind).

■ **PASS ON "DIET" TREATS** Studies show that overweight people who consume low-fat snacks take in twice as many calories as those who eat regular snacks. One explanation: Dieters think they can indulge in low-fat or sugar-free treats guilt free. Unfortunately, "sugar free" or "low fat" doesn't mean healthy. Rather, "low fat" often means "high sugar," and "sugar free" often means "lots of artificial sweeteners." (See "Ditch the Diet Soda" on page 146, for more on artificial sweeteners.) Plus, these "light" desserts may lack the rich taste you crave, so you end up eating more to feel satisfied. If you're searching for a healthier packaged dessert, look for one that doesn't contain high-fructose corn syrup and, ideally, uses whole grain flour. Kashi's cookies are a good place to start.

■ **AVOID GROCERY-STORE BAKED GOODS** Yes, those cream cheese raspberry scones look delicious. The problem is, foods that are prepared in-house—say, in the supermarket bakery—don't have to include nutritional information. So you have no idea how many calories or how much sugar and fat you're ingesting.

■ **MAKE SMART BAKING SUBSTITUTIONS** You don't have to give up baking while you're trying to lose weight. You just have to make clever swaps to cut calories and fat. For example, use applesauce, Sunsweet Lighter Bake, or pureed pumpkin instead of oil in your baked goods. Try substituting a cup of whey protein powder for a cup of flour in your cookies or muffins. Or when making a cheesecake, swap in cottage cheese (whipped in a food processor) for the cream cheese.

■ **BRUSH AND FLOSS AFTER DINNER** Trying to resist that brownie à la mode? Make a trip to the bathroom sink. If you brush and floss after your main course, your mouth will taste minty—a flavor that doesn't pair well with most desserts. Plus, who wants to brush twice in one night? If you're nowhere near your sink, pop a piece of sugar-free mint gum instead.

■ **TAKE A BUBBLE BATH** Instead of eating dessert, find another indulgence that doesn't involve food. Soak in a bubble bath for half an hour, paint your nails, or browse your favorite online store. Your urge to eat will likely pass with the distraction.

Dinner

20 tips for building a slimmer dinner

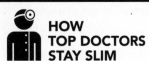
You've heard it before: Dinner should not be your largest meal of the day. Yet large dinnertime meals are ingrained in our culture. Suppertime is when we typically have the most time to prepare a meal and sit down to eat with family over a leisurely feast. So it tends to be the biggest and heaviest of our daily meals. Problem is, if we're stuffing our stomachs at dinnertime, we have very few hours to burn off those calories before our furnaces slow down for a night of sleep.

A National Institute on Aging study found that middle-aged people who packed their daily number of calories into one super-size supper pumped out more ghrelin, a hunger hormone, than when they spread the same amount of calories over three meals. It's far more logical to frontload your calories at breakfast, when you're about to embark on a new day full of activity and exercise. Stop thinking of dinner as an evening binge and think of it as a small but nutrient-dense end to a healthy day (or a way to make up for any areas you missed out on at breakfast and lunch). Cap it off at 450 calories, and follow these rules to make the most of your evening meal:

■ **SPICE THINGS UP** Want a metabolic jolt before bed? Add hot sauce to your meal. (Warning: Don't do this if you're prone to heartburn.) Australian scientists recently showed that overweight folks are more likely to burn fat after eating a meal that contains chile peppers than after one that isn't spicy. One reason: After the heat-infused meal, the diners' average level of insulin—a hormone that tells your body to store fat—was 32 percent lower. The scientists credit capsaicin, the compound that makes peppers hot. It's thought to improve your body's ability to shuttle insulin out of your bloodstream after a meal. Douse your dinner with as much Tabasco sauce as you can handle. (For more spicy tips, see "The Heat Index" on page 258.)

■ **SNACK BEFORE DINNER** Your parents probably told you, "Don't eat a snack. It will ruin your dinner." Turns out, that may not be bad thing. If you munch on a protein-rich snack a couple of hours before dinner, you may be less inclined to gorge yourself at the table, since you're not feeling dangerously ravenous. Eat a few sticks of celery with almond butter, a fistful of nuts, or low-fat Greek yogurt with fruit a couple of hours before diner. Limit your intake to about 150 calories—otherwise, you'll need to scale back the size of your meal.

■ **DON'T DRINK THEN DINE** A glass of wine before dinner isn't as harmless as it seems. In a British study, people who drank alcohol 30 minutes before a meal ate 15 percent more food than juice drinkers. As you start to feel a buzz, your inhibitions drop, which may make you more likely to go back for seconds. Plus, alcohol is thought to ramp up

your appetite, leading you to eat more. Save your alcohol for dessert.

■ **START WITH SALAD** Before you dive into that salmon fillet, stick your fork into a pile of leafy greens. A Penn State study found that eating a 100-calorie salad before your main course can reduce your overall food intake by up to 12 percent (even without trying to cut back). The fiber in the greens helps you feel fuller faster. You can also eat salad as your entrée, as long as you incorporate a source of protein, like lean meat, hard-cooked eggs, or legumes.

■ **. . . OR SOUP** Your favorite comfort food may also help you lose weight. Penn State scientists found that eating soup as an appetizer can significantly cut your calorie intake. In their study, people who ate a 150-calorie broth-based vegetable soup before a pasta meal consumed about 135 fewer calories than when they didn't hit the bowl. "Eating soup forces you to slow down, allowing your body to recognize that it's becoming full before moving to the second course," say the researchers. This can curb cravings and help prevent overeating. If you're dining at home, stick to low-sodium soups with a vegetable base or a low-calorie portion of creamy soups.

■ **CHILL YOUR SPUDS** This may sound strange, but consider popping your cooked potatoes into the fridge before dinner. The reason: Baked and roasted spuds contain a special type of starch that crystallizes when exposed to cool temperatures. When this happens, your body is no longer able to digest it, so it can actually prevent absorption of the carbs. Just don't reheat your potatoes: That breaks up the crystals, causing resistant starch levels to drop. Try serving cold potato salad as a side dish, or add chilled, chunked red potatoes to a salad. You can even puree cooked white potatoes and make chilled garlic potato soup.

■ **CALCULATE YOUR GRAINS** If you choose a carbohydrate-rich entrée, make sure to select nonstarchy sides. For example, if you're eating a whole-grain sandwich as your main course—which contains about two servings of carbs—skip the baked potato or green peas. (Ideally, carbs will occupy only a quarter of your plate.) Instead, steam a cup of nonstarchy broccoli, Brussels sprouts, or cauliflower.

■ **LOAD UP THE FRUIT AND VEGETABLES** Fill half of your dinner plate with produce, focusing primarily on nonstarchy vegetables: artichokes, asparagus, green beans, beets, broccoli, Brussels sprouts, cabbage, carrots, cauliflower, celery, cucumber, eggplant, green onions, leafy greens, leeks, mushrooms, okra, onions, peppers, radishes, snap peas, spinach, tomatoes, or zucchini. Then work in low-sugar fruits, such as apples, raspberries, and strawberries. Switch things up by eating salads, slow-braised or flash-sautéed vegetables, raw vegetables dipped in olive oil, or whole fruits. Diversity is the key to avoiding food fatigue.

■ **PACK IN THE PROTEIN** Although produce is your priority at dinner, you also need to work in belly-filling protein. Lean meats and fish are, of course, on your list of healthy choices. But you can also build your plate around legumes. Which variety offers the biggest protein impact? Canned white beans—a cup contains 19 grams of the stuff! Other top picks: pinto beans, kidney beans, and black beans, all of which pack 15 grams of protein per cup. Plus, beans are rich in fiber, a superfilling nutrient you should work into every meal. Protein should make up about a quarter of your plate.

■ **RETHINK YOUR PASTA** Vegetarian, whole-grain pasta is a no-brainer. But you can also safely enjoy meat-lovers' Italian food. The key: Think meat marinara, not meatball. With pasta dishes, you don't have to include large amounts of meat, since you can evenly distribute crumbled or thinly sliced pieces throughout the sauce. Try stirring chopped ham or diced grilled chicken into your pasta sauce. Hint: If you're using a bottled sauce, look for one that's low in added sugars, such as Ragú Light No Sugar Added Tomato & Basil.

■ **INCORPORATE DAIRY** Aim for at least one serving of low-fat dairy with every meal—dinner included. The calcium in dairy has been shown to enhance fat burning, plus the extra shot of protein makes your meal more filling. Dinner is the prime time to eat a slice of low-fat cheese or even sip a glass of milk on the side.

■ **ADD A LITTLE FAT** Fold in high-quality fats, such as those found in fatty fish like salmon and mackerel, nuts, and olive oil, at dinner. Scientists think that your body prefers fat to carbohydrates as fuel in the evening, plus good-for-you fats (unsaturated) will help keep you full until bedtime.

■ **TWEAK YOUR DINNER FORMULA** In a Penn State study, researchers found that people who keep a steady weight tend to eat the same basic foods, but vary the *way* they eat them. For example, they make grilled chicken a staple in their diet, but one night they eat it on mixed greens with mustard vinaigrette and on another they pair it with spinach and raspberry vinaigrette. They might also switch up the fruits and vegetables they toss in that salad. A go-to healthy meal that you can modify helps you control your calories without being boring.

■ **DINE OUT WITH A PLAN** When the waiter is staring you down, it's easy to panic and order the first thing to see. Unfortunately, that's often a burger and fries or some other waistline-threatening meal. Your strategy: Don't even look at the menu at the table. "Most people choose with their eyes and not with their heads," says personal nutrition consultant Christopher Mohr, PhD, RD. Check out the restaurant's menu and nutrition facts beforehand (when you're not hungry), and decide which nutritious option you're going to order. That way, you won't be tempted to choose with your eyes instead of your head.

■ **DOWNSIZE YOUR DINNERWARE** Rather than eating from a Frisbee-size platter, dish out your dinner on a salad plate. It's a mind trick: If your food fills up more of the plate, you'll think you're eating more—perhaps the simplest way to shrink your portions, says Brian Wansink, PhD, director of the Cornell University Food and Brand Lab.

■ **STICK TO THE SAME DINNERTIME** For years, doctors have said to pick a bedtime and stick to it. The same should be said about dinnertime. If dinner becomes a consistent part of your schedule, you're more inclined to do it right, rather than swinging by the pizza joint or grazing on junk all afternoon. An early dinner is preferable, since you don't want to go to bed on an overly full stomach. So choose a time between 5:30 and 7:30 p.m., and make it a can't-miss appointment at your dinner table.

■ **COOK ON THE WEEKENDS** If you regularly find yourself digging through the pantry for something—anything—to eat, consider planning your weekly dinner menu ahead of time. Then cook in big batches on the weekends. An easy place to start? Grilled chicken, brown rice, and veggies (either keep diced fresh veggies on hand or stock up on frozen ones). If you have a dinner strategy, you're less likely to succumb to the drive-thru when you're tired and hungry after work.

■ **AVOID DINNERTIME DISTRACTIONS** How often do you multitask during your meal: Watch TV? Eat dinner at your desk on a late night? Down a burger while you drive? These mealtime distractions can prevent your brain from registering fullness, often compelling you to overeat. So turn off the tube, pull up a chair, and sit down for dinner. Better yet, go all out and set the table. If you use real dinnerware, you'll feel like you've eaten a full meal, making that late-night cookie a little less tempting.

■ **KEEP SPLURGING UNDER CONTROL** Weekend dinners are perhaps your most vulnerable time for cheating—you're away from work, ready to unwind, and often at a restaurant with friends. If you so choose, you can schedule your weekly cheat meal for Friday or Saturday night. Just make sure you don't make the critical mistake of letting a big dinner turn into an all-weekend feed fest. To prevent this, plan the first meal you'll have after your cheat meal. For example, buy the ingredients for a healthy Sunday-morning breakfast of eggs and Greek yogurt with berries. That way, you're not as vulnerable to the "I've already overdone it, so why not do it again" cycle.

■ **FIRE UP THE BLENDER** There's nothing wrong with slurping a smoothie for dinner—as long as you (1) toss the right ingredients into the blender and (2) cover your nutritional bases the rest of the day. First, consider your liquid base: Skip sugar-filled, fiber-deficient juices and build your shake around 1% milk. Next, your thickeners: To make your smoothie more filling and flavorful, bolster it with a tablespoon of natural nut butter—almond, peanut, cashew—or low-fat plain Greek yogurt. Choose your frozen fruit according to your tastes—bananas, strawberries, or even avocados are all good options. You can also incorporate vegetables, such as carrots or spinach. Finally, add a couple of tablespoons of whey protein powder to boost the filling factor, since liquid foods tend to be less satisfying than solids. If need be, pair a reasonably sized smoothie with a side salad and low-fat dressing.

Fat

Use it to lose it

Fat isn't the dietary demon you may think it is. In fact, you may need to fatten up to slim down. Healthy fats—the monounsaturated fats found in olive oil, nuts, and avocados—have little to do with making you fat, since they don't raise your levels of insulin, the fat-storage hormone. The real culprit behind your inflating waistline is high amounts of carbs coupled with high amounts of fat. The carbs spike your insulin levels, and *bam,* your body starts absorbing more fat. The proof is in the science: A recent study from the United Arab Emirates found that people who cut carbs lost more weight and had lower insulin levels than those who scaled back the fat. Another study found that people who consumed moderate amounts of fat lost about 10½ pounds in a year—60 percent more than low-fat dieters dropped.

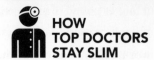

HOW TOP DOCTORS STAY SLIM

"I follow a carb-restricted diet that's moderate in protein and high in fat. A daily menu: a three-egg cheese-and-mushroom omelet, roast beef slices wrapped around Colby cheese, baked salmon, broccoli with butter, and a salad with dressing."

—JEFF VOLEK, PhD, RD, an associate professor of kinesiology at the Human Performance Laboratory at the University of Connecticut

The reason: Healthy fats may help curb your desire to overeat. "Fat is filling and it adds flavor to your meals, so it helps you avoid feeling deprived," says Alan Aragon, MS, a nutritionist based in Thousand Oaks, California. His rule of thumb: Aim to eat half a gram of fat per pound of your goal body weight. Just make sure you're eating natural fats, not trans fats, which have been linked to obesity. So go ahead, eat an avocado, a salmon fillet, a handful of nuts, or have olive oil on your salad. And don't worry about eating animal fats like butter, cheese, or beef, either. As long as your portions are reasonable, your waistline—and your heart—will be fine. Here's how to make sure you work the right fats into your diet:

■ **CALCULATE YOUR FATS** The majority of the fats you consume should be mono- or poly-unsaturated fats. To keep your fats in balance, follow this basic formula: Add up a food's mono- and polyunsaturated fats and calculate what percentage of the total fat they make up. Ideally, they'll equal about 75 percent of the total fat. (If the label only lists saturated and trans fats, subtract them from the total to determine the unsaturated fat count.) As for trans fats, shoot for as close to zero as possible. Altogether, fat should account for 20 to 30 percent of your daily calories.

■ **BITE INTO DARK CHOCOLATE** Dark chocolate is good for more than a fleeting sugar high. An ounce of the stuff contains nearly 4 grams of monounsaturated fat—the same healthy, filling fat that you'll find in nuts and olive oil. Limit yourself to a 100-calorie serving (one 2-inch square), and choose a bar that's at least 70 percent cacao, the source of antioxidants in chocolate. Try Chocolove Strong Dark Chocolate Bar, 70% Cocoa. It's dark enough to confer cacao's benefits but sweet enough to taste like dessert. Another delightful bar: the fruity Jacques Torres Midnight Soul (80 percent cacao).

■ **ADD FAT TO YOUR FRUIT** Pairing your fruit with fat won't make you pear shaped. It may actually help you lose weight. Fruit is a perfect source of instant energy (thanks to its natural sugars), but your midmorning or afternoon snack should also contain healthy fats and protein for more sustained energy. The perfect duo: a piece of fresh fruit plus a small chunk of cheese or a tablespoon of nut butter.

■ **MUNCH ON NUTS** Nuts are notoriously high in calories. However, they're not to be feared. The fatty acids in nuts can actually elevate your metabolism, protecting against weight gain, while stamping out your appetite.

Since you're cutting calories, limit yourself to an ounce of unsalted nuts per sitting—that's about 35 peanuts, 24 almonds, or 18 cashews. If portion control is a problem, buy shelled pistachios; all that cracking will force you to slow down, saving you as much as 86 calories per sitting, according to Eastern Illinois University research. You can also try pouring an ounce onto a plate and eating one at a time.

BONUS BENEFIT!

Walnuts may ease your anxiety. A study in the *Journal of the American College of Nutrition* found that their good-for-you polyunsaturated fats may help counteract your body's natural reaction to stress.

■ **EMBRACE NUT BUTTERS** Peanut butter may be the go-to food of preschoolers, but it's also the dieter's ideal spread. Like nuts, peanut butter is loaded with healthy monounsaturated fats, shown to prevent the accumulation of fat around the midsection, to boost calorie burn, and to help keep you full. "Peanut butter is convenient, and you don't need a lot to feel satisfied," says dietitian Katrina Seidman, RD. "It's a perfect food—it has fat, protein, carbohydrates, fiber, antioxidants, even resveratrol." People who eat a serving of peanut butter at least twice a week are less susceptible to weight gain than folks who rarely eat the spread, according to recent Harvard University research. And a study in the *International Journal of Obesity* found that dieters who included peanut butter in their plan lost an average of 9 pounds in 18 months.

Don't stop with peanut butter. Diversify your diet with almond, cashew, or macadamia nut butters, adding them to smoothies, sandwiches, or sauces. Choose a nut butter that has only two ingredients: nuts and salt. There's no need for added sugars, fillers, or hydrogenated oils, which add dangerous trans fats. And always choose the full-fat version. Reduced-fat nut butters replace healthy fats with empty carbohydrates and sugar. Make sure to stick with a 2-tablespoon portion (about the size of a golf ball). (For a more extensive buying guide, see "Pick the Perfect Nut Butter" on page 159.)

A study in the *Journal of the American Medical Association* found that consuming just 1 ounce of nuts or peanut butter at least 5 days a week may reduce your risk of diabetes by almost 30 percent!

■ **DITCH "DIET" FOODS** Don't assume that "low fat" equals healthy. Labels are all about marketing—which means food manufacturers fail to advertise that reduced-fat foods are often high in sodium, empty-carb fillers, and sugar. In other words, fat-free or reduced-fat foods are no less fattening than regular foods. That's scary, considering we tend to consume more calories when eating foods labeled "low fat," since we don't experience the same guilt as we munch, a study in the *Journal of Marketing Research* found. A better approach: Stick with whole foods (those that don't have a label), and if you do buy packaged foods, seek out those with heart-healthy omega-3s and monounsaturated fats.

■ **SWAP PORK RINDS FOR POTATO CHIPS** A recent Harvard University study identified potato chips as the primary food causing American weight gain. If you're craving a crispy snack, choose fried pork skins instead. Yes, they're fried, but 43 percent of the pork rind's fat is unsaturated, and most of that is oleic acid—the same healthy fat as in olive oil. Plus, a 1-ounce serving contains zero carbs and 17 grams of protein!

■ **SWITCH TO GRASS-FED BEEF** Unlike grain-fed products, grass-feed beef is rich in the same essential omega-3 fats you find in fish. This is noteworthy, because your body can't produce omega-3s from other fats; you have to eat the fatty acids in order to meet your needs. When picking cuts of beef, prioritize sirloin, which contains less of the bad fats than rib eye or porterhouse. For an ideal on-the-go snack, grab Gourmet Natural Beef Jerky (www.americangrassfedbeef.com). It's preservative free and made from grass-fed beef.

■ **CHOOSE LEAN MEATS** The number one rule of the meat and fish counter: Leaner is always better. You should select protein sources with primarily unsaturated fats, such as salmon, chicken breast, turkey breast, tenderloin, or round-cut beef, over those high in saturated fats. (For a primer on meats, see page 202.)

■ **AVOID FAT-FREE DAIRY** Whole milk and other types of full-fat dairy are loaded with unnecessary calories. (If dairy contains more than 4 grams of fat per serving, it probably contains whole milk or cream.) But you shouldn't go to the opposite extreme and buy fat-free dairy. Many of fortified milk's nutrients—vitamins A and D, for example—require fat to be absorbed. So rather than going skim, load up your cart with low-fat milk and yogurt; the nutritional difference is only 20 to 30 calories per serving. When it comes to cheese, select naturally light varieties, such as mozzarella (rather than the rubbery, fat-free stuff), and stick to 2-ounce portions.

■ **ADD AVOCADO TO YOUR CART** A single avocado packs nearly 20 grams of monoun-

saturated fat. That sounds like a surefire way to wreck your waistline—until you consider the science behind these fats. Research shows that monounsaturated fats, or MUFAs, can help lower your LDL "bad" cholesterol and may even enhance your fat burning. Avocados are particularly high in oleic acid, a type of MUFA that helps send hunger-curbing signals to your brain during digestion, according to a study in the journal *Cell Metabolism*. Plus, avocados are rich in folate, a nutrient linked to lower body weight. Try making homemade guacamole, add avocado slices to your sandwich, or toss the superfilling fruit with your salad. You can also whip up a quick salsa: Simply dice avocado with mango, onions, and cilantro.

■ **EAT MUFAS FOR BREAKFAST** A study found that eating a breakfast high in MUFAs may boost your calorie burn for 5 hours—especially if you have lots of belly fat. Avocados are one source of the fats; you'll also find MUFAs in plant foods such as olives and nuts. Try stirring almonds into low-fat Greek yogurt, or add diced avocado to your omelet.

■ **LOSE THE FAT-FREE DRESSING** Fat-free salad dressings are often packed with sugar—and that means lots of empty calories. Besides, you need a little fat in your dressing so you can absorb the vitamins A, D, E, and K found in your leafy greens. A smarter pick: oil-based dressings, such as those made with olive oil, vinegar, and herbs. They contain healthy fats and coat your salad more easily than thick, creamy dressings (which are often high in unwanted saturated fat), so you can use less. Try Newman's Own Olive Oil & Vinegar Dressing. As with any higher-calorie food, you should still control your portions by measuring out a 1- or 2-tablespoon serving.

Healthy fats may preserve your brainpower. In a Rush Institute study, people who took in a daily 24 grams of monounsaturated fat had an 80 percent lower risk of Alzheimer's disease than those who consumed 15 grams. One reason: Unsaturated fats improve your cholesterol profile, which can help keep brain cells healthy.

■ **DON'T FEAR BUTTER** Coating every meal in a thick layer of butter *will* make you fat. But

PICK THE PERFECT NUT BUTTER

Although high in calories, nut butters are loaded with waistline-friendly, heart-healthy mono-unsaturated fats and plant protein, making them super satisfying. To enjoy the tasty spreads' full benefit, you have to choose the right jar. Start shopping.

Ingredients: Nut butters should have no more than two ingredients: nuts and salt. (To make your search easier, limit yourself to "natural" nut butters.) If you see partially or fully hydrogenated oils on the ingredients list, shelve it. These scary oils are a source of heart-damaging trans fats.

Fat: Skip the reduced-fat stuff. The only thing you gain by cutting fat is a load of quick-burning carbs, often in the form of maltodextrin.

Sodium: This is one of the most highly variable aspects of nut butters—levels can range from 40 to 250 milligrams per serving! Look for a lower-sodium option. (Hint: Organic versions tend to have less.) The less sodium, the nuttier the spread will taste.

Sugar: Select a spread with 2 grams of sugars or less—any more, and it most likely contains added, and unnecessary, sweeteners. Natural brands are generally lower in sugar than commercial brands.

Smart picks

Smucker's Natural Chunky Peanut Butter
200 calories, 16 g fat (4.5 g polyunsaturated, 8 g monounsaturated), 90 mg sodium, 2 g fiber, 1 g sugars, 7 g protein*

Cream-Nut Natural Peanut Butter
190 calories, 16 g fat (13.5 g unsaturated), 35 mg sodium, 2 g fiber, 1 g sugars, 8 g protein

MaraNatha Natural Raw Almond Butter
195 calories, 16 g fat (15 g unsaturated), 0 mg sodium, 4 g fiber, 2 g sugars, 7 g protein

*Nutrition info is for 2 tablespoons.

in moderation, butter has a place in your fridge. "The health scare surrounding saturated fat and cholesterol was overblown," says Walter Willett, MD, chair of the department of nutrition at Harvard School of Public Health. In fact, the saturated fat in butter is composed primarily of palmitic and stearic acids, neither of which will impact your cholesterol.

Butter is also an excellent source of conjugated linoleic acid (CLA), a natural fat linked to lower levels of abdominal fat. Besides, alternatives like vegetable oil–based margarine and shortening contain hydrogenated or partially hydrogenated oils, which are weighed down with artery-clogging trans fats. Butter, on the other hand, contains less-threatening (and natural) dairy fats. Limit yourself to a portion of butter no bigger than the tip of your thumb, or try a whipped butter spread, which is less calorie-dense than stick butter.

■ **RETHINK YOUR OILS** Corn, soybean, and other vegetable oils are high in omega-6 fatty acids, a type of polyunsaturated fat. Unless balanced by a high intake of omega-3s (like those found in fish), omega-6s can trigger inflammation, potentially increasing your risk of heart disease. "We now consume 20 to 1 omega-6s to omega-3s," says certified nutrition specialist and weight-loss coach Jonny Bowden, PhD. "Our inflammatory factory is overstaffed, and our anti-inflammatory factory is understaffed." Skip the vegetable oil in favor or olive or canola oils, which have plenty of omega-3 fatty acids to offset their omega-6 content.

Canola oil is a perfect option for everyday cooking, since it has a neutral flavor and can withstand relatively high heat. Regular or light olive oils are also ideal for day-to-day meal prep. ("Light" refers to color, flavor, and aroma, not nutritional content.) Reserve extra-virgin olive oil for salads, vegetables, and cooked side dishes. To make your oil go a long way, pour it into a spray can or mister, such as the Misto Olive Oil Sprayer. That way, you can flavor foods for a fraction of the calories you add when pouring oil from the bottle.

BONUS BENEFIT!

A 3-year Italian study found that a diet high in monounsaturated fats from olive oil and nuts can reduce your markers of inflammation—a known trigger for disease and aging!

■ **CUT OUT BAD FATS** You don't want to overdo it on saturated fat, often found in animal products, such as butter, cheese, and fatty meats. However, a little saturated fat—fewer than 10 percent of your calories—isn't dangerous, according to the National Institutes of Health. But trans fats, which form when vegetable oil hardens, should be avoided entirely, since they can raise your bad cholesterol and lower your good. The scary part: You may not know they're even lurking in your foods. If a food contains less than 0.5 gram trans fats, manufacturers can legally claim "0 grams trans fats." So instead of relying on the nutrition panel, scan the ingredient list of every packaged food for hydrogenated or partially

WHY DID THE CHICKEN CROSS THE ROAD?
Answer: To Avoid the Deep Fryer

Deep-frying chicken or fish fills the breading up with tons of fat calories. "Whoa, but I'm from south of the Mason-Dixon Line and grew up on fried chicken. I can't live without the crispiness!" you scream. That's okay, there is a healthier way to enjoy the classic southern food without the heavy caloric toll. Simply coat a pan with a tablespoon of olive or canola oil and pan-fry the meat for 10 minutes per side. Blot up extra grease with paper towels, then transfer to a 250°F oven. Bake for 15 to 20 minutes.

hydrogenated oils—a dead giveaway that trans fats are hiding inside that box. Shelve any items that contain the oils.

■ **WATCH OUT FOR PALM OIL** Unfortunately, hydrogenated oils aren't the only scary oils making their way into your food. As food manufacturers work to eliminate trans fats, they've begun replacing them with tropical oils, like palm. Although palm oil was once praised for its high vitamin E content, the research is turning rancid: For one, it's 51 percent saturated fat, and, even scarier, it has been shown to act similarly to trans fats in your body, possibly raising your bad cholesterol. Scan ingredient lists for olive or canola oils instead, says Sally Kuzemchak, RD, a nutrition instructor at Ohio University Lancaster.

■ **DIP INTO HUMMUS** This Middle Eastern staple is the perfect veggie dip or sandwich spread. It's made from chickpeas, a type of belly-flattening legume, and offers a healthy dose of both mono- and polyunsaturated fats. Look for hummus made with traditional olive oil rather than soybean oil, such as Athenos Hummus. The dip is also a smart starter when dining out, especially if you dive into the basket of complimentary bread. The healthy fats will help nix the blood sugar spike-and-crash caused by refined carbs. (Even better, avoid the breadbasket altogether.)

■ **SNACK CAREFULLY** Grab-and-go snacks often come in a box or bag—with a dose of unhealthy fats. Make sure your munchies contain no more than 3 grams of saturated fat and no trans fats (or hydrogenated oils); look for heart-healthy unsaturated fats (8 grams or less) from nuts, seeds, and peanut butter. These enhance flavor and satisfy your stomach without clogging your arteries. Practice extra caution when buying salty snacks, as they can be particularly packed with oil and trans fats. An easy swap: Instead of scarfing potato chips, even the baked kind, snack on popcorn made with olive or canola oil. It's a source of fibrous whole grains, and the little bit of healthy fat will help slow digestion.

■ **GO FISH** Today's fresh catch could add years to your life. Fatty fish—salmon, tuna, sardines, mackerel, and trout—are high in omega-3 fatty acids, a type of polyunsaturated fat. These healthy fats not only help your body absorb vitamin D, boost your heart health, and enhance your brainpower, they've been linked to lower levels of abdominal fat, too!

Although a fish oil supplement will provide the omega-3s you need, you miss out on the protein, vitamins, and minerals of seafood when you pop a pill. Aim to eat fatty fish at least three times per week.

■ **PRIORITIZE FAT AT DINNER** Although you should have healthy fats at every meal, dinner is the time to focus on the stuff. The reason: Your body prefers fat to carbohydrates as fuel in the evening, since your insulin-carb system is less efficient late in the day. Try whipping up a healthy veggie and chicken stir-fry, and pair it with greens lightly dressed with olive oil. The combination of protein, fat, and fiber will keep you full until bedtime.

■ **REPLACE CARBS WITH HEALTHY FATS** Swapping in healthy fats for a few hundred calories' worth of carbs may help you drop pounds, according to University of Alabama research. That's because refined carbs cause your blood sugar to shoot up and then crash, leading to hunger and overeating. Healthy fats, on the other hand, keep you satisfied for hours, since they take much longer to digest. Start with this easy swap: Spread butter instead of sugary jelly on your toast. Adding a pat of butter to a slice of whole-wheat bread will help your blood sugar rise steadily in response to the carbs, instead of all at once.

■ **BEFRIEND FLAXSEED** Flaxseed is rich in omega-3 fatty acids and fiber—an ideal combination for boosting fullness. In a 2008 study in the journal *Appetite*, scientists found that a diet rich in omega-3s helps promote satiety in diet-

ers, while other research suggests that the good guys help fight abdominal fat. Add a tablespoon of flaxseed to your protein shake, yogurt, soup, salad, or oatmeal.

BONUS BENEFIT!

The fatty acids in flaxseed help your skin stay hydrated, according to recent German research.

■ **BLAST FAT WITH SOUP** Chowder has a bad reputation, thanks to its high calorie and fat toll. However, if you limit yourself to a small bowl, you can make the fatty soup work to your weight-loss advantage. In a University of Texas study, people who consumed fatty soups before eating pizza consumed 227 fewer calories overall. The reason: When your small intestine absorbs fat, it releases fullness hormones, says study author Jiande Chen, PhD. Plus, eating soup forces you to slow down, so you avoid scarfing 1,000 calories in a 10-minute span. To rev up your fullness factor, eat a 100-calorie serving of bisque, chowder, or cream soup, then wait 20 to 30 minutes before eating your main course.

■ **CUT REFINED CARBS** Refined carbs and unhealthy fats are partners in crime: If you find one in a food, you'll often face the other. That means cutting useless carbs—white bread, pasta, and sweets—from your diet can also help you eliminate scary saturated and trans fats. Start by eliminating processed foods wherever possible, and replace them with whole grains, fruit, and vegetables.

Fiber

18 tips for harnessing its weight-loss power

When you're trying to lose weight, cutting calories and carbs is most likely your top priority. But you should also focus on consuming more fiber. "Fiber is the best food you can eat when you're trying to lose weight," says Gay Riley, RD, a nutritionist based in Dallas. The rough stuff is a type of carbohydrate, yes, but it's different from those that low-carb dieters avoid or that make bagels your enemy. In fact, fiber can actually help lower your overall carb intake. Case in point: If you're noshing on cereal with 44 grams of carbs per serving, but 10 of those come from dietary fiber, your body will only absorb the 34 grams of nonfiber carbs.

There are two basic types of fiber. First is insoluble fiber—the kind you'll find in wheat bran, nuts, and many vegetables. It's usually found on the outside and skins of foods, giving them a chewy, tough texture. Since insoluble fiber doesn't dissolve in water, it contributes zero calories and speeds through your digestive system, giving fiber its bowel-stirring reputation. On its way out, it may bind to other foods, helping hustle calories out of your body. "With a very high-fiber diet, say 60 grams a day, you might lose as much as

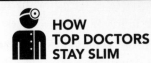

HOW TOP DOCTORS STAY SLIM

"My go-to snack is blueberries mixed into plain Greek yogurt, topped with homemade granola. Yes, it's filling and energizing, but eating something natural also helps bring inner calm."

—**WILLIAM POLLACK, PhD,** an associate clinical professor in the psychiatry department at Harvard Medical School

20 percent of the calories you consume," says Wanda Howell, PhD, a professor of nutritional sciences at the University of Arizona. A study in the *Journal of Nutrition* found that a high-fiber diet leaves roughly twice as many calories undigested as a low-fiber diet does, while USDA research revealed that people who consume 24 grams of fiber per day earn a 90-calorie free pass. And fewer calories means less flab.

The second type is soluble fiber, which tends to hide inside foods. It's found, for example, in the flesh of apples and inside a grain of rice. Soluble fiber dissolves in water, forming a gummy gel in your GI tract. This slows the rate at which food exits your stomach (so you feel full and satisfied longer) and puts the brakes on the absorption of sugar and carbs into your bloodstream (so you feel energized without a crash). As a result, it doesn't raise your blood sugar like starch or sugar do. Unlike insoluble fiber, a gram of soluble fiber contributes about 4 calories.

Why does all of this matter? Simple: People who add fiber to their diets lose more weight than those who don't. In a Brigham Young University study, women who ate an additional 8 grams of fiber for every 1,000 calories they consumed lost nearly 4½ pounds. The reverse is also true: Taking in less than 25 grams a day raises your risk of being overweight by up to 80 percent, according to a study in the *Journal of the American Dietetic Association*. Not only does fiber keep you fuller longer, it also requires more chewing

THE WORLD'S BEST SOURCES OF FIBER*

Pearled barley = 31 grams of fiber

Navy beans = 26 g

Lentils = 16 g

Split peas = 16 g

Black beans = 15 g

Pinto beans = 15 g

Artichokes (cooked) = 14 g

Dates = 14 g

Kidney beans = 13 g

Lima beans = 13 g

White beans = 13 g

Chickpeas = 12.5 g

Great northern beans = 12 g

*Nutrition info is per cup.

than fiber-free foods, notes Joanne Slavin, PhD, RD, a professor of nutrition at the University of Minnesota. And the more you chew, the fuller you feel, the less food you eat, and the more calories you burn!

The only bad thing about fiber is that we don't eat enough of it. According to Institute of Medicine recommendations, the average man should eat 38 grams of fiber per day, and the average woman 25 grams. Unfortunately, most of us take in a measly 15 grams. Ready to fill your fiber void? Get your fix from a mix of whole grains, vegetables, fruit, and nuts, since different types of fiber have different benefits. Caution: Up your intake gradually, as a drastic increase can leave you bloated and gassy.

■ **EAT FIBER AT EVERY MEAL** To keep hunger pangs from derailing your day, work fiber-rich foods into every meal. "Fiber is the secret to losing weight without hunger," says Tanya Zuckerbrot, RD, author of *The F-Factor Diet*. That's because the nutrient slows down digestion, so you'll fell fuller longer. Shoot for at least 5 grams of fiber per meal.

■ **BOOST YOUR BEAN COUNT** Beans are cheaper than almost any supermarket staple— and they're filled with weight-loss friendly fiber, says certified nutrition specialist and weight-loss coach Jonny Bowden, PhD. In fact, research shows that bean eaters have smaller waists and a 22 percent lower risk of obesity than folks who don't eat the legumes. (For a bean breakdown, see "The World's Best Sources of Fiber.") Don't confine your beans to chili: Add them to a salad, toss them with whole-grain pasta, make them a base for soup, or eat them as a meat substitute.

■ **CHOOSE THE RIGHT CEREAL** Fiber is the building block of a healthy cereal—it's what helps keep you full throughout the morning, and it is also a mark of whole-grain cereal. So before you toss that box into your cart, check the label to make sure it contains at least 3, but ideally 10, grams of fiber per serving. This will help balance out the effect of any sugar it may contain (although no amount of fiber justifies more than 8 grams of sugars per serving), while boosting the satiety of your morning meal. Shredded wheat cereals are usually a good start, or if you prefer something

hot, make it oat bran or steel-cut oatmeal, which contains beta-glucan. This type of fiber can dampen your appetite for up to 4 hours. On the go? Throw a packet of instant oatmeal into your bag.

■ **EMBELLISH YOUR EGGS** A plain omelet is an excellent source of protein. But why stop there? Fold in diced veggies, such as peppers, broccoli, or onions, for a hit of much-needed fiber with your breakfast. If you're short on time in the a.m., do your prep work ahead of time: Chop up enough veggies for a week and store them in a container in your refrigerator.

■ **LOAD UP ON WHOLE GRAINS** Refined carbohydrates—those that have been stripped of their fiber—spike your blood sugar and awaken your appetite. But whole grains, which still have their natural fiber intact, are extremely satiating and fight off hunger pangs. They can also blast fat: In a Penn State study, dieters who opted for whole grains shed two times as much belly fat as those who stuck with refined carbs. The study authors say the extra fiber found in whole grains helps you cut calories and keeps your blood sugar steady.

Unfortunately, not many of use are making the whole-grain grade: A 2010 Louisiana State University study reported that less than 5 percent of adults consume three or more servings of fiber-filled grains per day. Make the switch: Choose 100 percent whole-grain bread, pasta, even frozen waffles (they make them!) over their refined-carb alternatives. And remember, unless "whole-grain flour" or "whole-wheat flour" is the first and only flour on the ingredient list, it isn't 100 percent whole grain. A sign of a true whole-grain food: at least 3 grams of fiber per serving.

■ **EAT JUICY FRUITS** Foods that contain both fiber and water are superfilling and usually low in calories. This makes them a key weight-loss weapon. A medium-size grapefruit, for example, boasts 3 grams of the rough stuff, plus 320 grams of water (nearly 11 ounces). This makes the fruit extremely satisfying—and may explain why it can help you lose weight, according to a study in the *Journal of Medicinal Food.* Just make sure to eat the thin skin between grapefruit segments, where most of the fiber is found. Grapefruit isn't the only food with the water/fiber combo. You'll also find it in oatmeal, brown rice, tomatoes, raw veggies, and broth-based soups.

■ **SNACK ON FIBER** You should, of course, work fiber into every meal. But have you considered adding it to your snacks? As one of the most satisfying nutrients, fiber will stave off any hunger pangs between major meals, helping you avoid a binge once you do sit down for lunch or dinner. This is especially important if you're eating a late dinner or going out for drinks—fiber wards off hunger and helps absorb alcohol. In between meals, pick up a fresh piece of fruit or half of a Thomas' 100% Whole Wheat Mini Bagel. Pair it with a little protein, such as a tablespoon of peanut butter or a string cheese.

■ **START WITH SALAD** Unlike the complimentary bread at restaurants, your predinner salad isn't a waste of stomach space. In a Penn State study, people who ate a 100-calorie salad as an appetizer consumed 12 percent fewer calories during the meal—without even trying to control their intake. The reason: Leafy greens are full of fiber, which helps stamp out appetite.

■ **EAT WHOLE FRUIT** Drinking a glass of orange juice is not the same as eating an orange. Consider the nutritional stack-up: A cup of OJ contains 122 calories, 21 grams of sugars, and less than 1 gram of fiber, while a medium orange has 62 calories, 12 grams of sugars, and 3 grams of fiber. Fiber helps slow the absorption of sugar into your body, thus blunting a dangerous spike in blood sugar. This makes whole fruit a smarter choice than any juice on the shelf, even if it's 100 percent juice. Prioritize fruits that are high in pectin, a type of soluble fiber known to promote weight loss. Apples, apricots, grapefruit, and citrus fruits are all good sources of the stuff.

■ **DRINK LOTS OF WATER** When you increase your fiber consumption, you need to drink more water to avoid digestive problems. Aim to drink at least one glass with every meal or snack. If you still experience discomfort, consider taking Gas-X or a supplement like Beano, which contains enzymes that help your body break down complex carbohydrates.

■ **ADD AVOCADO TO YOUR DIET** Avocado is perhaps best known for its heart-healthy monounsaturated fats. But it's also an incredible source of fiber. Half an avocado contains nearly 7 grams! Guacamole isn't the only way to fold the green fruit into your diet. You can also add avocado slices to a sandwich, chop it up in homemade salsa (add corn, another great source of fiber), or toss it into your salad.

■ **LOAD UP ON VEGETABLES** Focusing on veggies may be the ultimate diet cliché—but it works. In a study of 2,000 low-carb dieters, those who ate four servings of nonstarchy vegetables per day lost the most weight. That includes virtually any vegetable of your choice, other than potatoes and corn. One explanation: Eating more produce increases the amount of fiber in your diet, which helps keep you full.

IS ADDED FIBER AS GOOD AS THE REAL STUFF?

Foods that contain "added fiber," such as Fiber One bars and Kashi GoLean, often contain inulin, a type of fiber produced from chicory root (it may also be called chicory root fiber). Although it's not bad for you, it can aggravate your stomach, resulting in bloating and discomfort, and it lacks the cholesterol-lowering effect of natural fiber. Another fake fiber is polydextrose, made from glucose, sorbitol (a sugar alcohol), and citric acid. According to the FDA, it can be called fiber, since it isn't absorbed in the small intestine and increases stool weight. However, there's no research proving that it's as beneficial as the real stuff. Your best bet? Fill up on whole foods, such as fruits, veggies, whole grains, nuts, and legumes, rather than relying on added-fiber foods.

■ **GO NUTTY** Although nuts are usually praised for their protein, they're also an excellent source of fiber. Almonds, pistachios, and pecans all contain 3 grams of fiber per ounce—as much as an entire grapefruit! Take the edge off your appetite by eating a handful (¼ cup) per day. According to Loma Linda University research, the trio of nutrients—fiber, protein, and healthy fats—in nuts makes them especially filling.

■ **REPLACE RICE WITH QUINOA** White rice is nothing more than a sticky glob of refined carbs. Instead, eat quinoa, a South American grain with more fiber and fewer carbs than most other whole grains (including brown rice). You can find it in the rice aisle or the health food section of most supermarkets. To prepare your quinoa, rinse it well, add a serving to boiling water, turn the heat down to low, and cook until tender, about 20 minutes. Drain the water and allow the quinoa to cool. You can also cook it in bulk, then store it in an airtight container in your refrigerator to eat throughout the week. Try this tasty combination: Toss quinoa with roasted peppers, cubed mozzarella, and chopped basil. Quinoa also makes a great alternative to oatmeal or can even be used to make a creamier version of rice pudding.

■ **SWAP IN POPCORN** Craving something salty? Grab a bowl of popcorn instead of potato chips. You'll enjoy the salt and crunch of chips while adding a significant dose of fiber to your snack. Choose either oil-free microwave popcorn or a variety popped in good-for-you oil, such as olive or canola. You can also opt for plain, lightly salted popcorn, such as Orville Redenbacher's Natural Simply Salted.

■ **DRINK YOUR ROUGHAGE** If you struggle to work enough fiber into your day, add a fiber supplement to your morning coffee. It's not as gross as it sounds: Fibersure, a supplement from the makers of Metamucil, dissolves flavorlessly into your drink, contributing 5 grams of fiber per teaspoon. You can also stir it into a smoothie or add it to a glass of milk.

■ **ADD FIBER TO DESSERT** It's your cheat day. So what do you do? Grab a piece of chocolate cake, naturally. But before you dive in, sprinkle it with a few fresh raspberries, blackberries, or strawberries. Berries are among the most fiber-rich fruits—raspberries lead the pack with 8 grams per cup—which means they can help control the blood sugar spike you would normally experience when downing a dessert. Better yet, fill a bowl with a cup of berries and top them with low-fat yogurt and toasted wheat germ, a great source of fiber. You may find you don't need that cake after all.

GO FOR THE GARBANZO BONANZA You probably think of fruit first when you think of fiber. But garbanzo beans (aka "chickpeas")—the legume that hummus is made from—are also an excellent source of roughage. (Half a cup of chickpeas contains 17 grams of fiber!) Whip up your own homemade hummus, or for fiber on the fly, toss some canned garbanzo beans into a Mediterranean-inspired salad, soup, or stir-fry.

Fish

6 ways to shed fat with seafood

If the only fish you eat is the Swedish kind that causes cavities, you're missing out on one of nature's most nutritious foods. Fish is packed with "complete" protein, meaning it contains all of the essential amino acids, which your body can't produce on its own. It's also one of the richest sources of omega-3 fatty acids, a healthy polyunsaturated fat linked to improved heart health and lower levels of abdominal fat. This nutritional duo forces your body to take its time when digesting fish, making it an extremely satisfying food. In fact, one study found that fish is more satisfying, per calorie, than lean chicken or beef! Follow these rules to make the most of your fresh catch:

■ **EAT THE FATTY KIND** Fatty fish (also known as oily fish) may sound like the last thing a diet-conscious person should eat, but they're actually an important weight-loss tool. That's because the fat content of salmon, tuna, trout, herring, sardines, anchovies, and mackerel is primarily omega-3 fatty acids. These heart-healthy fats not only help you absorb essential vitamins like D and E, but they also promote the rapid transfer of "I'm full" signals to

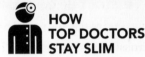

HOW TOP DOCTORS STAY SLIM

"I eat fish that are rich in omega-3 fatty acids, like salmon and trout, three times a week. I also exercise 4 days a week for 30 minutes each session. I either do intense intervals on my elliptical trainer or walk up 103 steps two or three times a day at work."

—PREDIMAN KRISHAN SHAH, MD, director of the cardiology division at Cedars-Sinai Hospital in Los Angeles your brain, according to the National Institutes of Health. Plus, compared to lean fish, fatty varieties contain up to four times more vitamin D, which partners with omega-3s to promote weight loss. Make a point to eat fatty fish at least three times per week.

■ **STOCK UP ON SALMON** If you add just one type of fish to your diet, make it wild Alaskan salmon. The pink fish blows other fish out of the water: It's higher in omega-3s than almost any other seafood. Plus, it is low in contaminants and is an environmentally friendly option, according to the Environmental Defense Fund. Avoid farmed salmon, which may contain contaminates from polluted water and offers just 25 percent as much vitamin D as its wild cousins. Other smart, omega-3-packed seafood picks: farmed mussels and wild sardines.

■ **DRESS FISH WITH SALSA** The fastest way to ruin fish: Smother it with tartar sauce. The classic seafood sauce is made primarily with fatty mayo, making it a gut bomb waiting to happen. For an instant flavor boost, top your grilled fish with fresh salsa instead—it's an excellent, low-calorie source of antioxidants and an easy way to work more produce into your diet. Whip up this simple corn salsa: Toss together fresh corn kernels; finely chopped jalapeño chile pepper; chopped fresh cilantro, tomato, and onion; and a pinch of chili powder.

■ **COAT WITH CARE** If you love the satisfying crunch of breaded fish, swap your usual bread crumbs with flaxseed or even crushed nuts. Bread crumbs are loaded with nothing more than empty carbs, but flaxseed and nuts contribute a shot of belly-blasting omega-3s and protein. Just make sure not to go overboard, since both are high in calories (albeit good-for-you calories). Limit yourself to a 2-tablespoon serving.

■ **OBSERVE PROPER SERVING SIZES** Portion control is an important part of your new lifestyle, even if you're eating the healthiest of foods. So skip the paddle-size fillet and bake or broil a piece of fish that's about the size of a checkbook. You'll consume about 3 ounces, or one serving.

■ **CHOOSE CANNED SEAFOOD CAREFULLY** Canned fish is an easy, healthy way to add more seafood to your diet—as long as you

CAN I TAKE A FISH OIL SUPPLEMENT INSTEAD OF EATING FISH?

Fish oil supplements are the perfect way to protect your heart and brain, especially if you hate eating seafood. In fact, a recent review in the *American Journal of Clinical Nutrition* found that increased consumption of omega-3s, even from a supplement, may reduce your risk of a cardiac catastrophe. However, don't expect to enjoy the weight-loss benefits of the real deal. In a recent trial, Texas researchers found that fish oil supplements don't significantly speed fat loss. You're missing out on seafood's protein and vitamin D—two weight-loss nutrients—when you pop a pill. If it's cardio protection you're after, look for a fish oil supplement that delivers about 500 milligrams each of EPA and DHA, such as those by Nordic Naturals and Coromega.

crack open the right can. Start by limiting your search to fish canned in water rather than oil. This will ensure that the calories you're consuming are from actual fish and not an unnecessary coating of fat. To cut down your mercury intake, choose canned light tuna (as long as it doesn't contain yellowfin tuna) instead of canned albacore or, even better, opt for canned salmon, which has significantly less mercury than tuna. (As a general rule, the larger the fish, the higher its mercury content.) Try Bumble Bee Wild Alaska Pink Salmon.

TAKE THE BAIT: AN EAT-MORE-FISH PRIMER

People will eat more fish if they know how to cook it, says Kate Geagan, MS, RD, author of *Go Green Get Lean*. Here's how to incorporate more low-mercury, nutrient-rich fish into your diet.

Salmon

This pink-fleshed fish is perhaps most famous for its high level of omega-3s, but it's also an amazing source of vitamin D. Opt for wild species, such as Alaskan king. "Its varied diet makes it more flavorful than farmed varieties," says Geagan.

Flavor: Mildly to moderately rich

Best with: Light flavors such as citrus or soy to balance its strong flavor. It pairs nicely with slightly acidic greens like bok choy or spinach, which offset its richness.

Try it: Broiled with lemon vinaigrette; poached in a salad with dill yogurt dressing; grilled with a maple-soy-orange sauce

Barramundi

If you like cod, halibut, or sea bass, you'll love this Australian whitefish, which is loaded with omega-3s. Barramundi is low in calories and mercury—in fact, some U.S. farmed varieties have no detectable amounts of the metal.

Flavor: Delicate and slightly buttery

Best with: Bold Latin spices, mild Asian lemongrass-soy flavors, Mediterranean tomatoes and capers

Try it: On the grill. Since it's high in fat, it won't dry out under direct heat. Skewer 1-inch pieces of barramundi, red peppers, and scallions, and serve the grilled kebabs over sweet-potato puree. Or try it in fish tacos.

Sardines

"Sardines are health food in a can," says Geagan. Since sardines consume a mostly vegetarian diet of plankton, their mercury content is low, and like most oily fish, they're chock full of omega-3s.

Flavor: Salty and slightly mineral tasting

Best with: Equally bold flavors, such as olives, capers, Parmesan, and sherry vinegar

Try them: Grilled with lemon and olive oil, for about 2 minutes per side (use fresh sardines); on top of whole-grain pasta or salad

Fruit

9 ways to work more into your weight-loss plan

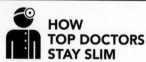
Although popular low-carb diets advise eliminating fruit because of the sugar content, there are smart reasons to make fruit a part of your plan. It contains the natural sugar fructose, but it doesn't raise your blood sugar like table sugar does, thanks to its punch of fiber. Plus, fruit is high in water and low in calories, provides carbs to fuel your muscles, and will satisfy your sweet cravings. Sounds like the perfect diet food, right? Science agrees: A review of 16 studies in the journal *Obesity Reviews* concluded that eating fruit is associated with weighing less. And in a recent Brazilian study, women who added three small apples to their normal meals and snacks lost 2 pounds in 10 weeks—without dieting. Another study found that eating fruit before a meal can reduce your overall calorie intake by 15 percent.

Aim to eat at least two daily servings of fruit—the amount most normal-weight people eat, according to research from the University of California at Los Angeles. Overweight folks eat an average of one serving per day. Here's how to work in more of nature's most colorful food group:

■ **ADD FROZEN FRUIT TO YOUR SMOOTHIE** Scooping ice cream into your smoothie isn't the only mistake you can make. Using a juice base or a fruit syrup adds unnecessary calories and sugars to your liquid concoction. So build your smoothie around low-fat Greek yogurt and frozen fruit. The fruit will chill your smoothie while also adding bulk and texture. And don't worry—you're not missing out on nutrients by choosing frozen varieties. Since the fruit is frozen just hours after harvest, it may actually retain more of its nutrients than fresh produce! Make sure to select the varieties that contain no added sugars.

■ **GO FRESH** Think of it this way: You can eat 20 raisins or 20 grapes. Which sounds more filling? Fresh fruit's water content is high, which means it's more satisfying and less concentrated with sugar than dried varieties. Stock your fridge with fresh fruit, and carry a piece with you at all times in case you need a snack. If only chewy fruit will do, munch on Stretch Island Fruit Co. Original Fruit Strips, which are less sugar filled than regular dried fruit.

■ **PAIR FRUIT WITH PROTEIN** The perfect midafternoon snack is one that is filling but not too high in calories. Your go-to

THE PERFECT FRUIT SALAD

The more colorful your fruit salad, the more healthy it is. That's because the pigments in fruits often confer valuable body benefits. Red fruits are generally loaded with lycopene, a red-colored antioxidant that may help protect your skin from the sun's UV rays, decrease prostate cancer risk, and reduce the threat of heart disease. Blue and purple fruits are colored by anthocyanins, shown to boost your brain and improve heart health. Green fruits get their hue from chlorophyll, thought to hinder bacterial growth, while yellow and orange fruits are loaded with vision-protecting, immune-boosting beta-carotene. Choose at least one fruit from each of the following categories, and cut them into similar-size pieces.

Red
Watermelon, persimmon, guava, pink or ruby red grapefruit

Blue
Blackberries, blueberries, plums, grapes

Green
Grapes, kiwifruit, honeydew melon, Granny Smith apples

Yellow/orange
Cantaloupe, pineapple, peaches, apricots, oranges, bananas

HOW SUGARY IS YOUR FRUIT?

MOST SUGARY

Pomegranate (4") = 53 g carbs; 39 g sugars

Mango (1 cup, pieces) = 25 g carbs; 23 g sugars

Sweet cherries (1 cup, with pits) = 25 g carbs; 20 g sugars

Apple (medium) = 25 g carbs; 19 g sugars

Pear (medium) = 28 g carbs; 17 g sugars

Pineapple (1 cup, chunks) = 22 g carbs; 16 g sugars

Blueberries (1 cup) = 21 g carbs; 15 g sugars

Grapes (1 cup) = 16 g carbs; 15 g sugars

Banana (medium) = 27 g carbs; 14 g sugars

Honeydew melon (1 cup, diced) = 15 g carbs; 14 g sugars

Sour red cherries (1 cup, with pits) = 19 g carbs; 13 g sugars

Peach (medium) = 14 g carbs; 13 g sugars

Papaya (small) = 17 g carbs; 12 g sugars

Orange (medium) = 15 g carbs; 12 g sugars

Cantaloupe (1 cup, diced) = 13 g carbs; 12 g sugars

Nectarine (medium) = 15 g carbs; 11 g sugars

Tangerine (medium) = 12 g carbs; 9 g sugars

Watermelon (1 cup, diced) = 11 g carbs; 9 g sugars

Grapefruit (medium) = 10 g carbs; 9 g sugars

Strawberries (1 cup, sliced) = 13 g carbs; 8 g sugars

Blackberries (1 cup) = 14 g carbs; 7 g sugars

Plum (2⅛") = 7.5 g carbs; 6.5 g sugars

Kiwifruit (green) = 10 g carbs; 6 g sugars

Raspberries (1 cup) = 15 g carbs; 5 g sugars

Tomato (medium) = 5 g carbs; 3 g sugars

Apricot = 4 g carbs; 3 g sugars

Lime (medium) = 7 g carbs; 1 g sugars

Lemon (medium) = 5 g carbs; 1 g sugars

LEAST SUGARY

combination: a piece of fruit, which offers lots of fiber, plus a source of protein, such as a tablespoon of nut butter, string cheese, or low-fat Greek yogurt. Fiber and protein are perhaps the most satiating of nutrients, so you won't face a growling tummy between meals. If you're a regular exerciser (which we hope you are), make sure apples have a place in your diet. They're exceptionally high in antioxidants, which can help offset the damage caused by free radicals that are produced during daily exercise.

■ **CUT OUT THE JUICE** It'd seem that all juice is good for you since it comes from fruit. Unfortunately, that's not the case. Most juices contain not only the natural sugar from the fruit but also outrageous amounts of added sugars to keep them from tasting tart. The result is something more akin to sugar water than juice. Even 100 percent juices aren't as good as whole fruit—most lack the fiber to counterbalance the natural sugars, plus they're more caloric. Eat whole fruit with the skin (when possible) instead of drinking juice. In a study in the *International Journal of Obesity*, people who simply substituted whole fruit for fruit juice reduced their lunchtime calorie intake by 20 percent! If you really want your fruit in liquid form, sip on no more than 2 or 3 ounces of 100 percent juice per sitting. Try diluting it with water to make it last longer.

■ **EAT A GRAPEFRUIT A DAY** There's a reason the grapefruit diet was hugely popular.

The citrus fruit is full of water and fiber, and its acidity can help slow your rate of digestion. Both qualities help you feel fuller longer. Grapefruit may also lower your postmeal levels of insulin, a hormone that triggers fat storage, says Ken Fujioka, MD, an internal medicine practitioner at Scripps Clinic Center for Weight Management who has extensively studied the fruit. In his 2006 study in a *Journal of Medicinal Food*, folks who ate half of a grapefruit before each meal lost 3.6 pounds in 12 weeks, compared to less than a pound among nongrapefruit eaters. Kick off every meal with a half of a ruby red grapefruit, making sure to eat the thin, fiber-rich skin between segments. You can also transform the fruit into a delicious, low-calorie dessert: Drizzle it with honey, sprinkle it with cardamom, and broil for 2 to 3 minutes.

BONUS BENEFIT!

In the same *Journal of Medicinal Food* study, the people who ate grapefruit before each meal lowered their blood pressure by 6 points, thus reducing their stroke risk by 40 percent!

■ **COOK YOUR TOMATOES** Believe it or not, tomatoes are a fruit, not a vegetable. And unlike most produce, their nutritional power only multiplies when they're cooked. That's because lycopene—a disease-fighting antioxidant that gives tomatoes their red color—is activated when heated. So sauté or roast the red fruit, or puree cooked tomatoes to make a delicious, low-calorie soup.

■ **EAT THE RAINBOW** You love apples, but have you tried plums? Or maybe you eat an orange a day, but have you considered tangerines? And why stop at a lemon with your water? Why not try a lime, too? By broadening the range of fruits in your diets, you'll also expand your spectrum of vitamins and antioxidants. Plus, research shows that when presented with a variety of foods, people tend to eat more. This is one case where that's a good thing, since most people don't meet the daily recommended intake of fruit. Color your plate with a fresh fruit salad rather than limiting yourself to the same fruits day after day. See "The Perfect Fruit Salad" on page 173 for an easy recipe.

■ **BUY A FRUIT BOWL** You eat what you see, especially when you're famished. That means if you store your fruit in a tabletop bowl, you'll be more inclined to snack on it when hunger strikes. Try keeping a bowl on your desk at work, too.

■ **CONTROL YOUR CARBS** Not all fruits are created equal. Sure, bananas and pears are good for you, but they offer relatively few nutrients for the carbs they contain. You don't have to eliminate them from your diet entirely, but when given the choice, opt for lower-carb, high-fiber picks, such as blackberries, raspberries, and papaya.

SHOP BY THE SEASON

The supermarket is consistently stocked with every fruit you could imagine. But just because a fruit is available doesn't mean you should buy it. If you purchase produce that's in season, you'll not only save money—you'll take home the most nutrient-dense fruit on the shelf. It's a win-win.

Apples: September to May

Apricots: June to July

Bananas: Year-round

Blueberries: June to August

Cantaloupe: May to September

Cherries: May to June

Figs: July to September

Grapefruit: October to June

Grapes: June to December

Honeydew melons: February to October

Kiwifruit: June to August

Lemons: Year-round

Limes: May to October

Mangoes: April to August

Nectarines: June to September

Oranges: November to June

Papayas: Year-round

Peaches: June to September

Pears: August to February

Pineapple: March to July

Plums: June to September

Raspberries: May to November

Strawberries: June to August

Watermelons: May to August

Glycemic Index

How to use it to eat smarter

The glycemic index (GI) ranks foods by how they affect your blood sugar levels. The theory goes like this: The higher a food's GI score, the more it elevates your blood sugar; this glucose overload triggers a spike-crash cycle, ultimately causing you to eat more carbs and signaling your body to release more insulin. That rush of insulin causes you to store more fat. Low–glycemic index foods (less than 55) trigger a more gradual rise in blood sugar that is healthier for the body.

The idea is interesting, but the science is flawed, since GI studies are most often conducted in unrealistic conditions. To test a food's GI, researchers have people fast overnight, then give them a portion of the food that contains 50 grams of digestible carbohydrates, which includes starch and glucose, but not fiber. Although this may be similar to a real-world portion for junk foods, which are often high in starch and sugar, the test portion is grossly inflated for healthier foods, like fruit or vegetables.

For example, to hit the 50-gram mark, you'd have to eat only about a cup and a half of chocolate ice cream, compared to nearly two 9-inch-long parsnips. This is why, according to the glycemic index, chocolate ice cream is preferable to a parsnip. Or pound cake is better than watermelon. A heaping pile of parsnips or

HOW TOP DOCTORS STAY SLIM

"My favorite vegetable stew: a 15-ounce can of unsalted stewed tomatoes and a pound of frozen vegetables. I combine them with whole-grain rice and pasta."

—ALLEN LEVINE, PhD, dean of the College of Food, Agricultural, and Natural Resource Sciences at the University of Minnesota watermelon *will* significantly spike your blood sugar. But a single, real-world serving of either will have less of a blood sugar impact on your body than a bowl of ice cream or a slice of pound cake. Forget the glycemic index and follow these rules instead:

■ **PRIORITIZE WHOLE FOODS** A food's glycemic index rating doesn't necessarily indicate whether it's a good or bad choice. A better way to classify foods: whole or processed. Whole foods—fruits, vegetables, low-fat dairy, lean meats, and whole grains—are always superior

8 "HEALTH FOODS" THAT SPIKE BLOOD SUGAR

Fruit-on-the-bottom yogurt

Individually, fruit and yogurt should have a prominent place in your fridge. But when combined by food manufacturers, they're a deadly duo. Fruit-on-the-bottom yogurt is more corn syrup and sugar than actual fruit—for example, 96 percent of the carbs in Dannon's fruit-on-the-bottom yogurt are sugars! A healthier option: stirring real fruit into low-fat plain Greek yogurt.

Baked beans

Research shows that bean eaters have smaller waists than those who forego the legumes. However, any weight-loss benefit is negated once you top 'em with the sugary sauce found in most baked beans. Since the fiber and protein is *inside* the bean, it's unable to slow the speed at which the sugar-packed glaze is absorbed into your bloodstream. Trade baked beans for red kidney beans (drained and rinsed). Try tossing them in hot sauce, which can boost your metabolism.

California roll

This sushi crime is essentially a Japanese sugar cube. It consists of white rice and imitation crab—both of which are loaded with simple, fast-burning carbohydrates. Stick to authentic sushi made with tuna or salmon, which are packed with protein, or better yet, switch from rolls to sashimi, a rice-free option.

Granola bars

Don't let the oats distract you. Granola bars are glued together with a glut of sugar, high-fructose corn syrup, and other blood sugar–spiking ingredients. Look for a protein bar that contains no more than 5 grams of digestible carbs and at least 15 grams of protein.

to processed foods. Whole foods are any item that has one ingredient: the food itself.

■ **FOCUS ON DIGESTIBLE CARBS** If you're concerned about a food's impact on your blood sugar, all you need to know is the amount of digestible carbs (starch and sugar) that it con-tains. The higher this number, the higher your blood sugar will rise. To determine the digestible carb content, simply subtract the fiber content from the total carbohydrate content. Generally speaking, any amount over 40 grams will send your blood sugar through

English muffins

Sure, classic English muffins save you calories over the majority of sandwich breads. But these refined-carb rounds offer little fiber or protein to deter a postmeal rise in blood sugar. Switch to 100 percent whole-grain English muffins.

Fat-free salad dressing

The sad truth about fat-free foods: They often remove healthy fats and replace them with unhealthy sugars. Not only do you tack on empty calories, but you reduce your ability to absorb fat-soluble vitamins. An Ohio State University study found that people who ate a salad topped with fat-containing dressing absorbed 15 times more beta-carotene than those who munched on greens dressed in fat-free stuff. Ditch the "diet" junk in favor of an olive- or canola-oil-based salad dressing. Choose one with less than 2 grams of carbs per serving.

Reduced-fat peanut butter

This is yet another case of good fats being replaced by cheap carbs. Peter Pan's Reduced Fat Peanut Butter, for example, has 33 percent more sugar per serving than the full-fat version. Stick to full-fat, natural peanut butter that has no added sugars. (For a peanut butter buying guide, see page 159.)

Pretzels

Dieters have been deceived by these empty-carb snacks for years. They're low in fat and calories, yes, but they also have zero nutritional value. With little or no accompanying fiber, their fast-burning carbs will send your blood sugar soaring. If you're craving a salty snack, munch on popcorn, which is rich in fiber and counts as a whole grain.

the roof. Hint: Whole grains contain fewer digestible carbs than refined!

■ **HIT THE GYM** The glycemic index of a food can vary according to your recent workout habits (yet another flaw with the system). After you exercise, your body shuttles glucose out of your bloodstream at a rapid rate to replenish carb stores you burned during your workout. In fact, in a recent Syracuse University study, people who lifted weights experienced a reduced blood sugar response to sugary drinks for the next 12 hours. Incorporate resistance training into your workout three times per week. Since muscle stores glucose, the more lean muscle you have, the more sugar your body will remove from your bloodstream.

■ **PAIR CARBS WITH FAT** You can avoid a blood sugar surge by pairing carbs with fat, which slows the absorption of sugar into your bloodstream. In a recent Finnish study, researchers found that adding fat to mashed potatoes reduced people's blood sugar response to the starchy vegetable. So go ahead, smear a pat of butter on your whole-wheat toast, or stir some nuts into your cereal. This will ensure that your blood sugar rises steadily, rather than suddenly, after your meal. A word of caution: This is not a license to overindulge in butter, cheese, and sour cream. You should still control your portion sizes, since controlling overall calories also plays a large role in weight loss.

■ **PUMP UP THE PROTEIN AND FIBER** The same Finnish study found that adding a high-protein food, such as chicken breast, to mashed potatoes significantly reduced people's blood sugar response to the starchy meal. That means spreading peanut butter on bread or adding lean meat to pasta will slow your body's absorption of the carbs. Another sugar-stopping nutrient: fiber. Try to incorporate a shot of roughage at every meal, whether in the form of fresh veggies, fruit, or whole grains, to help blunt your blood sugar response.

High-Fructose Corn Syrup

4 ways to banish HFCS from your diet

More than half of Americans say they're concerned with the high-fructose corn syrup (HFCS) content of foods, a 2011 Harris Poll reports. That makes us sound like a health-conscious bunch, but there's one problem: The average American is still consuming 36 pounds of the sweetener every year. See, HFCS is sneaky. It makes its way into lunchmeats and hot dogs (to keep ingredients evenly dispersed), salad dressings and condiments (to make them viscous), bakery products (to make them look browned), and ice cream (to prevent freezer burn). High-fructose corn syrup is used to enhance texture and color, to mask natural flavors, and to extend shelf life. And here's what food manufacturers love most: It's cheaper than table sugar. That means it's everywhere.

Like table sugar, high-fructose corn syrup contains both glucose and sucrose and in roughly the same proportions. As a result, the two sweeteners are equally caloric, and your body breaks them down in essentially the same way, says Michael Jacobson, PhD,

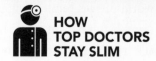

HOW TOP DOCTORS STAY SLIM

"The key to eating well boils down to avoiding life's daily little temptations. To avoid fatty, sugary snacks, I keep a drawer full of foil pouches of tuna for when I get the munchies."

—MARK S. LITWIN, MD, MPH, a professor of health services and urology at the David Geffen School of Medicine at UCLA executive director of the Center for Science in the Public Interest. "There's no evidence that high-fructose corn syrup is worse than sugar once it's in your body," he says.

So how has HCFS earned its evil reputation? For one, it's a relative newcomer to the world of sweeteners. Sugar has been plaguing foods for centuries, but it wasn't until the 1970s that high-fructose corn syrup gained ground as a food additive. This also happens to coincide with the rise in American obesity, which is why researchers have speculated that HFCS is directly related to obesity. The science isn't conclusive, but the message is clear: Consume less of both HFCS and sugar. If you eat any source of empty calories in mass amounts, you *will* pack on the pounds. Plus, since high-fructose corn syrup is sweeter than sugar, you can enhance your cravings for super-sweet foods by eating it. As you can imagine, that will also lead to weight gain.

■ **PRIORITIZE WHOLE FOODS** Foods that have one ingredient—the food itself—won't contain high-fructose corn syrup (or any other additives, for that matter). So focus on whole foods: fruits, veggies, lean meats, and fish.

When you do purchase packaged foods, look for those that list whole-food ingredients, such as whole grain flour, oats, nuts, and real fruit, in the first line of ingredients.

■ **ALWAYS CHECK THE LABEL** Processed products that you don't think of as sweet—pasta sauce, salad dressing, crackers—may still contain high-fructose corn syrup. So before you buy any food that comes in a box, bag, or bottle, check the ingredient list for the sweetener. This is perhaps the simplest way to slash excess calories.

■ **SKIP SOFT DRINKS** High-fructose corn syrup is the primary sweetener in nondiet soda, and it's often lurking in flavored waters, too. If you're craving something fizzy or flavored, mix soda water with a jigger of juice. (Note: Diet soda isn't much better than regular. See page 245.)

■ **WATCH YOUR YOGURT** Research shows that calcium-rich dairy can help you lose weight. The caveat: It can be weighed down with a glut of high-fructose corn syrup. Steer clear of yogurts that are sweetened with the stuff, such as the fruit-on-the-bottom kind. You're much better off with low-fat plain Greek yogurt.

High-Volume Foods

10 belly-filling tactics to help you eat less

When you're famished, you want to eat—and you want to eat a lot. Here's the good news: If you choose the right foods, you can. In fact, you can eat large amounts of food at every meal and still lose weight, as long as you choose low-calorie fare that's full of water and fiber, or "high-volume foods." It's a proven strategy: A study in the *American Journal of Clinical Nutrition* found that dieters who cut back on fat and folded in more water-rich, low-cal foods lost more weight than those who only trimmed the fat. The best part is that the folks who added high-volume foods to their diet consumed 25 percent *more* food (by weight) than those who didn't. And they still shed an extra 5 pounds. "Water-rich foods allow you to eat satisfying portions while still providing few calories," explains study author Julia Ello-Martin, PhD.

■ **SIDLE UP TO THE SALAD BAR** Lettuce and other leafy greens contain virtually no calories and are loaded with nutrients and

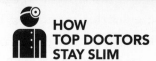

HOW TOP DOCTORS STAY SLIM

"I make an entrée salad with arugula, shredded cabbage, chopped tomatoes, carrots, cucumbers, roasted kale chips, and then topped with a protein source, such as heart-healthy barbecue salmon or leftover veggie stir-fry. For salad dressing, I use the Olive Tap's basil olive oil and their highest quality balsamic vinegar. This is a 'volumetric' type meal— a satisfying meal that's low in calories and high in fiber and disease-fighting phytochemicals."

—**ROBERT KUSHNER, MD,** clinical director of the Northwestern Comprehensive Center on Obesity water. Iceberg lettuce, for example, is 96 percent water, while raw spinach is 91 percent water! That means you can eat a lot, feel full, and shed flab at the same time. The key: Avoid weighing your greens down with salad bar no-no's like shredded Cheddar cheese and croutons. Stick to fresh veggies, fruit, less-dense cheeses (like mozzarella), and a small sprinkling of nuts.

■ **STOCK UP ON FRUIT** What makes fruit so juicy? Water! Fruit is about 80 to 95 percent water, with papayas, watermelon, and tomatoes (yes, they're fruit) leading the water-rich pack, according to USDA data. Try keeping a bowl of fruit on your kitchen counter, or even at your desk, so you grab a piece in a pinch, rather than less-filling convenience snacks like dried fruit. For around the same amount of calories, you can down an entire cup of grapes or a measly 3 tablespoons of raisins.

■ **FILL YOUR CART WITH VEGETABLES** Like fruit, vegetables consist primarily of water and a substantial load of essential vitamins and minerals. Any produce you add to your plate is a positive, but if it's water-rich picks you're after, look no further than cucumbers, cooked butternut squash, and spinach. Boost the volume of a rice or pasta dish by replacing half of it with water-rich vegetables.

■ **SWITCH TO PUFFED CEREALS** Cornflakes and bran flakes are flat and dense. Not exactly filling. But puffed cereal is pumped full of air, and that air fills up your belly without making you feel bloated. Plus, when a food is puffed, it looks bigger, so you'll likely pour—and feel satisfied eating—a smaller portion. Trade your cornflakes or Raisin Bran for puffed, whole grain cereals, such as Kashi 7 Whole Grain Puffs cereal.

■ **NUKE A BOWL OF OATMEAL** Think about it: What do you mix oatmeal with? Water or milk. This combination of moisture and fiber makes oatmeal the perfect high-volume food to add to your breakfast. (For easy ways to pump up the flavor of your oats, see "10 Ways to Upgrade Your Oatmeal" on page 109.)

■ **DRESS UP YOUR POPCORN** Cheese and crackers aren't necessarily a *bad* snack. However, before you start slicing, consider this: Six Cheddar-cracker stacks could easily cost you 330 calories—and snacks should contain 200 calories, max. If you're craving the cheesy/salty combo, switch to popcorn sprinkled lightly with Parmesan cheese. Popcorn is high in volume and low in calories and is loaded with belly-filling fiber. You'll be able to eat more without noticing the effects on your belly.

■ **SLURP BROTH-BASED SOUPS** Soup appears time and again on the USDA's list of the most water-rich foods. Not only is the appetizer built around water, but it's also the perfect vessel for veggies, another high-volume food. To fill up for relatively few calories, look for low-sodium, broth-based soup, such as tomato or vegetable soup. In a study of 150 overweight people, those who ate soup every day for a year dropped 50 percent more weight than those who didn't.

■ **ADD ICE TO YOUR DRINK** This one's a no-brainer. Ice, of course, has zero calories, and it adds serious volume to your drink. Translation: You can enjoy your occasional flavored beverage longer. Plus, research shows that ice-cold drinks may elevate your metabolism, since your body burns calories bringing the chilly beverages up to body temperature.

■ **MAKE THE PERFECT SHAKE** Protein shakes are, of course, based around liquid, so they have a high water content. But you can still enhance the satiety of your shake—without adding any extra calories. Let your blender work a little longer, allowing your smoothie to be whipped into a froth. When Penn State researchers had people drink blended shakes of various volumes, they found that those who drank the more-aerated shakes ate 12 percent less food at their next meal. The frothy appearance of the shakes may have tricked them into thinking they were drinking more, so they felt fuller, the scientists said.

■ **STICK A SPOON IN YOGURT** Studies suggest that the calcium in low-fat dairy can help blast belly fat. To ensure you get the most bang for your caloric buck, choose yogurt over cheese. Yogurt contains more water than cheese, especially the hard, aged varieties. That means yogurt more quickly activates stretch receptors in your stomach, which then fire "full" signals to your brain.

Juice

8 strategies for avoiding juice-induced weight gain

**HOW
TOP DOCTORS
STAY SLIM**

"A few years ago, I would frequently have one or two glasses of wine at night with dinner, at about 120 calories per glass. Not coincidentally, I weighed 10 pounds more than I do now. I never drink soda, but I make sure I kick fruit juice and alcohol, too. Liquid sugar is not satiating, and your brain doesn't register that you've consumed calories the way it would if you actually ate food. Cutting it out is the quickest, easiest fix I know."

—**CAROLINE APOVIAN, MD,** director of the Nutrition and Weight Management Center at Boston Medical Center

Nearly half of Americans rate juice as "healthy" or "very healthy," a recent Harris Interactive poll revealed. They're sadly mistaken. In most cases, juice is to fruit as refined grains are to whole grains—often high in sugar and totally stripped of any redeeming fiber. Since it's so concentrated with calories and sugar, juice is more of a weight-loss enemy than ally. Even 100 percent juice isn't as nutritious as the fruit that it came from, so stick to whole fruit whenever possible. Control your sipping with these smart strategies:

■ **SWITCH YOUR GLASSES** Research shows that we perceive objects that are tall as being larger than short, squat ones. What that means: You're more likely to fill a low, wide juice glass to the brim, but you'll stop halfway when filling a tall glass—even if they hold the same volume. Trade your short tumblers for tall, slender glasses, and you'll find it easier to limit your liquid portions.

■ **CAN THE JUICE** Even the purest of juices can be high in calories. Take, for example, Welch's 100% Grape Juice—a single 8-ounce serving costs you 140 calories, not to mention 36 grams of sugars. That's the calorie equivalent of 70 grapes! Even more dangerous are fruit juice "cocktails," which contain minimal amounts of actual juice and lots of added sugars. You're better off snacking on whole fruits. They're full of belly-filling fiber, which most juices are not, and they're naturally portion controlled. In a study in the *International Journal of Obesity*, people who swapped in whole fruit for fruit juice with lunch slashed their calorie intake by 20 percent. If you really love the occasional glass of juice, limit yourself to a 2- or 3-ounce serving. To make it last longer, try diluting it with water or plain seltzer water, which adds a satisfying fizz to your drink.

■ **MAKE GRAPEFRUIT JUICE THE EXCEPTION** There's one fruit juice that you can feel good about drinking: grapefruit juice. The whole fruit has been shown to promote weight loss, and researchers say that 8 ounces of grapefruit juice is just as effective for belly trimming. Try Tropicana Pure Premium Ruby Red Grapefruit Juice. A recent study found that it packs more heart-healthy antioxidants than any other brand tested.

ARE FRUIT JUICE GUMMIES A HEALTHY SNACK?

The short answer: No. Sure, these fruity bites contain a trace amount of actual juice. Even so, they're more closely related to candy than to whole fruit. The reason: Fruit gummies are often infused with high-fructose corn syrup and partially hydrogenated oils, a source of heart-clogging trans fats. If you're craving a chewy, fruity snack, try Stretch Island Fruit Co. Original Fruit Strips. They're made from real fruit puree and contain no added sugars or artificial additives.

■ **SIP ON VEGETABLE JUICE** Unlike sugar-packed fruit juices, vegetable-based juices are low in calories and extremely nutritious. If you're not eating enough veggies, consider adding a glass of low-sodium vegetable juice, such as V8 Spicy Hot Low Sodium Vegetable Juice, to your meal. It may even help you lose weight: Penn State scientists found that drinking a glass of vegetable juice before meals can reduce your calorie intake by 135 calories later in the day.

■ **SKIP THE JUICE FASTS** If you're considering a juice fast in an attempt to fast-track your weight loss, don't do it. You will, of course, drop a few pounds on a liquid diet. But as soon as you resume normal eating, you'll gain it all back. (You may even tack on a few pounds, since you have been feeling deprived for days and will therefore overeat.) A better kind of cleanse: Cut out refined sugars, carbs, alcohol, and processed foods. Replace them with healthy whole food, such as fruits, vegetables, lean meats, whole grains, and healthy fats.

■ **DRINK MORE WATER** A study from the Obesity Society shows that switching from juice to water can help you lose weight in more ways than one. Researchers analyzed data from 277 women on one of several weight-loss plans who'd averaged two cans of sugary beverages before starting to diet. Those who traded juice and soda for water dropped 3 pounds more than dieters who didn't. And those who drank more than four glasses of water daily lost an additional 2 pounds.

Choosing water slashes calories but may also boost your metabolism—when your cells are well hydrated, you burn calories more efficiently. So stop swigging sweet stuff and down at least four glasses of water per day.

■ **SWAP IN MILK** Water isn't your only liquid option. Low-fat milk is an ideal weight-loss drink, since it contains both fat-burning calcium and protein. In an Australian study, people who drank milk in the a.m. instead of the calorie equivalent in juice took in 8.5 percent fewer calories throughout the day.

■ **TURN JUICE INTO DESSERT** Milk may be better than juice, but juice bars always prevail over ice cream. Stock your freezer with whole-fruit and juice bars, such as Edy's Fruit Bars, which contain just 80 calories. Or make your own juice pops: Puree strawberries, bananas, and blueberries with low-fat vanilla yogurt and freeze the mixture in molds.

THE TRUTH ABOUT SUPERMARKET JUICES

Ocean Spray Cran-Apple Juice Drink

130 calories, 30 g sugars*

If the word "drink" is tacked onto a juice's name, it's a sign that the actual fruit juice content is alarmingly low. This Ocean Spray crime contains 130 calories per serving and is only 15 percent fruit juice.

Welch's Mountain Berry Cocktail

140 calories, 33 g sugars*

"Cocktail" is another sign of trouble—it's generally attached to a drink that's more sugar water than fruit. Welch's berry blend is only a quarter juice.

Tropicana Grape Juice Beverage

150 calories, 38 g sugars*

Before you sip this juice impostor, check the label: High-fructose corn syrup appears in the ingredients list before grape juice concentrate.

Ocean Spray Cranberry Juice Cocktail

120 calories, 30 g sugars*

How does one of nature's tartest juices house so much sugar? Simple: The guys at Ocean Spray dumped in lots of added sugars.

*Nutrition info is for 8 ounces.

Legumes

7 ways peas and beans can keep you lean

Don't forget to show some love to legumes. A 2009 study in the *Journal of Nutrition* reported that people who eat diets high in vegetables, seafood, legumes, fruits, nuts, and cereal grains have slimmer waists. A study in the *Journal of the American College of Nutrition* found that bean eaters have smaller waists and lower blood pressure than those who don't eat them. In other words, legumes—chickpeas, beans, lentils, and yellow peas—are an essential part of a healthy diet. And not just because they're good for your heart. They're packed with belly-filling protein, fiber, and antioxidants, plus they're cheaper than most supermarket staples. One problem: Most of us neglect them entirely. Here's how to fold more legumes into your diet:

■ **COOK A BATCH OF CHILI** Chili is perhaps the most common delivery system for legumes—and one of the best. It not only contains a hearty serving of beans, which provide complex carbs, fiber, and protein, but it also features a range of vegetables. For a healthy

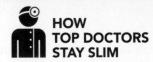

HOW TOP DOCTORS STAY SLIM

"My mother is part Mexican, and she introduced me to pinto beans early on. Now I enjoy dozens of varieties of beans, from Tongue of Fire to black garbanzos. They promote healthy digestion and have lots of fiber to keep me full."

—**CHRISTINE GERBSTADT, MD, RD,** a spokesperson for the Acadamy of Nutrition and Dietetics chili recipe, see "The Perfect Weight-Loss Chili." If you're not much of a cook, heat up a can of Eden Foods chili. Unlike most makers of canned goods, Eden strictly uses BPA-free cans.

■ **TOP YOUR SALAD WITH LEGUMES**
Legumes are the perfect, meatless way to up the protein content of your salad. Try pumping up your greens with half a cup of chickpeas, or black, kidney, or lima beans. A study in the journal *Appetite* found that people who added chickpeas to their diet felt more satiated and ate fewer processed foods, while another study showed that legume eaters have a 22 percent lower risk of obesity than those who don't eat beans.

THE PERFECT WEIGHT-LOSS CHILI

Makes 6 servings

1 pound ground turkey*

1 large onion, peeled and finely chopped

1 can (15 ounces) kidney beans

1 can (15 ounces) pinto beans

2 red bell peppers, seeded and finely chopped

1 green bell pepper, seeded and finely chopped

1 habanero (or jalapeño) chile pepper, seeded and finely chopped

2 stalks celery, finely chopped

1 can (15 ounces) diced tomatoes

1½ tablespoons chili powder

2 teaspoons ground cumin

1½ teaspoons sea salt

1 tablespoon fresh oregano, finely chopped, or 1 teaspoon dried oregano

½ cup Cheddar cheese, grated

*You can omit the meat for a vegetarian version.

1. Lightly brown the turkey in a skillet over medium-low heat, breaking it into small pieces. Drain and set aside.

2. Combine the onion, beans, peppers, celery, tomatoes, chili powder, cumin, salt, and oregano in a 5½-quart slow cooker.

3. Layer the browned meat on top of the other ingredients in the cooker.

4. Cook on high for 6 hours or on low for 8 to 10 hours.

5. Serve in individual bowls, topping each with 1 to 2 tablespoons of cheese.

PER SERVING: 300 calories, 4 g fat (1 g saturated), 37 g carbs, 12 g fiber, 1,050 mg sodium, 29 g protein

Beans are rich in soluble fiber, which forms a gel-like substance in your digestive tract. The effect: Food exits your stomach more slowly, and you don't experience a blood sugar surge after eating. Plus, when eaten regularly, soluble fiber has been shown to lower bad cholesterol levels.

■ **TOSS PASTA WITH BEANS** Instead of eating a heaping plate of pasta—even the whole grain kind—cut your portion in half and fill out your meal with beans. Although beans contain carbs (like pasta), you'll gain a significant amount of protein and fiber by making the substitution.

■ **COMBINE BEANS WITH OTHER PROTEIN** Beans are a staple in any vegetarian diet. Unfortunately, unlike animal proteins, plant-based proteins are considered "incomplete"—that is, they don't contain all nine essential amino acids. If your diet is meat free, you can build complete protein from plant-based foods by pairing legumes with nuts, peanut butter, and whole grains. One caveat: You must consume 20 to 25 percent more plant-based protein to reap the benefits of animal sources. You can also stir beans into whole grains that boast complete proteins, such as buckwheat or quinoa.

■ **MAKE A BED OF LENTILS** Boiled lentils pack about 16 grams of fiber, a weight-loss-promoting nutrient, plus they have more folate than spinach. According to a yearlong study in the *British Journal of Nutrition*, dieters who consumed the highest amounts of folate were 8$\frac{1}{2}$ times more likely to shed significant weight than those who ate the least. Convinced? Use lentils as a bed for chicken, fish, or beef instead of your standard pasta or rice. Try the colored lentil varieties—black, orange, and red—to load up on disease-fighting antioxidants.

■ **DIP INTO BLACK BEAN SALSA** Salsa is the ultimate condiment—low in calories, loaded with flavor, and high in nutrients. Don't limit your dipping to strictly tomato-based varieties. Try a salsa that has beans thrown into the mix, such as Muir Glen Organic Black Bean & Corn Salsa, with just 10 calories per tablespoon. And instead of traditional Tostitos, dip into your salsa with fibrous black bean chips, like Garden of Eatin' Black Bean Tortilla Chips.

■ **ADD BEANS TO YOUR STEW** Beans take well to big flavors, which means they're the perfect addition to a hearty stew or soup. Toss $\frac{1}{2}$ cup of chickpeas or beans into your next hot pot.

Lunch

18 secrets to a leaner midday meal

HOW TOP DOCTORS STAY SLIM

"Salads—they're the perfect antidote to a week of no-holds-barred eating. I also ban desserts, so if my sweet tooth is aching, I'll eat strawberries, raspberries, kiwifruit, or melon, which curbs my cravings for rich, high-calorie desserts."

—KARA MOHR, PhD, co-owner of Mohr Results

Breakfast is the time for calorie loading. And dinner is the time to start winding down your day. But lunch? Your midday meal is the perfect time to feast on the essential, nutritious foods: fruit, vegetables, legumes, dairy, and whole grains. Unfortunately, it can also be a battlefield. Lunch is the meal you're most likely to purchase, which means you will often find yourself face-to-face with high-calorie, low-nutrition convenience foods. This is dangerous, because your lunch is what sustains you for the rest of the afternoon. Simple carbs simply won't cut it. Follow these instructions to construct the perfect lunch:

■ **PLAN FOR BUSY DAYS** Lunch can be unpredictable. You're most likely at work, running errands, or generally preoccupied—which can make you more prone to grabbing an unhealthy option on the go. If you anticipate an overscheduled day, toss a protein bar or an apple and almonds into your bag, in case you're starving with no time to piece together a healthy lunch. That way, you're not tempted (or forced) to hit the drive-thru.

■ **BULK UP YOUR LUNCH** Even a "light" lunch can be filling. Load up your lunchbox with lots of bite-size veggies—baby carrots or red bell pepper strips, for example. They're low in calories but full of water and fiber, both of which help fill your belly. This is especially important if you're eating a carb-based entrée, such as a sandwich or wrap, which often contains not one but two servings of grains. And, don't worry, a recent Cornell University study found that eating a small lunch won't drive you to chow down later in the day.

■ **WORK IN PROTEIN** You should also make sure to include a few ounces (10 to 20 grams) of protein, such as lean ham on whole grain bread or a chopped egg and a handful of sunflower seeds on a salad. This will help keep your stomach quiet through the afternoon hours. Plus, meals that are high in protein (and fiber) require more chewing, giving your brain time to send the "stop eating" signal.

■ **NEVER ASSUME "HEALTHY" IS HEALTHY** Beware the Subway diet: Diners tend to grossly underestimate the calorie counts in "healthy" fast food, a recent Cornell University study found. When people ate a Subway meal with as many calories as a McDonald's meal, they misjudged the Subway meal's load by 21 percent (159 calories). One way to be more accurate: Estimate the number of calories in your healthy fast-food meal, and double it, say Cornell researchers.

■ **ESCAPE YOUR DESK** Take a real lunch break. Recent British research suggests that eating at your desk can cause you to eat more later in the day. In the study, people who ate a meal in front of a computer consumed twice as many calories later than those who dined away from their desks. Distracted eating can cause you to

remember less about the meal, which may make you feel less full, explain the scientists. "Changing your surroundings, even if it's only for 20 minutes, not only gives your fatigued mind a break but also boosts your mood," says Bryan G. Robinson, PhD, author of *Chained to the Desk*. Your ideal move: Have lunch outside, soak up some sun, then take a short walk afterward.

■ **CHEW GUM BEFOREHAND** Pop a piece of sugar-free gum before lunch. In a University of Rhode Island study, people who chewed gum for an hour in the morning took in 67 fewer calories at lunch and didn't compensate by eating more later on. Chewing may stimulate nerves in your jaw that are linked to the brain region responsible for satiety, explains study author Kathleen Melanson, PhD, RD. Plus, chewing burns an extra 11 calories an hour!

■ **FILL UP ON WATER** Before you sidle up to the deli counter, chug a glass of water. A Virginia Polytechnic Institute study found that drinking water before a meal can help you consume fewer calories. Then sip on another glass with your meal—try taking a swig after every bite. This will not only help fill you up faster but it will also slow down your shoveling.

■ **HEAT THINGS UP** Sprinkle a little red pepper on your soup or salad. In a Canadian study, people who ate appetizers that contained red pepper before lunch took in an average of 189 fewer calories later. The scientists credit capsaicin, a chemical in chiles that gives them their heat and helps tame your appetite. If you can't handle it straight, try

(continued on page 196)

4 SUPER SINGLE-SERVING LUNCH SALADS

TUNA SALAD

- 3 ounces light tuna (canned in water, unsalted), drained
- 1 tablespoon olive oil mayonnaise
- 1 medium apple, chopped
- 3 cups baby spinach
- 2 tablespoons Newman's Own Olive Oil & Vinegar Dressing

Combine the tuna, mayo, and apple. Serve on the spinach and drizzle with the dressing.

Bonus! Pectin, a type of fiber found in high amounts in apples, has been shown to boost satiety.

PER SERVING: 423 calories, 22 g fat (3.5 g saturated), 34 g carbs, 8 g fiber, 430 mg sodium, 24 g protein

GRILLED CHICKEN CRANBERRY SALAD

- 7 walnut halves
- 1½ cups baby spinach
- ½ cup chopped beets
- 1 tablespoon dried cranberries
- 1 tablespoon balsamic vinegar
- ½ grilled chicken breast
- 1 ounce semisoft goat cheese

Preheat oven to 350°F. Roast walnuts on an ungreased baking sheet until golden brown, about 6 minutes, stirring occasionally. Combine walnuts, greens, beets, and cranberries in a salad bowl. Toss with balsamic vinegar, then top salad with sliced chicken breast and goat cheese.

Bonus! The acetic acid in vinegar is thought to help reduce the accumulation of body fat.

PER SERVING: 420 calories, 21 g fat (8 g saturated), 22 g carbs, 5 g fiber, 325 mg sodium, 37 g protein

ASIAN CHICKEN SALAD

1 cup shredded red cabbage

1 cup chopped raw spinach

½ grilled chicken breast

½ cup fresh mandarin orange slices

1 tablespoon pine nuts

1 ounce soft goat cheese

1½ teaspoons olive oil

2 tablespoons balsamic vinegar

Combine all ingredients in a large salad bowl.

Bonus! Dutch researchers found that a polyunsaturated fat in pine nuts stimulates the release of cholecystokinin (CCK), a hormone that slows the emptying of your stomach. Translation: You'll feel fuller longer!

PER SERVING: 371 calories, 21 g fat (6 g saturated), 26 g carbs, 4 g fiber, 188 mg sodium, 23 g protein

MOZZARELLA AND TOMATO SALAD

1 medium tomato, cubed

1 ounce fresh part-skim mozzarella cheese, cubed

1 cup fresh spinach leaves

1 clove garlic, pressed

1½ teaspoons olive oil

2 tablespoons balsamic vinegar

2 teaspoons sunflower seeds

¼ teaspoon freshly ground black pepper

Combine all ingredients in a large salad bowl.

Bonus! An Australian study review concluded that garlic reduces blood pressure in people with hypertension.

PER SERVING: 243 calories, 16 g fat (4 g saturated), 15 g carbs, 3 g fiber, 188 mg sodium, 11 g protein

stirring red pepper into hummus or low-fat salad dressing. Or whip up a pot of chili that will last you all week long. It's the perfect vessel for spicy flavor—and it's full of complex carbs, produce, and a sizable shot of protein.

■ **BROWN BAG IT FREQUENTLY** The more often you make your lunch, the more calories you'll save. When you prepare your own food, you control the quality, the portion sizes, and the amount of sugar, salt, and fat you consume. (Make it a policy to resist anything that's not in your lunch sack throughout the day.) Even the most innocent-seeming restaurant fare can be loaded down with unwanted calories, and research shows that the nutrition information restaurants post is not always accurate. It's okay to grab the occasional lunch out, but it should be the exception rather than the rule.

■ **PACK YOUR LUNCH AFTER DINNER** If you pack your lunch first thing in the morning, when you're hungry, that last slice of chocolate cake on the kitchen counter could easily end up in your sack. Instead, assemble your meal the night before, shortly after you finish dinner. Since you're full, your stomach will carry less influence over your food choices.

■ **CONSIDER YOUR DINNER PLANS** Have a big night out ahead of you? Lunch is the perfect time to trim back. When you dine with friends, you consume about 50 percent more than you do alone, according to Penn State scientists. In other words, you can count on dinner being more indulgent than normal. To give yourself a little wiggle room, choose a low-cal yet filling lunch, such as soup or salad. (Note: If you can, make lunch your time to eat with friends. It's easier to go light at lunch, when sit-down restaurants often shrink their meal portions.)

■ **RETHINK LUNCHMEAT** Sure, packaged lunchmeat is convenient. But consider its nutritional makeup: These presliced meats are swamped with sodium, which can cause you to retain water and experience a boost in blood pressure. Perhaps more concerning is the nitrates they contain. These compounds are added for flavor and color—and have been linked to a heightened risk of heart attack, diabetes, and cancer. The easiest way to spot processed meats is by their shape: Each slice is nearly uniform, designed to fit perfectly on a bun.

Ditch the funky stuff and instead fill your sandwich with grilled chicken, roasted turkey breast, or tuna. Or shop for nitrate-free, low-sodium lunchmeat. (Hint: Hormel's Natural Choice line is blissfully free of nitrates and preservatives.) Keep in mind, honey- and maple-flavored meats will have more calories per serving than plain or spiced varieties.

■ **STUFF YOUR SANDWICH WITH GREENS** Don't stop with meat and cheese when building your sandwich. Load your bread with fresh or roasted veggies—spinach, alfalfa, tomatoes, or roasted red peppers, for example. You can even create an open-faced creation, which will allow you to pile the produce higher. Vegetables are low in calories and high in nutrients and, thanks to their water content, make your sandwich seem more substantial.

■ **CHOOSE YOUR CHEESE WISELY** A slice of cheese is the perfect way to fold calcium-rich dairy into your lunch. But, remember, some slices are better than others. Swiss cheese, for example, has 83 percent less sodium and significantly more calcium than the processed American stuff. As a general rule, softer cheeses, such as mozzarella, are less fat- and calorie-dense than hard varieties, since they contain more moisture. If you're buying your cheese from the deli counter, ask for it to be thinly sliced. You'll save a few calories without even noticing the difference.

■ **MEDITATE DURING LUNCH** Before you take your first bite, spend 2 minutes doing absolutely nothing. Just relax and forget about the project back at your desk. Once you've cleared your head, slowly unwrap your lunch, and inhale its aroma, imagine where it came from (a farm, hopefully), then take a small bite. Chew slowly, so you can pay attention to the food's taste, texture, and temperature. This turns your lunch break into a mental break—and helps you eat at a slower pace, so you feel satisfied longer.

■ **END YOUR MEAL WITH FRUIT** If you crave sweets after lunch, it may be because your meal was overwhelmed by savory foods. Rather than diving into the candy dish, eat a piece of fresh fruit or a cup of fruit salad. (See "The Perfect Fruit Salad" on page 173.)

■ **CONCLUDE WITH COFFEE** Make afternoon joe a part of your routine. "Whenever possible, finish lunch and dinner with a hot beverage (preferably not loaded with sugar, fat, and calories), and sip it slowly," says David Katz, MD, MPH, director of the Yale-Griffin Prevention Research Center. "It gives your brain time to register that you're full and satisfied and provides a nice sense of closure." Not a fan of coffee? Try unsweetened hot tea, or even low-calorie hot chocolate, as long as you skip dessert.

■ **CHANNEL YOUR LUNCH LATER** Don't down your sandwich and then immediately forget about it. British research suggests that thinking about your lunch later in the afternoon can help you resist those tempting vending machine snacks. Recalling a recent meal may boost your awareness of how satisfying the food was, so you eat less, the scientists explain.

Reorganize Your Refrigerator

Science suggests that the way you arrange your groceries and how you stock your fridge may shape the way you eat.

1 SHELVE STRATEGICALLY

The refrigerator shelf closest to eye level should house your fruits, vegetables, and other healthy snacks. You're 2.7 times more likely to eat healthy food if it's in your line of sight, according to a Cornell University study. Stash less-healthy foods in the crisper, in the back of the fridge, or on the bottom shelf, out of view.

2 DIVIDE AND CONQUER

To avoid overeating, divide your leftovers into meal-size portions and store them in individual containers. That way, you're not tempted to heat up a heaping portion when mealtime comes around and your tummy is growling.

3 SHOP MORE, BUY LESS

Rather than stocking up for an entire week, stop by the supermarket every 2 or 3 days and buy enough only for the next few meals. A 2008 study in the *Journal of Consumer Psychology* found that having too many choices in the fridge may undermine your willpower.

4 TOSS THE JUNK

You probably won't drive to the store at midnight to quiet a craving for chocolate chip cookies. But you *will* raid the fridge—you're far more likely to cave to a craving when the object of your desire is close by. So make sure it's not: Dispose of any tempting foods in your fridge, and restock it with healthy options, such as cheese, fruit and vegetables, and lean meats.

Meal Frequency

Learn how to eat more and weigh less

One day, diet experts tell you to eat several small meals a day. The next, they recommend adhering to the standard three. Both are good advice. When it comes to meal frequency, consistency—not number—is key; it doesn't matter if you eat three, four, or six meals a day, as long as you follow a regular schedule. According to a recent Australian study review, there's no substantial evidence that your frequency of eating really matters.

So why is the mini-meal approach so popular? The "graze, don't gorge" strategy is built around the idea that frequent eating keeps your blood sugar stable, your metabolism burning hot, and your appetite in check. Only one part of that is true: Eating several small meals doesn't stoke your calorie burn or steady your blood sugar, according to a recent Syracuse University study. It simply keeps you from becoming crazy hungry and pigging out. There's a downside to the approach: Some studies have revealed a link between obesity and eating more than three times per day, particularly in women. The reason is simple. The more often you eat, the greater your number of opportunities to overdo it. Plus, if you're an emotional eater, constantly worrying about what you're going to eat can create unnecessary stress, and that anxiety can fuel belly-fat storage.

HOW TOP DOCTORS STAY SLIM

"Structured eating instead of stressed snacking. I make sure I'm sitting down to three complete meals, at more or less the same time each day, and two small snacks. Spreading out my food intake throughout the day means I'm never ravenous. Because I'm a night eater, I try to give myself a bit of a treat every night so that I don't feel deprived."

—**MADELYN FERNSTROM, PhD,** founding director of the University of Pittsburgh Medical Center Weight Management Center

The bottom line is that you should find an eating schedule that works for you. Then make it a policy never to skip a meal or a planned snack. Straying from your feeding schedule disrupts your normal hunger cues. This may put you at risk of eating foods you'd normally resist or of overeating once you do finally get around to a meal. When building your plan, consider these factors:

■ **NEVER SKIP BREAKFAST** There's one time when eating is nonnegotiable: first thing in the morning. A study in the *American Journal of Epidemiology* found that breakfast skippers have a 450 percent greater risk of obesity than people who regularly eat in the a.m. It's okay to grab an Egg McMuffin in a pinch, but you should aim to eat breakfast at home as often as possible. In the study, frequently going out for breakfast was also associated with a higher risk of obesity. Why? Breakfasts eaten away from home packed more calories and saturated fat and less fiber than home-cooked meals. Aim to consume at least a quarter of your calories at breakfast, ideally from protein, healthy fats, and slow-burning carbs.

■ **STICK TO YOUR PLAN** Let's say you've scaled back your daily intake to 1,200 calories. Now divide that by six. That's only 200 calories—the equivalent of 29 almonds—per meal on a six-meal schedule! If you're seriously cutting calories, you may find that the mini-meal approach leaves you feeling deprived, making you susceptible to cheating. When building your meal plan, start by determining the daily number of calories you want to consume. Then experiment with different strategies, all while keeping your calorie intake constant. You can try three full-size meals, three medium meals plus two snacks, or five mini-meals—whatever works for you. Once you find a plan you like, adhere to it day in and day out. A British study found that women who ate the same number of meals each day consumed fewer calories than those who switched it up.

■ **FILL UP ON FIBER AND PROTEIN** Foods that keep you fuller longer make it easier to stay consistent. The best nutrients for enhancing fullness are fiber and protein, since they're slow digesting. In one Penn State study, women ate 30 percent fewer calories when they prioritized fiber in their diet without changing the overall weight of the food they consumed. A University of Missouri study found that dieters who ate 25 percent of their calories from protein at breakfast, lunch, and dinner felt fuller than those who spread it over six small meals. Aim to incorporate both fiber and protein into every meal or snack, whether in the form of a hard-cooked egg and veggies, low-fat yogurt and fresh fruit, or peanut butter on celery sticks.

■ **KEEP MEAL SIZE IN CHECK** If the mini-meal approach works for you, make sure to, well, keep your meals mini. A Purdue University study found that the average American's "snacks" have morphed into meals, and meals into feasts. In fact, over the past 30 years, we've tacked on an extra 220 calories to every snack we consume! As a general rule, limit your snacks to 200 calories, and don't allow yourself to stray from the nutritional guidelines you abide by at meals. Protein, fiber, slow-digesting carbs, and healthy fats should still be king—not the empty carbs and sugar you find in so many snack foods.

■ **EAT BY THE CLOCK** Set your meal and snack times, and treat them like can't-miss appointments. In a study in the *American Journal of Clinical Nutrition,* women who ate at regular, fixed times burned more calories after eating than those who divided their usual amount of food into unscheduled meals throughout the day. Plus, scheduling your meals, rather than mindlessly grazing, helps you stay in control of your calorie intake.

■ **FOCUS ON HOW YOU FEEL** There's no such thing as a one-size-fits-all approach to losing weight. This may explain why in a recent University of Texas at Austin study, women who fixated on diet rules (for example, eating a certain number of meals or snacks) and external cues to stop eating (like cleaning their plate) lost *less* weight than those who learned to be mindful of their behavior and hunger. Rather than following a trendy diet, tune in to what works for your own body. How hungry do you feel shortly after eating? Do you feel energized or lethargic after exercise? If you're perpetually hungry or tired, you may need to increase your calorie intake slightly.

Meat

21 ways to trim your waistline with meat

Forget what you heard about meat in the '90s. Eating beef, chicken, turkey, and pork may actually help keep you lean, according to Danish researchers. They tracked the diets of more than 42,000 people for 5 years and found that those who consumed the most animal protein experienced the smallest increases in waist size. A British study found that people who boosted the percentage of protein-based calories in their diet burned 71 more calories per day than those who stuck to low-protein diets. One reason: High-quality protein from meat may help you feel full longer while also boosting your metabolism.

Unlike the protein from plant sources, such as nuts and whole grains, animal products provide "complete" protein. It contains the perfect proportions of the essential amino acids your body can't synthesize on its own. In other words, you can eat less of it and still reap the muscle-building, weight-loss benefits of protein. Maximize the power of your meats by following these guidelines:

■ CHOOSE YOUR CUT

POULTRY

Leanest cuts:

Skinless turkey or chicken breast

BEEF

Leanest cuts:

Eye of round roast and steak

Top round roast and steak

Bottom round roast and steak

Sirloin tip side steak

Top sirloin steak

Tenderloin

Chuck

PORK

Leanest cuts:

Tenderloin

Chops

■ CHECK YOUR GROUND POULTRY

Ground chicken or turkey can be a great addition to a pot of chili, especially if you hate beef—but don't assume it's lean. Ground poultry can be just as caloric as ground beef, since it often contains dark meat and skin. If you're going ground, make sure to select a cut that's strictly made with breast meat, which is the leanest part of the bird. Always drain ground meat after cooking to remove liquefied fat.

■ REMOVE THE SKIN
You can leave the skin on when roasting a whole chicken or turkey. Just make sure to remove it once you're ready to chow down, since the skin is a sneaky source of fat.

> **BONUS BENEFIT!**
>
> Lean meats are rich in iron, which women lose each month during menstruation. Replenishing your stores of the mineral helps keep your energy levels high and your metabolism burning hot.

■ SKIP THE FRYER
Dunking your chicken in the fryer is essentially bathing it in empty carbs and unhealthy fats. Sound healthy? Didn't think so. Grilling is the obvious low-calorie cooking method, but you can also experiment with roasting, baking, and broiling your meats. When you cook your meat in the oven, place it on a rack to ensure that the fat drips away rather than being reabsorbed.

■ PREPARE MEAT IN ADVANCE
You're more likely to skip the drive-thru if you have a cooked chicken breast or roasted turkey waiting for you at home. Make Sunday your day of meal prep, and cook up a batch of lean meat to eat throughout the week. Store it in a zipper-lock bag in your refrigerator, then pop a piece in the microwave for an instant dinner. Likewise, if a dish calls for boiled meat, prepare your protein a day or two ahead of time, then stick it in the fridge. An easy way to cut calories: Once the meat cools, remove the fat that hardens on top.

■ APPROACH LUNCHMEAT WITH CAUTION
If you've lived on lunchmeat for years, you may be in trouble: These packaged meats are often dangerously high in sodium and contain

nitrates, compounds thought to raise your risk of heart attack, cancer, and diabetes. Thankfully, you don't have to sacrifice your turkey sandwiches just yet: Some food manufacturers are coming out with no-preservative, nitrate-free options, such as Hormel's Natural Choice line.

■ **PLAY WITH MARINADES** Not only do marinades add flavor to your meat—which is especially important when you're trimming fat—but they also help tenderize and moisten it during cooking. Skip the gooey, high-calorie marinades and opt for one that's based around low-sodium soy sauce, wine, or lemon juice. (See "5 Tasty, Healthy Marinades" on page 206 for inspiration.)

■ **WATCH THE WORDING** Before you buy beef, check the label. If you see the word "prime," put it back in the cold case, since prime cuts are some of the fattiest. Choose cuts that are labeled "choice" or "select" instead.

■ **CHECK YOUR GROUND BEEF** Craving a burger? That's fine—just make sure to select the leanest ground beef possible. Pick a package that contains at least 90 percent lean meat. If you stick to the skinny kind, it can actually be leaner than turkey or ground pork! As with any ground meat, make sure to drain after cooking.

■ **RETHINK YOUR MEAT SAUCE** If your pasta sauce is normally more meat than tomato, flip that ratio to instantly save calories. Don't worry about losing flavor: Ground meat or thinly sliced pieces are easy to evenly distribute throughout the sauce, so you'll still enjoy meat in every bite. If you want to add more texture, toss grated carrots into your sauce and let it simmer. The veggies will soften up to the consistency of meat.

■ **DON'T FEAR JERKY** Most people think of beef jerky as a fattening, high-sodium snack that's to be avoided. That is sometimes the case, but you can also find chemical-free, lean beef jerky, which is high in protein and perfect for on-the-go eating. Try Gourmet Natural Beef Jerky (www.americangrassfedbeef.com). It contains no preservatives and is made from lean, grass-fed beef. Research shows that grass-fed beef contains more heart-healthy omega-3 fatty acids than grain-fed beef.

■ **TREAT MEAT LIKE A GARNISH** You don't have to eliminate meat entirely to lose weight. However, meat shouldn't be the star of your plate, either. Use chicken, beef, pork, or turkey to accent dishes rather than to define them. That means adding meat to salads, whole grain pastas, stir-fried vegetables, or soups instead of serving it as a stand-alone dish.

BONUS BENEFIT!

You'll save on your grocery bill, since meat tends to be one of the priciest items in the supermarket.

■ **WATCH SERVING SIZES** Even the leanest of meats can be high in calories if your portions are bloated. According to USDA recommendations, a serving of meat is 3 ounces—about the size of a standard deck of cards or the palm of your hand (not including your fingers). That's half of a small boneless, skinless chicken breast; two thin slices of roast beef; or a small lean hamburger. If you struggle to gauge proper serving sizes, consider investing in a food scale, so you can easily divide your meat into 3-ounce slabs.

■ **CHEW ON THIS** Chewy foods, like lean meats, force your body to work hard during digestion. All of that protein takes time and effort to break down, and that process burns calories! To maximize the chew factor, eat your meat in its whole state whenever possible—for example, a sirloin steak instead of ground beef. Japanese scientists found that people who ate the foods that required the most work had slimmer waistlines than those who filled up on softer, easy-to-eat foods.

■ **BEEF UP YOUR SALAD** Don't confine salads to the first course. If you pile sirloin,

SHOULD I BANISH BACON?

Breaking bacon news: The breakfast staple won't give you a heart attack. A recent Harvard University study review concluded that there's no link between saturated fat and heart disease. Besides, the fat content of bacon is actually pretty reasonable, if you choose the right brand and watch your portions. Try Applegate Farms Organic Sunday Bacon. Each thick-cut slice contains just 1 gram of saturated fat (2.5 grams total fat) and 30 calories, plus adds 2 grams of protein to your plate. So go ahead, fry up a couple of slices, drain off most of the fat, and enjoy—it's always a smarter choice than sausage. Oh, and those little red pebbles Betty Crocker calls Bac-Os? They're soy and trans-fatty partially hydrogenated oil, not bacon.

grilled chicken, or turkey breast onto your greens, you'll significantly boost the protein content of your salad as well as the meal's satiety factor. Think of it as sandwich built on veggies instead of bread. To make your salad seem more like a meal, heat up the meat first. Hot food tends to be more satiating, so you'll need less of it to feel full.

■ **SWITCH YOUR SAUSAGE** Sausage has a fatty reputation—and rightfully so. Take, for example, Hillshire Farm Beef Smoked Sausage. A single 2-ounce serving packs 170 calories, and 76 percent of those calories come from fat! However, you don't have to eliminate sausage from your breakfast table entirely. If you switch to turkey sausage, you can save a significant amount of calories and fat. Hillshire Farm Turkey Smoked Sausage contains 90 calories per 2-ounce serving, with only half of the calories coming from fat.

■ **BEWARE OF MEAT IMPOSTORS** Watch out for processed meats that pose as the real thing but actually contain very little meat. What they do contain: empty-calorie fillers. The primary offenders are breaded chicken patties, chicken nuggets, burgers that aren't 100 percent beef or turkey, bologna, salami, hot dogs, and pepperoni.

■ **GO ORGANIC** When it comes to meats, going organic is well worth the extra cost. USDA-certified organic meats are free of hormones and antibiotics. Why that matters: According to a report in the *International Journal of Obesity*, the use of hormones in

(continued on page 208)

5 TASTY, HEALTHY MARINADES

Marinades and spice rubs do more than kick up the flavor of your meat. Many spices have anticancer compounds, and some can even rev up your metabolism! These simple recipes are the perfect dressing for whatever meat is on your menu.

COFFEE BUZZ

Makes 4 servings

½ cup strong coffee
Juice of 1 lime
Juice of ½ orange
1 tablespoon sriracha sauce
1 tablespoon canola oil

1 tablespoon minced cilantro
¼ teaspoon cinnamon
¼ teaspoon cumin
Salt and pepper to taste

Combine all ingredients in a medium bowl.

PER SERVING: 48 calories, 4 g fat (0 g saturated), 4 g carbs, 0 g fiber, 115 mg sodium, 0 g protein

CURRIED YOGURT

Makes 4 servings

1 cup low-fat Greek yogurt
1 teaspoon curry powder

1 teaspoon salt
½ teaspoon ground pepper

Combine all ingredients in a medium bowl.

PER SERVING: 35 calories, 1 g fat (1 g saturated), 2 g carbs, 0 g fiber, 598 mg sodium, 4 g protein

SPICY MOROCCAN

Makes 4 servings

1 jar roasted red peppers

3 tablespoons olive oil

3 garlic cloves

2 teaspoons red-pepper flakes

1 teaspoon salt

1 teaspoon ground cumin

1 teaspoon coriander

Puree all the ingredients in a blender.

PER SERVING: 121 calories, 11 g fat (2 g saturated), 7 g carbs, 2 g fiber, 637 mg sodium, 0 g protein

LEMON PEPPER

Makes 4 servings

⅓ cup olive oil

1 teaspoon grated lemon peel

¼ cup freshly squeezed lemon juice

2 finely chopped garlic cloves

1 teaspoon salt

1 teaspoon ground pepper

Combine all ingredients in a medium bowl.

PER SERVING: 176 calories, 19 g fat (3 g saturated), 2 g carbs, 0 g fiber, 582 mg sodium, 0 g protein

BALSAMIC RED WINE

Makes 4 servings

¼ cup red wine

2 tablespoons balsamic vinegar

1 tablespoon Worcestershire sauce

1 garlic clove, minced

1 tablespoon fresh rosemary, chopped

Combine all ingredients in a medium bowl.

PER SERVING: 99 calories, 0 g fat, 12 g carbs, 0 g fiber, 177 mg sodium, 0 g protein meat may be a contributing factor to the obesity epidemic. Don't be led astray by "natural" claims—the government doesn't strictly regulate this term, which means that "natural" meats may still contain preservatives and artificial colors or flavors. Only organic should make your grade.

■ **AVOID PLASTIC-WRAPPED MEATS** It's not just chemicals inside meat that you have to worry about. The plastic wrap used at supermarkets is made primarily with PVC, a type of plastic that's laden with phthalates, says Frederick vom Saal, PhD, a professor of biological sciences at the University of Missouri–Columbia. These chemicals can interfere with your hormone levels (particularly testosterone), potentially leading to weight gain. Ask your butcher to wrap your meat in paper instead.

■ **WATCH THE SODIUM** Your meat may be injected with a sodium-rich solution to enhance moisture and flavor. In fact, an estimated 30 percent of poultry, 15 percent of beef, and 90 percent of pork fall victim to such saline injections! To keep your sodium intake (and blood pressure) in check, scan the nutrition label on your meat. Any more than 50 to 75 milligrams of sodium per 4 ounces is a red flag.

■ **BREAD WITH CAUTION** The best meat is naked—no skin, no breading. However, if you crave the crunch of breaded meat, you can coat your cut in flaxseed or ground nuts instead of traditional bread crumbs. That way, you're adding protein and healthy fats, rather than empty carbs, to your meat dish. Limit yourself to a 2-tablespoon portion of the stuff, and dunk your fillets in water instead of beaten eggs or milk.

Mediterranean Diet

Eating for heart health is also good for your waistline

The Mediterranean diet isn't a trendy weight-loss plan that requires expensive shakes, the elimination of entire food groups, or weekly counseling sessions. It's an eating style based on the traditional diet of Southern Europe: vegetables and legumes, along with fruits, whole grain breads, dates, olives, olive oil, nuts, red wine, and small infrequent portions of meats and fish. The main source of fat in the diet comes from monounsaturated fats from olives and olive oil rather than saturated fats from animal foods.

Being physically active is also a major component of the traditional lifestyle along the Mediterranean coastlines of Greece, France, Italy, and Spain. Recently, an analysis of 50 studies linked the Mediterranean diet to reduced risk of heart disease, diabetes, and stroke by lowering blood pressure, cholesterol, and blood sugar and even reducing abdominal fat.

■ **FEEL FULL WITH VEGETABLES** Studies of Mediterranean-style diets suggest that there may be a strong healthy-weight advantage, too. Whole foods like vegetables are fiber- and water-dense, which makes them filling and satisfying, so you're less likely to overeat.

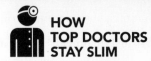

HOW TOP DOCTORS STAY SLIM

"I am picky about what meat I buy and cook. I try to buy free-range chicken, organic beef—I'd rather buy more expensive organic meat and just eat less meat."

—NAOMI STOTLAND, MD, a doctor at the Center for Obesity Assessment, Study, and Treatment at the University of California, San Francisco

■ **GET MORE MUFAS** The acronym stands for monounsaturated fats, the heart-healthy fats that make up the bulk of Mediterranean-style diets. Like fruits and whole grains, these fats are highly satisfying. They taste good, digest slowly, and don't trigger blood sugar spikes. Top sources of MUFAs include vegetable oils, such as olive, canola, and safflower oil; two fruits, olives and avocados; and nuts and nut butters made from almonds, peanuts, hazelnuts, pecans, pistachios, and cashews.

■ **ORDER THE SANGIOVESE** Red wine in moderation is a big part of the Mediterranean meal culture. While wine, like any alcohol, can lead to weight gain if not consumed carefully, red wine appears to offer health benefits other varieties lack. Wine contains compounds called polyphenols that help prevent LDL cholesterol from sticking to artery walls. One such phenol in red wine is resveratrol, a powerful anti-inflammatory that may reduce the risk of cancers like breast and colon cancer, heart disease, stroke, and Alzheimer's disease. "Resveratrol is an antioxidant and can help slow

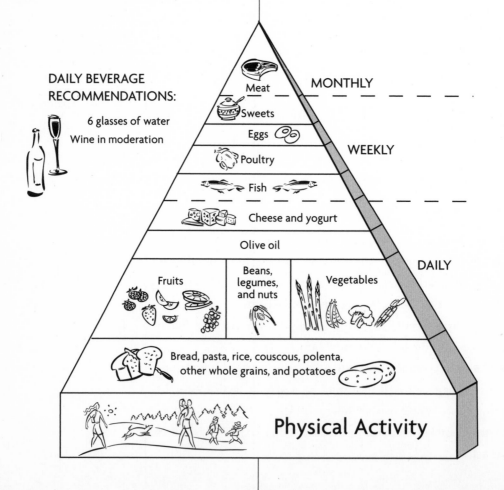

DAILY BEVERAGE
RECOMMENDATIONS:

6 glasses of water
Wine in moderation

Meat — MONTHLY

Sweets

Eggs

Poultry — WEEKLY

Fish

Cheese and yogurt

Olive oil

Fruits — Beans, legumes, and nuts — Vegetables — DAILY

Bread, pasta, rice, couscous, polenta, other whole grains, and potatoes

Physical Activity

down aging, maintain DNA repair, and even have an effect on carbohydrate metabolism, which can help insulin sensitivity in diabetes," says Joseph Maroon, MD, a neurosurgeon at the University of Pittsburgh Medical Center and author of *The Longevity Factor: How Resveratrol and Red Wine Activate Genes for a Longer, Healthier Life.*

■ **VISIT THE PYRAMID** The Mediterranean Diet Pyramid is different from the USDA's "MyPlate" recommmendations, which recently replaced the food pyramid of the 1990s.

Unlike MyPlate, which includes meats as a way of consuming enough protein every day, the Mediterranean pyramid depends on legumes, fish, and nuts to supply the necessary protein. Red meat is reserved for a few times a month. The makeup of the daily meals in the traditional Mediterranean Diet Pyramid are found at the base of the illustration (opposite page) and include whole grains, fruits, vegetables, beans, legumes and nuts, and large amounts of olive oil, as well as daily doses of cheese and yogurt, and, of course, red wine.

Nutrition Labels and Claims

Learn to decode the hype on supermarket foods

Food labels are all about marketing. But the nutrition panel and ingredients list are about content. Ignore the billboard on the front of the box entirely, so you avoid being fooled by misleading label claims. Think you're immune? Consider this: In a University of South Carolina study, dieters shown a meal that consisted of vegetables, salami, and pasta rated it as healthier when it was called "salad" instead of "pasta." And a study in the *Journal of Consumer Research* found that people—especially those with a history of dieting—tended to eat more of a sweet treat when it was called a "fruit chew" instead of a "candy chew." By labeling foods with healthy-sounding names, manufacturers convince you to eat more, regardless of how nutritious (or not) the snack may be. Skip the bold-faced claims and head for the nutrition and ingredient panel on the side or back of the package.

CLAIMS TO IGNORE

■ **"NATURAL"** The FDA doesn't regulate this label claim—which is why Cheetos, 7UP, and other unhealthy packaged foods can freely slap the word on their label. Never assume that *natural* means healthy.

■ **"LOW FAT," "REDUCED FAT," "FAT FREE"** A study in the *Journal of Marketing Research* found that people consume more calories when foods are labeled low fat. The most likely reason is that we feel less guilt when eating these foods, so we're less inclined to control our portions. The problem: When fat is taken out, it's often replaced with sugar and empty carbs to maintain the flavor.

■ **"TRANS FAT FREE"** Artery-clogging trans fats *are* to be avoided. However, "trans fat free" or "0 grams trans fats" isn't a surefire sign of a health food. Manufacturers can legally make the claim if a food has less than half a gram of trans fats per serving. Even trace amounts can be enough to do your arteries damage.

■ **"HIGH IN ANTIOXIDANTS"** This only means that the product contains some plant-based ingredients. You're better off eating whole foods than antioxidant-fortified packaged foods.

■ **"MADE WITH WHOLE GRAINS"** Whole grains are always preferable to refined. However, this label claim doesn't mean that *every* grain is the heart-healthy, belly-flattening kind. Unless it's 100 percent whole grain, there may be enriched flour lurking inside the package.

■ **"NO HIGH-FRUCTOSE CORN SYRUP"** Sure, it's free of HFCS—but it may still contain sugar. That's not a big improvement. All types of sugar need to be limited and consumed in moderation, not just HFCS.

■ **"A GOOD SOURCE OF CALCIUM"** Even Cookie Crisp cereal boasts 10 percent of your calcium needs. And no nutritionist would tell you it's your best option.

WHAT TO WATCH

■ **SERVING SIZE** Even if a food appears to be in a portion-controlled package, it may contain more than one serving. (Case in point: Campbell's Chunky Soup.) The amount listed also may not represent how much you'd actually eat. Determine how much of the food you'd eat per sitting, then judge the nutritional impact accordingly.

■ **CALORIES** Ninety-one percent of shoppers often bypass the calorie count when buying an item, according to a University of Minnesota study. Make the calorie information the first place you look.

■ **SODIUM** Your rule of thumb: Avoid any foods that have higher sodium levels than calories. Lots of sodium generally indicates overly processed foods.

■ **FAT** Add up the amount of mono- and polyunsaturated fats in a food, then calculate what percentage of the total fat they account for. (If the label only lists saturated and trans fats, subtract them from the total to determine the amount of unsaturated fats.) If less than 75 percent of the fat is unsaturated, put it back. Next, look for zero grams trans fats by scanning for hydrogenated or partially hydrogenated oils on the ingredient lists. If these dangerous oils make the list, the food contains trans fats, whether or not the nutrition panel says it does.

■ **PROTEIN** This one's simple: The more protein, the better. Protein-rich foods keep you fuller longer, so they can help prevent overeating.

■ **FIBER** The Institute of Medicine recommends that men consume 38 grams of fiber per day and that women take in 25 grams. When choosing grain products, select those that have at least 2 grams of fiber per 100 calories.

■ **SUGAR** Sugars should make up no more than 10 percent of the total calories. That's

7 SHOPPING STRATEGIES TO HELP YOU LOSE WEIGHT

Avoid lines
The longer you stare at that Twix in the checkout line, the more likely you are to toss it into your cart, say University of Arizona scientists. To reduce your wait, shop during off-peak hours, such as Wednesdays or any day after 9:00 p.m.

Leave the kids at home
If you hope to keep the junk out of your cart, you're better off shopping alone. A 2011 Mintel report found that 80 percent of parents said they'd probably buy snacks or frozen desserts at the supermarket if their children asked for them. If taking your little ones with you is unavoidable, try this strategy: Pretend you can't understand what your child is whining for, then steer the cart in the opposite direction.

Write a list
Never go into a supermarket unarmed. If you don't have a list, you're more likely to succumb to junky packaged foods. Try planning your menu for the next few days, write down what you need, and stick to the list.

Check yourself out
You're less likely to make impulse purchases if you use a self-checkout station. A study of more than 500 US shoppers found that impulse sales declined by about 43 percent when peo-

2.5 grams per 100 calories. (Beverages should provide little or no sugar.) Remember, every 4 grams of the sweet stuff is the equivalent of one sugar cube.

■ **INGREDIENTS LIST** Whole foods should be the bulk of your diet—and they don't have ingredients lists. However, when buying the occasional packaged food, look for those that list whole foods, such as oats, nuts, and real fruit, in the first line of ingredients. Make sure that every grain is whole—that means no enriched flour, white flour, or even wheat flour if it doesn't have the word "whole" in front of it—and avoid sneaky sources of sugar, such as high-fructose corn syrup, barley malt, brown rice syrup, fructose, evaporated cane juice, maltodextrin, and molasses. Your rule of thumb: The fewer ingredients found in any packaged food, the better it probably is for you.

ple rang up their own groceries. Scanning your own items distracts you from temptations, the scientists say. Plus, self-checkout lines are generally about 66 percent shorter, so you have less time to grab last-minute items.

Look high and low

Eye-level shelves are prime supermarket real estate. That means they're occupied by highly profitable foods—popular, often heavily processed fare—that you generally want to avoid. Healthier foods tend to be on the top and bottom shelves.

Eat before you shop

Before you head to the supermarket, grab a healthy snack, such as a handful of almonds or a piece of string cheese. Those potato chips and sugary cereals will seem less alluring if you're not hungry.

Shop the perimeter

Spend more time shopping the perimeter of your supermarket—where you'll find the produce, fresh lean meats, seafood, and low-fat dairy—and less in the center aisles, where the packaged junk lurks.

Nuts

8 ways to tap into their fat-blasting power

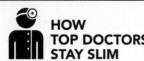

HOW TOP DOCTORS STAY SLIM

"For long workouts, I pack dried fruit and nuts in the pocket of my bike jersey. I mix dried mangoes, apricots, and dates with salted roasted almonds. The high-fiber dried fruits keep my blood sugar levels up and provide a slow, steady burn; the almonds provide healthy fats and replace the sodium I lose through sweat. I order big bags from nuts.com, so I'm always stocked up."

—JORDAN METZL, MD, a sports medicine physician at the Hospital for Special Surgery in New York City

Nuts are a prime example of why calories aren't the only thing that matters on the nutrition panel. Half a cup of pistachios packs 346 calories, and the same amount of almonds costs you 411 calories. That sounds sky-high—and for many dieters, it is enough reason to banish nuts entirely. But before you send nuts to the supermarket graveyard, consider this: In a recent Swedish study, people who snacked on 1,360 calories' worth of peanuts every day for 2 weeks didn't gain any weight around their waists and actually saw an increase in their resting metabolic rate. The fatty acids in peanuts elevate metabolism, protecting against weight gain.

Nuts are especially rich in an unsaturated fat called oleic acid, shown to fight off hunger, as well as superfilling protein. It's no wonder that dieters who snacked on pistachios lost more weight than pretzel eaters in a recent study. Keep in mind: This isn't a license to eat nuts with abandon, since your overall calorie intake still matters. But we are giving you permission—even encouraging you—to add unsalted nuts to your daily diet.

■ **TAKE YOUR NUTS TO GO** To avoid grabbing convenience-store snacks, plan ahead and pack a handful of unsalted nuts to carry on the go. You can even stash a zipper-lock bag of nuts in your glove box for on-the-road eating or in your desk drawer for office emergencies.

BONUS BENEFIT!

Some nuts, such as peanuts, almonds, pecans, and cashews, are rich in plant sterols, which have been shown to help lower cholesterol. Nuts also contain fiber, another cholesterol-taming agent.

■ **CONTROL YOUR PORTIONS** Since nuts are high in calories, it's essential that you monitor your portion sizes. According to the USDA, a serving of nuts is 1 ounce, or about a handful. If you struggle to keep your snacking under control, use the chart on page 218 and physically count out an ounce of nuts. Pour them onto a plate, and eat them one at a time.

■ **STOCK UP ON NUT BUTTERS** Calling nut butter a diet food may seem crazy, since it's high in fat and calories. However, it has the perfect combination of fiber and protein to fill you up for hours, so you end up eating less overall. Plus, nut butters taste indulgent, which can help you fight cravings and stick to your plan. If you choose a natural nut butter, the spreadable stuff is just as healthy as actual nuts. That makes it the ideal addition to your sandwich, a perfect partner for sliced fruit, or even a healthy snack by itself. In fact, a snack that includes peanut butter can help you stay full for 2½ hours, compared to only 30 minutes for a carb-heavy snack, a recent Purdue University study found. Stick to 2-tablespoon portions, about the size of a golf ball, to keep your calories in check. If you struggle with spoon-to-mouth syndrome, try single-serve packs. (For a nut butter buying guide, see page 159.)

■ **ADD NUTS TO EVERYTHING!** Nuts are a great snack on their own. But they're also the perfect way to ramp up the protein and fiber content of other foods. A few ideas: Stir chopped nuts into oatmeal or yogurt, pair peanut butter with an apple or banana, sprinkle nuts on a salad, or add nuts to the occasional baked good. If you do work them into your meal, make sure to limit your consumption of other high-fat foods.

■ **EAT THEM BOILED** A recent Alabama A&M University study compared the antioxidant content of boiled, roasted, and raw nuts and found that boiled peanuts pack four times the antioxidant punch of other varieties. Boiling transfers antioxidants from the shell to the nut, explains study author Lloyd Walker, PhD. To make your own boiled nuts, simply drop raw peanuts (in the shell) in boiling water for 30 minutes.

■ **PAIR NUTS WITH OTHER PROTEIN** Nuts are an excellent source of protein. However, they contain plant protein, which is "incomplete." That means it doesn't contain all of the

NUT (RAW)	NUMBER OF NUTS (1-OUNCE SERVING)	NUTRITION
Pistachios	49	159 calories 13 g fat (2 g saturated) 3 g fiber 6 g protein
Almonds	23	163 calories 14 g fat (1 g saturated) 3.5 g fiber 6 g protein
Hazelnuts	21	178 calories 17 g fat (1 g saturated) 3 g fiber 4 g protein
Peanuts	35	161 calories 14 g fat (2 g saturated) 2 g fiber 7 g protein
Brazil nuts	6	186 calories 19 g fat (4 g saturated) 2 g fiber 4 g protein
Walnuts	14 halves	185 calories 18 g fat (2 g saturated) 2 g fiber 4 g protein
Macadamia nuts	11	204 calories 21 g fat (3 g saturated) 2 g fiber 2 g protein
Pine nuts	167	191 calories 19 g fat (1 g saturated) 1 g fiber 4 g protein
Cashews	18	157 calories 12 g fat (2 g saturated) 1 g fiber 5 g protein
Pecans	19 halves	196 calories 20 g fat (2 g saturated) 3 g fiber 3 g protein

essential amino acids, as animal protein does. The simple fix is to make sure you eat meat, eggs, and dairy along with your nuts. Or pair nuts with other sources of plant protein, such as beans and whole grains, to expand your range of amino acids.

■ **BUY IN-SHELL VARIETIES** To slow your snacking, munch on nuts that you have to crack one by one. Eastern Illinois University scientists found that people ate only 125 calo-ries' worth of pistachios when given the in-shell variety, compared to 211 calories when given naked pistachios. Cracking nuts slows you down, thus giving you more time to realize you're full, the scientists say.

■ **SAVOR YOUR NUTS** Chew slowly: Research shows this can help boost your satiety. In fact, one study found that the longer you chew almonds, the more satisfying their healthy fats become.

DOES POURING THE OIL OFF OF NATURAL NUT BUTTER CUT SIGNIFICANT CALORIES?

This will slash a few calories, but probably not enough to make a noticeable difference on the scale, says Keri Glassman, RD, founder of NutritiousLife.com. Besides, the fats in nut butters are the healthy unsaturated kind, which not only add flavor to your spoonful but also help keep you full. Your best bet is simple portion control: Measure out a single 2-tablespoon serving (or half serving) of nut butter, since it's tough to judge by sight alone.

Super Snack Alert!

How can you make a handful of nuts instantly more satisfying? It's easy: Roast and season them. Spray an ounce of nuts—almonds are especially delicious prepared this way—with non-stick cooking spray, and bake at 400°F for 5 to 10 minutes. Remove and sprinkle with one of these tongue-teasing combinations:

Spicy: chili powder + cayenne + black pepper
Sweet: unsweetened cocoa powder + ground cinnamon + a little brown sugar

Portion Control

22 tips to avoid overeating

Is the pat of butter on your toast no bigger than the tip of your thumb? Do you eat your lunch on a salad plate? Are you able to stop after one fist-size serving of spaghetti? If you answered no to any of these questions, your portion sizes may be derailing your diet.

As kids, we're taught to clean our plates at every meal. So it's no small wonder that we grow up to believe we have to finish whatever's in front of us, even if it's supersize. That's a tough habit to break—and a scary one, considering the inflated portions we're now facing. Fortunately, you don't have to rely on your resolve alone. Simple strategies—for example, switching your dishes or even painting your dining room—can help you push back the plate. Watch as the weight falls off: A study in the journal *Obesity Research* found that practicing portion control is the most effective strategy to help you shed the pounds.

■ **PLATE IT** If you eat straight out of the box or bag—especially while standing at the kitchen counter—you're more likely to overdo it. Even if you're just snacking, serve your food on a plate or in a bowl. That way, you can more easily gauge how much you're eating.

■ **CUT IT IN HALF** Slice that sandwich in half. In a recent French study, researchers found that people who were given the same snack, either whole or cut into halves, consumed half as much when eating the sliced-up snack. One explanation: People may consider the *number* of items, not the size of them, on their plate.

■ **SWITCH HANDS** Eating with your non-dominant hand sounds silly (and messy). But it can actually help you pay attention to what—and how much of it—is going down your gullet. When you're mindful of what you eat, you'll probably consume less.

■ **SHRINK YOUR MENU** Call it the buffet effect. When there are a variety of foods on your plate, you may eat up to 40 percent more than when given a single dish, a study in the *Journal of Consumer Research* found. Color, smell, and taste—all the sensory input can prevent you from noticing that you're full. "When exposed to different types of foods, you actually eat more because of all the different tastes and textures," says Marjorie

12 EASY WAYS TO ESTIMATE SERVING SIZE

ONE SERVING OF . . .

Cooked pasta/rice = a tight fist

Chicken breast = the palm of your hand + 4 of your fingers

Fruit/starchy vegetables = a tight fist

Sausage link = a shotgun shell

Butter/mayo = the tip of your thumb

Mashed potatoes = half an apple

Cheese cubes = 4 dice

Ice cream = a tennis ball

Chicken soup = a baseball

Salad dressing = a golf ball

Lasagna = 2 hockey pucks

Beef = deck of cards

Freedman, PhD, an associate professor of nutrition at San José State University. Stock your pantry with only one "cheat" food, then load up on a variety of fruits and veggies. That way, you'll be less inclined to binge on junk and more inclined to fill your plate with a rainbow of produce.

■ **MAKE YOUR OWN SNACK PACKS** What do Oreos, Pringles, and Twinkies have in common? They're sold in bite-size, 100-calorie portions. Don't be sucked in: A study in the *Journal of Consumer Research* found that restrained eaters—those who consciously control what they eat—consumed 91 percent more calories when given mini cookies packaged in small bags compared to larger cookies in bigger bags. One reason: Small bites in portion-controlled containers seem like "diet" food—even if they're junk—which may compel you to overeat, says study author Maura Scott, PhD. Dole out small portions of your favorite snacks into zipper-lock bags instead. Since the food isn't deceptively small, you won't experience the 100-calorie snack pack effect. A perfect combination: ⅓ cup Kashi GoLean cereal, 1 teaspoon dried berries, plus 1 tablespoon of slivered almonds.

■ **WRITE IT DOWN** Keeping a food log makes you more aware of how much you're putting into your mouth. And that makes it easier to keep your portions in check. Think about it: Who wants to write down "half a pan of brownies"? That's embarrassing, even if it's for your eyes only.

■ **OPT FOR WHOLE FRUIT** A cup of orange juice costs you 122 calories. Grape juice contains even more. That's not to mention the total lack of fiber and overload of sugar you'll find in most juices. Switch to whole fruit: It's not only more nutritious than juice, since it contains fiber, but is also preportioned so you don't overdo it.

■ **WATCH WHAT YOU EAT** Don't clear the table after each course. The sight of messy plates may help you stop eating, a recent Cornell University study suggests. The researchers watched people as they ate chicken wings at a Super Bowl party and found that when the bones were left on the table, the diners downed 27 percent fewer wings. Evidence of the damage you've done may sound your internal "I've had enough" alarm, the scientists say.

■ **FORGET FAMILY STYLE** Fill your plate from the stovetop. This may help you eat up to 35 percent less than if you shovel from a serving dish on the table, say Cornell University researchers. "It makes people think twice about whether they want to have that second, third, or fourth helping," says study author Brian Wansink, PhD. It's simple: If you can see food, you're more likely to eat it.

■ **GRAB A MEASURING CUP** Always measure these foods: rice, cereal, peanut butter, oil, dried fruit, and hummus. They're tough to eyeball, plus they can be pretty dense with calories. For foods you eat every day, like cereal, try keeping a measuring cup in the box to remind you. If you can't keep your spoon out of the peanut butter or overdo it on dried fruit, buy individual packets.

■ **ASK FOR A DOGGIE BAG** Restaurant meals aren't designed with your diet in mind. In fact, you're most likely receiving two full servings of food—sometimes as many as three or four. As soon as your meal arrives, divide it into reasonable portions, leave one on your plate, and put the rest in a to-go box. (If you're easily tempted, ask the server to put half in a doggie bag before he or she even brings out your plate.) Chances are, the food that remains will be enough to fill you up.

OUR INFLATED PORTIONS

GRAINS

Bagel (4.5") = 4 servings

Muffin (3.5") = 3 servings

English muffin = 2 servings

Bakery cinnamon bun = 4 servings

Pancakes (four 5" cakes) = 6 servings

Tortilla (9") = 2 servings

Individual bag of tortilla chips (1.75 oz) = 2 servings

Popcorn (movie theater, medium) = 8 servings

Hamburger bun = 2 servings

STARCHY VEGETABLES

Baked potato (large) = 3 servings

French fries (medium order) = 4 servings

MEAT

Sirloin steak (8 oz) = 3 servings

Prime rib (13 oz) = 5 servings

Ham or roast beef (in deli sandwich) = 2 servings

■ **DOWNSIZE YOUR BOWLS** An oversize bowl may tempt you to inflate your portions—even if you're a healthy eater! In a Cornell University study, nutritionists who were given large bowls and scoops dished out about 50 percent more ice cream than those given smaller bowls and scoops. That's scary, since an 8-inch bowl can hold up to 1,000 more calories' worth of food than a 6-inch bowl, according to a 2011 Australian study. Your move: Use soup cups or mugs for foods you tend to gulp down, like cereal and ice cream. Save the cereal bowls for salads and broth-based soups.

■ **SHRINK YOUR SERVING DISHES** Beware the giant-size chip bowl. One study found that people eat 56 percent more when they serve themselves from a gallon-size bowl than from a half-gallon bowl. And choose ceramic over glass: Transparent containers can tempt you to eat more, compared to opaque dishes, according to a study in the *International Journal of Obesity*.

■ **SWITCH TO SMALLER PLATES** Since the 1970s, dinner plates have grown by 25 percent to an average of 12 inches in diameter. Eat off of a plate about 2 inches smaller and you'll serve yourself 22 percent fewer calories per meal, research shows.

■ **DRINK FROM A TALL GLASS** Dust off the highballs. Research shows we tend to pour less liquid into tall, narrow glasses than into short, squat ones. It's an optical illusion: Equal amounts of liquid appear more voluminous in thin glasses than in wide ones.

■ **DON'T SHOP AT WAREHOUSE SUPER-MARKETS** Buying in bulk may save you a few bucks—but can cost you serious calories. One Cornell University study found that when given a large package of noodles, sauce, and meat, people prepared nearly 25 percent more food than those given medium packages!

■ **EXERCISE BEFORE YOU EAT** Working out may blunt your craving for a heaping plate of carbs. In a new study in the journal *Appetite*, people who exercised desired smaller portions of pasta, garlic bread, and chocolate an hour afterward than those who didn't hit the treadmill.

■ **READ NUTRITION LABELS CAREFULLY** "Don't assume the amount listed is an accurate serving size for you," says Chris D'Adamo, PhD, an assistant professor of epidemiology and public health at the University of Maryland School of Medicine. Determine how much you'll actually eat, and judge the nutritional cost accordingly. And keep in mind: Serving sizes aren't standardized from, say, cereal to cereal or chip to chip. For example, a serving of Cheerios is ¾ cup, while a serving of Raisin Bran is 1 cup.

■ **BROWN-BAG IT A FEW TIMES A WEEK** If you eat out, you run the risk of overdoing it, even if you think you're controlling your portions. Restaurant food tends to be more calorie-dense than homemade fare, so even a reasonable-looking portion could be off the charts. "When you make and eat your own food, you not only control the quality and portion sizes but also reduce the amount of sugar, salt, and fat that you're consuming, which can be significantly higher in restaurant fare," says Ashley Koff, RD, a nutrition consultant based in Los Angeles. Pack your lunch at least three times per week.

■ **DRAW THE LINE AS YOU IMBIBE** A glass of wine can be a nebulous thing. What looks like one glass may actually be two or three. Invest in Wine-Trax glasses (www.wine-trax.com), which discreetly mark off 4, 6, and 8 ounces, so you can easily practice portion control. One serving is 5 ounces.

■ **PAINT YOUR WALLS** A blue dining room may help you avoid overdoing it. The color is thought to suppress appetite—in fact, one study found that people who dined in a blue room ate 33 percent less than those who ate in a yellow or red room. "Blue lights make food look less appealing, while warmer colors, especially yellow, have the opposite effect," explains Val Jones, MD, president and CEO of Better Health. "Fast-food restaurants have known and used this fact for decades, which is why almost all of them have yellowish interiors—they want you to eat more."

■ **FIGHT THE 3 P.M. CRASH** You naturally feel sluggish a few hours after lunch, when your levels of the sleep hormone melatonin begin to rise. Unfortunately, this causes your dietary defenses to drop. "The worst time of day for mindless eating: 3 p.m., when energy dips and many people find themselves making a trip to the vending machine to fill up on lots of unnecessary calories," says Mehmet Oz, MD, host of TV's *The Dr. Oz Show*. "If you're really craving a specific food, practice portion control. Acknowledge to yourself that the first taste is the best taste. Have a few bites, and then wash them down with a big glass of water. Get the taste out of your mouth, or else that drive to have more will continue."

Potatoes

6 ways to make spuds a weight-loss food

Potatoes are perhaps the most misunderstood of foods. Since the arrival of the low-carb craze, we've written off spuds as the food of couch potatoes. But the veggie itself isn't evil; it's the way we eat potatoes that does our waistlines an injustice. We slice them up and fry them into crispy, fat-coated chips and fries. We mash them with whole milk and butter or dress them in a heaping pile of sour cream, Cheddar cheese, and butter. It's no wonder a recent Harvard University study pegged potatoes and potato chips as two of the worst foods for your waistline. Processed spuds are digested like simple sugars—in other words, your body absorbs the glucose quickly, leaving you hungrier faster, the scientists say.

But, here's the thing: Eating any food in its most processed form will do a number on your figure. When boiled, baked, roasted, or mashed—without a glut of unhealthy toppings—potatoes deserve a place on your plate. They take a while to break down, so they linger in your intestines and help delay hunger pangs, says Katherine Beals, PhD, RD, an associate professor of nutrition at the University of Utah. Not only are they incredibly filling, but

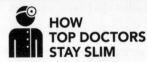

HOW TOP DOCTORS STAY SLIM

"I make veggie soup with a bag of frozen broccoli or cauliflower, a clove of garlic, a tablespoon of organic butter, sea salt, black pepper, curry powder, and a dollop of 2 percent Greek yogurt. It's also great with carrots or sweet potatoes. Vitamins in veggies are better absorbed when eaten with some fat, which is why I put butter in my soup. And it tastes great!"

—NAOMI STOTLAND, MD, a doctor at the Center for Obesity Assessment, Study, and Treatment at the University of California, San Francisco they also offer a payload of potassium, vitamin C, and fiber. University of California, Davis, researchers even found that dieters who ate five to seven servings of spuds per week dropped nearly 5 pounds in 3 months.

■ **RETHINK POTATO CHIPS** It's not just the grease that makes potato chips nutritionally costly. The salt awakens your taste buds and the crunch amplifies the flavor, so you crave more chips, explains Valerie Berkowitz, MS, RD, director of nutrition at the Center for Balanced Health in New York City. This trio of bad fats, salt, and crunchy texture is what makes it hard to stop after just a handful.

If you can't quit chips cold turkey, look for one with no more than 150 calories and 150 milligrams of sodium and at least 2 grams of fiber per ounce: Boulder Canyon Natural Foods Totally Natural Kettle Chips fit the bill. Even better, make your own at home: Lightly coat thin-sliced potatoes in olive oil, then toss them with a little salt and pepper. Roast in a 400°F oven until lightly browned and crispy. As with any snack, limit yourself to a 150- to 200-calorie portion, or about a handful.

■ **BALANCE YOUR SPUDS** Potatoes become perilous when they're the only vegetable in your diet. It's okay to eat the tubers in moderation—consider them one of your three daily servings of starch—but you also need to consume plenty of nonstarchy veggies. That's virtually any vegetable besides potatoes and corn. If you already have a grain on your plate,

consider swapping in a nonstarchy option for your side of potatoes. For example, trade in cauliflower for mashed potatoes. It tastes starchy but is actually low in carbs. Simply zap fresh or frozen cauliflower in the microwave, spritz it with olive oil, stir in a little half-and-half, and puree in a food processor. Season with salt, pepper, and roasted garlic to taste. Turnips and rutabagas are also perfect potato substitutes.

■ **SAVE THE SKIN** Set down the peeler: The majority of potatoes' nutrients—vitamin C, potassium, fiber—reside in the skin. In fact, the skin houses nearly 70 percent of the fiber! If you hate the taste, try lightly brushing your spuds with olive oil before baking or roasting. The oil will cause the skin to crisp, making it almost chiplike in texture.

■ **PAIR POTATOES WITH A LITTLE FAT** Loaded baked potatoes are inarguably dangerous—smothered with fatty bacon, cheese,

ARE BAKED POTATO CHIPS A HEALTHY SNACK?

Sure, they're lower in fat than regular potato chips, but switching to baked only saves you about 40 calories per serving and actually adds an extra gram of sugar. If you're craving something crunchy and low in calories, you're better off eating fiber-packed popcorn. Bonus: Popcorn eaters take in about two and a half times more whole grains than people who don't snack on the stuff, a study in the *Journal of the American Dietetic Association* reports.

THE PERFECT POTATO SALAD

Makes 7 servings

Potato salad usually consists of an unholy trinity of spuds, mayo, and sugar. Not this one. Make sure to chill your salad before serving, so you activate the potatoes' resistant starch, which can help block your body's absorption of carbs.

- 2 pounds red potatoes, quartered
- 3 tablespoons cider vinegar
- ½ cup chopped celery
- ½ cup chopped scallion (green and white parts)
- 2 tablespoons sweet pickle relish, drained
- 3 hard-cooked eggs, chopped (optional)
- ½ cup low-fat Greek yogurt
- 3 tablespoons Dijon-style mustard
- ½ teaspoon salt
- ¼ teaspoon freshly ground black pepper

1. In a medium saucepan, boil the potatoes until tender, about 15 minutes.

2. Drain the water, and while still warm, add the vinegar, celery, scallion, pickle relish, and eggs; toss gently.

3. In a separate bowl, combine the Greek yogurt, mustard, salt, and pepper. Fold into the potato mixture. Cover and chill before serving.

PER SERVING: 150 calories, 3 g fat (1 g saturated), 25 g carbs, 3 g fiber, 402 mg sodium, 7 g protein

sour cream, and butter, they're more a meal than a side dish (and an unhealthy one, at that). However, there's nothing wrong with dressing your baked potato, as long you do so in moderation. In fact, in 2011 a Finnish study showed that adding a little fat to your potatoes can help tame your body's blood sugar response to the starchy vegetable. So choose one topping for your baked potato—a small pat of butter, a conservative sprinkling of cheese, a dollop of sour cream (or Greek yogurt)—and stop there.

■ **CONTROL YOUR PORTIONS** One medium baked potato has only about 161 calories, plus 4 grams of belly-filling fiber. Problem is, when potatoes are diced, sliced, or mashed, it can be tough to tell exactly how many spuds you're consuming. Your guide: A serving of potatoes should be about the size of your fist.

Potatoes are loaded with kukoamines, a type of plant chemical that can help lower your blood pressure, according to USDA research. Plus, a medium-size potato offers 20 percent of your daily potassium, another known hypertension fighter.

■ **GOBBLE SWEET POTATOES** Unlike white potatoes, which we tend to fry and load up with butter, sweet potatoes are typically eaten in an unadulterated state. This may explain why the orange guys have a much healthier reputation than their white brethren. But, really, the two have complementary nutritional differences: Sweet potatoes have more fiber and vitamin A, while white potatoes are higher in iron, magnesium, and potassium. Your diet has room for both types of spud, as long as you keep 'em out of the fryer. (Yes, even sweet potato fries are bad for you.)

■ **GOBBLE PURPLE ONES, TOO** Early man ate about 800 different plant foods, compared to modern man's measly 20. "We evolved expecting a mix of vegetables from diverse sources," says Susan Bowerman, MS, RD, assistant director of the UCLA Center for Human Nutrition. "When you eat exotic vegetables, you introduce a wider range of health-promoting compounds to your antioxidant defense system." Switching from white to sweet potatoes isn't the only to way to expand your repertoire of spuds. Cook up a batch of Peruvian purple potatoes, which get their color from anthocyanins—the same brain-boosting antioxidants found in blueberries. To preserve the antioxidants and bold color, steam and dress your purple potatoes with olive oil and dill. Hint: Pair them with grilled salmon for a delicious dinner.

Protein

15 secrets to dropping the pounds with protein

The moment it leaves your fork, protein starts winnowing your waistline. First, you have to chew it—and that alone can boost the satisfaction factor of your meal. But the benefits of protein don't stop once you swallow: You burn more calories breaking down protein than you do carbs or fat. "The body has to work harder to process it because it contains nitrogen, which is metabolically expensive," says Ronald Deitrick, PhD, director of exercise science at the University of Scranton. The nitrogen has to be stripped away and eliminated by your liver—and that requires calories. Protein-rich fare also lingers in your stomach—it can take up to 4 hours to digest—so you feel fuller longer.

One problem: Most of us never consider the protein content of the foods we eat. In 2011, a study in the *Journal of the American Dietetic Association* reported that most people stop to read only the first five lines of the nutrition panel: servings, calories, total fat, saturated fat, and trans fat. Bad idea, since protein may be the most important factor in determining how full you feel after a meal. Fullness can prevent overeating, ultimately leading to weight

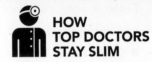

HOW TOP DOCTORS STAY SLIM

"I keep protein-packed energy bars in my briefcase and desk. I use these as quick snacks midmorning and midafternoon so I don't get overly hungry."

—DAVID SARWER, PhD, a psychologist at the University of Pennsylvania's Center for Weight and Eating Disorders loss. In a 12-week study in the journal *Nutrition Metabolism,* dieters who began consuming 30 percent of their calories from protein reduced their overall daily intake by nearly 450 calories and lost about 11 pounds—without taking any other dietary measures.

Make it your goal to include protein in every meal or snack, no matter the size. "We have separate appetites for protein, fat, and carbohydrates, and when we don't get enough protein, we keep eating in an attempt to attain our target level," says Alison Gosby, PhD, of the University of Sydney. Meeting your quota will not only satisfy you for hours but it will also give you a metabolic jolt. Research shows that protein can boost your postfeeding calo-

THE PROTEIN BAR PICKER

Protein bars sound like a healthy snack. But if you're not careful, you could end up with a bar that's nothing more than a glorified candy bar. "Energy bars are typically designed for athletic performance and contain around 300 calories and lots of sugar," says Cynthia Finley, RD, a clinical dietician at the Johns Hopkins Weight Management Center. Although 300 calories is reasonable for a meal-replacement bar, you should stick to fewer than 200 for a snack. Then check for . . .

Protein: 6 grams or more

Since most bars are formulated for athletes, protein is generally the primary ingredient. Athletes eat it to build muscle—but it has the side benefit of fueling your calorie-burning furnace and silencing a growling stomach. All good things, right? Prioritize whey protein, a dairy-derived protein thought to blast body fat more effectively than other types. Steer clear of soy.

Total fat: 8 grams of fat or less

A little healthy fat gives your bar some flavor and helps keep you full. Look for heart-healthy unsaturated fats from nuts, seeds, and peanut butter (also great sources of protein). Aim for 3 grams or less of saturated fat.

Trans fats: zero grams

Even if the nutrition panel says "0 g trans fats," scan the ingredient list for hydrogenated or partially hydrogenated oils. Food manufacturers aren't required to list trans fats if the amount is less than 0.5 gram per serving, so even those bars that claim to be free of the stuff may contain small (but still dangerous) amounts.

rie burn by as much as 35 percent! To reap protein's rewards, strive for at least 10 to 20 grams per meal, using these simple tips:

■ **FIND YOUR TARGET INTAKE** The USDA recommends that men eat 56 grams of protein per day and women 46 grams. However, most dieters will benefit from going above and beyond this, since protein helps preserve your muscle mass as you lose weight, says Donald Layman, PhD, a professor emeritus of nutrition at the University of Illinois.

Your target: Every day, consume between 0.4 and 0.8 gram per pound of your goal weight. (If you're extremely active, steer toward the higher end.) So if you want to weigh 130 pounds, you should be taking in

Carbohydrates: 35 grams or less
The carbs in your bar serve as instant energy, plus they help your body soak up the amino acids in protein. Ideally, they'll come from whole grains, such as oats or brown rice.

Sugars: 19 grams or less
The less sugar, the better. You also want to avoid high amounts of sugar alcohols, a common sugar stand-in that can cause gas and stomach pain.

Fiber: 2 grams or more
Most bars don't identify the type of fiber they contain, but many have some combination of insoluble and soluble fiber. Both take up space in your digestive tract to keep you full.

THE BEST OF THE BUNCH

Pure Organic Cranberry Orange Bar
190 calories, 8 g fat (0.5 g saturated, 0 g trans), 27 g carbs (19 g sugars, 3 g fiber), 6 g protein

Snickers Marathon Energy Crunchy Honey & Toasted Almond Bar
150 calories, 4.5 g fat (2 g saturated, 0 g trans), 22 g carbs (10 g sugars, 7 g fiber), 10 g protein

Smart for Life Green Tea Protein Bar
180 calories; 4 g fat (2 g saturated, 0 g trans); 18 g carbs (10 g sugars, 2 g fiber), 18 g protein

between 59 and 104 grams of protein per day. That sounds like a lot, but think of it this way: The more protein you eat, the fewer carbs you'll likely consume, since you still have a caloric bottom line. For more specific recommendations, see "Protein in Proportion."

■ **EMPHASIZE ANIMAL PROTEIN** Not all protein is created equal. Unlike plant protein, animal protein is "complete," so it contains all of the essential amino acids that your body can't produce on its own. (Nutritionists often refer to it as "high-quality" protein.) The best sources of animal protein are lean meats, fish, eggs, and low-fat dairy products—ideally, these foods will be your primary sources of

protein. However, you can—in fact, should— still eat sources of plant proteins, such as beans and nuts, since they confer additional nutritional benefits. If you're vegetarian, cover all of your amino acid bases by eating a combination of legumes, nuts, and grains. Keep in mind, you'll need to consume 20 to 25 percent more protein if your only sources of the nutrient are plant foods.

■ **LOAD UP AT BREAKFAST** The star of your morning meal should be protein. By replacing carb-heavy fare—think pancakes, waffles, bagels—with protein-rich foods, you'll feel fuller and satisfied longer. In fact, a study in the journal *Obesity* found that eating a protein-rich breakfast may help increase fullness and stifle cravings later in the day. One problem: Most of us consume the majority of our protein *after* 6:00 p.m., say University of Illinois scientists.

Sure, cereal and bagels are convenient. But so are eggs—perfect your technique, and you could whip up an omelet in just a couple of minutes. It's worth it: In a study in the *International Journal of Obesity*, dieters who ate eggs for breakfast at least five times a week for 5 weeks lost 65 percent more weight than bagel eaters. Any approach will do, whether it's an omelet, scrambled, or poached. (If you're on the go, you can even swing by McDonald's for an Egg McMuffin. Seriously.) Pump up your protein intake even more with lean breakfast meats, such as ham or Canadian bacon, and low-fat dairy. Ideally, you'll pack in

---

PROTEIN IN PROPORTION

Protein is an easy way to fill your belly—fast. But it also serves another important purpose that extends beyond your appetite: Protein repairs and creates skin, organ, and muscle cells. The amount your body requires depends on how often and intensely you damage those cells through exercise, says nutritionist Cassandra Forsythe, PhD.

GENERAL PROTEIN RECOMMENDATIONS BASED ON ACTIVITY
(grams per pound of goal body weight)

Sedentary adults:	0.4 g/lb
Recreational athletes:	0.5 g/lb
Strength athletes:	0.5–0.9 g/lb*
Endurance athletes:	0.5–0.6 g/lb

*Not all experts agree.

Source: Marie Dunford and J. Andrew Doyle, *Nutrition for Sport and Exercise*, 2nd edition

30 grams at breakfast, roughly the amount in two eggs and a cup of cottage cheese.

■ **SPREAD OUT YOUR INTAKE** Breakfast is an ideal time to load up on protein—but you shouldn't try to cram an entire day's worth of protein into a single meal. Your body can only process so much protein at a time. A recent University of Texas study found that eating 30 grams of protein in one meal confers just as much benefit as scarfing 90 grams. Your body is like a gas tank, says study author Douglas Paddon-Jones, PhD. "There's only so much you can put in to maximize performance." Make protein a priority every single time you eat, even if it's just a snack.

■ **STICK TO PROPER SERVING SIZES** You want to eat as much protein as possible, but remember, you still have to consider calories. A serving of meat is 3 ounces, about the size of a standard deck of cards. The same amount of fish is the size of a checkbook, and an ounce of cheese is about as big as your thumb.

■ **BULK UP YOUR BEAN COUNT** Beans may be best known for their gas-inducing effect. But there *is* a positive side to the legumes: They're loaded with appetite-taming protein (and fiber). Problem is, most of us neglect beans unless they're in the form of chili or sugary baked beans. With their meaty, satisfying texture, they're the perfect addition to whole grain pasta, brown rice, salad, or soup. The highest protein picks? White, pinto, and kidney beans.

■ **OFFSET CARBS WITH PROTEIN** Even if you don't follow the Atkins prescription and make protein the bulk of your diet, you can still use protein to your weight-loss advantage. If you're in a pinch where only refined carbs—white bread or pasta, for example—are available, offset the damage by pairing them with protein. This will help nix a blood sugar spike-and-crash. Likewise, you can upgrade even the healthiest of carbs, such as those in whole grains, by partnering them with protein. For example, you can boost the satiety of your whole-grain pasta by stirring extralean ground turkey into the sauce. Or complement the natural sugars in fruit with a dose of peanut butter. The carbs give you instant energy, while the protein helps sustain you for hours to come.

■ **STOCK UP ON CHICKEN BREAST** Chicken isn't the fastest dinner to prepare—which can be a problem when your stomach is complaining. However, boneless, skinless chicken breast is high in protein, superlean, and amazingly cheap, making it the perfect base for any meal. Your solution: Cook up a few grilled or roasted chicken breasts on Sunday to last you through the week; store them in a resealable container in your fridge and heat 'em as you need 'em. Need some inspiration? Try dicing your chicken up in a stir-fry, top it with salsa, rub it with spices, or coat it in crushed nuts. The options are endless, so you'll never fall into a dinner rut.

■ **BEFRIEND YOUR BLENDER** What's the difference between a milkshake and a smoothie? One word: protein. Whereas shakes rely on calorie-dense ice cream, healthy smoothies are based around low-fat, protein-rich yogurt. No need to stop at yogurt, though: Inject extra protein by adding a tablespoon of nut butter or a scoop of whey protein powder to your smoothie. USDA scientists recently found that consuming 55 grams of whey protein a day for 23 weeks can leave you 4 pounds lighter than if you'd eaten those calories in carbs. (For easy smoothie recipes, see page 416.)

■ **MUNCH ON NUTS** Don't be deterred by the calories in nuts. Those calories come largely from protein and healthy fats—both of which promote fullness and prevent overeating. In fact, USDA researchers recently found that eating pistachios may help you reach your weight-loss goal. For a simple, protein-packed snack, spray a handful of nuts with nonstick cooking spray, then bake at 400°F for 5 to 10 minutes. Remove and sprinkle with spices, such as cinnamon, chili powder, or even garlic powder.

■ **EAT PROTEIN BEFORE EXERCISE** Preworkout calories fuel your body for optimal performance. But not just any bite will do: You should eat a 150- to 200-calorie snack that contains both protein and carbs, such as peanut butter and fresh fruit. Not only will this energize you during your workout, but it may also boost your burn. In a Syracuse University study, people who sipped on a protein/carb shake before working out experienced a greater spike in their metabolism than when they only consumed carbs—and the effect lasted throughout the next day! One reason: Properly fueling up limits the effects of cortisol, a stress hormone released during intense exercise that tells your body to store fat.

Ideally, you'll eat your preworkout snack about an hour before you hit the gym. If you're crunched for time, grab a protein/carb shake, since your body can break down liquids more quickly than solids. Try mixing a single scoop of protein powder with low-fat milk or water, or sip on a premade shake.

■ **. . . AND AFTERWARD** Your postworkout snack should essentially match what you ate beforehand. The amino acids in protein help your body repair and build new muscle; carbs slow the breakdown of protein, also encouraging muscle growth. "When you work out, your muscles are primed to respond to protein," says Jeff Volek, PhD, RD, an exercise and nutrition scientist at the University of Connecticut, "and you have a window of opportunity to promote muscle growth." Remember, the more muscle you have, the more calories you burn, even while doing nothing.

Try sipping on a glass of low-fat chocolate milk—a study in the *Journal of the American College of Nutrition* found that the sweet stuff is a perfect postworkout drink. "It has the ideal ratio of carbs to protein for recovery," says Molly Kimball, RD, of Ochsner's Elmwood Fitness Center in New Orleans. Or if you want to make it a meal, grab a turkey

5 PROTEIN-PACKED SNACKS

Not big on bars? There are plenty of other protein-rich bites you can grab on the go.

Beef jerky

Forget whatever you think you know about beef jerky. It's packed with protein and won't raise your levels of insulin, a hormone that signals your body to store fat. Sure, some brands are full of high-sodium ingredients, but you can also find chemical-free, lower-sodium products, such as Gourmet Natural Beef Jerky. It's made with grass-fed beef, so it has higher levels of omega-3 fatty acids than most jerky. Or try turkey jerky, like Oh Boy! Oberto All Natural Teriyaki Turkey Jerky, which is minimally processed and offers 11 grams of protein per serving.

Pork rinds

Pork rinds are one of the most underappreciated snacks on the shelf. A single serving contains zero carbs, 17 grams of protein, and 9 grams of fat—a better nutritional profile than any bag of potato chips. What's more, 43 percent of the fat is unsaturated, and most of that is oleic acid—the same good-for-you fat in olive oil. Try J&J Critters Microwave Pork Rinds, which are cooked and puffed in a microwave instead of in a deep fryer, making them leaner than regular pork rinds.

Greek yogurt

Low-fat Greek yogurt is the stuff of the gods: It's loaded with protein, low in calories, and superportable. Stick to reduced-fat, plain varieties, and stir in fresh fruit or whole-grain cereal for a shot of flavor.

Hard-cooked eggs

They don't call it "the incredible, edible egg" for nothing. Hard-cooked eggs are not only convenient, but they pack 6 grams of protein and are only 78 calories apiece. Don't sweat the fat: It's primarily the healthy unsaturated kind.

String cheese

String cheese isn't just for kids. With lots of protein for very few calories, it's the perfect snack to hold you over between meals. Stick to reduced-fat string cheese, such as Weight Watchers Natural Light Smoked Mozzarella String Cheese.

sandwich on whole-wheat bread with a piece of fruit.

■ **STAVE OFF HUNGER BETWEEN MEALS** If you're starving at 10:00 a.m., it's perfectly acceptable to have a snack—as long as it includes protein. Pack an extra hard-cooked egg or string cheese in your bag, or store 1-ounce servings of nuts or individual peanut butter packets in your desk drawer. For extra hunger-fighting power, pair your protein-rich snack with fiber, such as a piece of fresh fruit or celery. The combo also makes an ideal afternoon snack.

■ **SLURP YOUR PROTEIN** Soup shouldn't be reserved for sick days. Often spiked with sources of lean protein, such as chicken and beans, it's the perfect addition to any meal. Choose a soup that's based around legumes, lean meat, and veggies, and make sure the amount of sodium isn't outrageous—no more than 300 milligrams.

■ **UPGRADE YOUR GRAINS** Did you know you can cover your carb *and* protein bases with a single whole grain? Meet quinoa, a South American grain that contains more hunger-taming protein (and fewer carbs) than almost any whole grain. Unlike most plant-based proteins, it's a complete protein, so it contains all of the essential amino acids. Try cooking up a batch of quinoa instead of run-of-the-mill brown rice or pasta. To deepen its flavor, toast it in a skillet in oil over low heat before cooking, says Carol Fenster, PhD, president of Savory Palate, a cookbook company. Hemp seed and buckwheat are also complete proteins.

Snacking

25 ways to manage your munchies

Americans love snacking. And we're doing it all wrong. In 2011, Americans dropped $3.65 billion on potato chips and $4.25 billion on cookies, while spending on apples and oranges totaled little more than $1 billion. "Everyone is constantly eating, especially foods that are convenient to buy and hold," says Phil Lempert, a food-industry analyst in Santa Monica, California. Unfortunately, it's these foods that are most often laden with bad fats, sugar, and sodium. No wonder the obesity rate among American adults has more than doubled in recent decades.

Snacking itself isn't to blame for the obesity crisis. In fact, if you choose the right between-meal bites, munching can actually elevate your weight loss. It can help you avoid feeling famished, reducing your risk of a pantry raid. Follow these guidelines to snack smartly and lose weight faster:

■ **CAP YOUR CALORIES** Snacking won't make you fat. What will? Allowing your snacks to morph into meals. Unfortunately, this is exactly what many of us are doing. According to a study in the *Journal of Nutrition*, Americans consume a quarter of their calories from snacks and drinks—a third more than in 1977. And

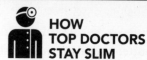

HOW TOP DOCTORS STAY SLIM

"Snacking on healthy foods between meals helps me not overeat at meals. I am always starving at 10:00 a.m. and want to eat my lunch. If I eat an apple or banana or a handful of nuts, I can wait until noon. I eat three meals a day and usually two or three snacks. I try not to snack at all after dinner, but I will occasionally have fruit if I'm really hungry before bed."

—**NAOMI STOTLAND, MD,** a doctor at the Center for Obesity Assessment, Study, and Treatment at the University of California, San Francisco as the size of our snacks grows, so do our waistlines. It's perfectly acceptable to snack throughout the day, as long as you limit your portions to 200 calories, two times a day.

■ **FOLD IN PROTEIN AND FIBER** A truly healthy snack is built around protein and fiber, a nutritional duo that helps you feel fuller longer. (Notice neither is found in that bag of Skittles.) The benefits extend well past snack time—research shows that eating protein can temporarily elevate your calorie burn by 35 percent. Step 1: Pick your protein. Natural peanut butter, nuts, low-fat cheese or Greek yogurt, hummus, and black bean dip are all smart choices. Step 2: Choose your fiber. Look to fruit, veggies, or whole grain crackers.

■ **SNACK BEFORE DINNER** If your parents forbade you from snacking before dinner, it's time to break their rules. Eating a few hours before mealtime can actually help you avoid overeating—especially if you plan to eat late or at a restaurant where temptations abound. Around 4:00 p.m., grab a healthy snack that contains fiber and protein to help hold you over. Try an apple with natural peanut butter or low-fat cheese. Likewise, if you're anticipating a late night with friends, grab a snack before you head out. That way, you'll be less tempted to indulge in greasy bar food.

■ **BANISH THE CANDY BOWL** The most dangerous way to snack is mindlessly—and nothing sets you up to do so like a candy dish. As your hand moves from bowl to mouth, your brain may not register that you're eating, so it fails to send out satiety signals. Before long, you've housed half a bowl of M&M's and don't even feel full. "We eat with our eyes," explains Brian Wansink, PhD, director of the Cornell University Food and Brand Lab. "Having food in plain sight tempts people to eat every time they look at it." That, as you'd imagine, will lead to weight gain. Ditch the candy dish and, instead, fill a bowl with fresh fruit—a much healthier, preportioned snack that's okay to eat lots of.

PICK YOUR POPCORN

Too often, microwave popcorn is loaded with calories, sodium, trans fats, and a slurry of preservatives. If you go the prepackaged route, choose popcorn made with olive or canola oil (and no hydrogenated oils), or pick a plain version, like Newman's Own 94% Fat Free Microwave Popcorn, and season it yourself. Even better, pop your own fresh batch on the stovetop:

1. Heat 2 tablespoons canola oil and a few popcorn kernels in a large pot over medium-high heat. When the kernels start popping, remove the pot and add ¼ cup kernels and ½ teaspoon kosher salt. Put on the lid, return to the heat, and count to 20, allowing the popcorn and oil to reach the same temperature; otherwise some of the kernels will burn.

2. Gently move the pot back and forth over the burner; with your free hand, hold the lid like a shield over the pot, leaving it slightly ajar. Heat the popcorn until you notice a delay of several seconds between pops, about 3 minutes total.

3. Add flavor. Try this delicious combination: ¼ cup grated Parmesan, 1 teaspoon fresh thyme leaves, 1 minced clove garlic, and ½ teaspoon freshly ground black pepper.

■ **REDEFINE SNACKING** If you think of snacks as indulgences, you're headed for trouble. Snack time isn't dessert, nor is it an excuse to stray from your normal nutritional rules, says Keri Glassman, RD, author of *The Snack Factor Diet*. Snacks should be real food—say, a packet of oatmeal with a few walnut halves or canned tuna on top of Triscuits—not the prepackaged junk so many of us resort to.

■ **SCHEDULE YOUR SNACKS** It sounds silly, but you can minimize mindless munching by booking snack appointments in your desktop calendar. When an e-reminder pops up, step away from your desk and enjoy your food. If you're aware of what you eat when, you'll be less likely to nibble all day.

■ **BE PICKY ABOUT PACKAGED FOODS** Call it the snack trap: Even the healthiest of eaters are vulnerable to packaged foods when they're in a pinch. What do we most often reach for? Chips, granola bars, pretzels, and candy. In other words, prepackaged empty carbs. Although the healthiest snacks are whole foods, which don't come in a box or bag, you can safely munch on packaged foods if you know what to choose. Look for snacks that list whole-food ingredients, such as oats, nuts, and real fruit, in the first line of ingredients. Your rule of thumb: The fewer the ingredients, the healthier the snack.

■ **DON'T BE A SUCKER FOR "DIET" SNACKS** Sugar-free pudding. Fat-free fruit chews. Reduced-fat peanut butter. By labeling foods with healthy-sounding names, manufacturers tempt you to eat more, regardless of how bad for you the snack may be. A study in the *Journal of Consumer Research* found that people consumed more of a snack described as "fruit chews" than when the identical item was labeled "candy chews." And when Cornell University scientists marked M&M's either "regular" or "low-fat," people downed 28 percent more of the "low-fat" candy. Skip the labeling hype on the front of the package and read the ingredients list and nutrition panel instead.

■ **STOCK UP ON FRUIT** What's not to love about fruit? It's portable, delicious, and preportioned. It also has an amazing nutritional profile: Fruit is high in fiber and water, which help keep you full, and offers a range of essential vitamins and minerals for relatively few calories. Don't worry about the sugars: Fruit contains the natural sugar fructose, which doesn't raise blood sugar levels like table sugar does. To avoid snacking on junk, fill your fridge with fresh fruit, and always keep a piece on hand at the office or in your purse. The more the better: In one study from Brazil, women who added three small apples to their day lost 2 pounds in 10 weeks without dieting.

■ **FOLD IN VEGETABLES** If you eat two snacks a day, make sure at least one of them features a veggie. Like fruit, vegetables are high in both water and fiber, so they fill you up for very few calories. To make your snack more satisfying, pair sliced veggies, such as cucumbers, carrots, or bell peppers, with hummus, salsa, or even a Greek yogurt–based dip.

■ **MUNCH ON NUTS** Nuts contain a righteous combination of healthy fats and protein that will keep you full and satisfied for hours. Though they may be high in calories, they're preferable to other savory snacks: In a study in the *Journal of the American College of Nutri-* *tion*, dieters who snacked on pistachios had lower body mass indexes after 12 weeks than those who munched on pretzels. Whatever nut you choose, opt for unsalted, and make sure to practice portion control. A single serving is 1 ounce, or about a handful. If you're going the

CALM SNACK CRAVINGS

Dieters have a tendency to eat around their cravings—a bite of cottage cheese here, a handful of nuts there. In other words, they eat anything but the food they desire. When all is said and done, they've racked up a 500-calorie debt, and their craving for salt or sugar or chocolate is still nagging at them. Whatever your taste buds desire, we have your solution—and you won't feel even a trace of guilt.

Chocolate
Country Choice Organic Soft Baked Double Fudge Brownie Cookie
This soft, chewy treat is made with antioxidant-rich dark chocolate chips.
Per cookie: 90 calories, 3 g fat (0.5 g saturated), 16 g carbs, 1 g fiber, 80 mg sodium, 1 g protein

Skinny Cow Low-Fat Mini Fudge Pop
Forget Fudgsicles. These delectable pops pack big fudge flavor in a portion-controlled vessel.
Per bar: 50 calories, 1 g fat (0.5 g saturated), 10 g carbs, 0 g fiber, 15 mg sodium, 1 g protein

Emerald Cocoa Roast Dark Chocolate Almonds
These nuts taste like candy, but each serving has only 1 gram of sugars.
Per serving: 100 calories, 8 g fat (0.5 g saturated), 4 g carbs, 2 g fiber, 15 mg sodium, 3 g protein

Salt
Kalamata olives
Their meaty texture and briny bite are just as satisfying as potato chips, but way better for you. Three-quarters of the fat in olives is the heart-healthy monounsaturated kind.
Per 10 olives: 90 calories, 8 g fat (1 g saturated), 4 g carbs, 2 g fiber, 460 mg sodium, 1 g protein

nut butter route, which is just as healthy as eating whole nuts, buy preportioned packs of natural peanut butter, such as Barney Butter Squeeze Packs.

■ **ADD AIR** Are you a sucker for cereal? Or salty snacks? It's okay to eat both—as long as you follow two rules: (1) Go whole grain. (2) Choose air-filled versions. For example, if you love to crunch on plain cereal, look for a puffed cereal, like Kashi 7 Whole Grain Puffs. Or if salt is what you crave, grab popcorn or Popchips instead of pretzels or potato chips.

Newman's Own 94% Fat Free Microwave Popcorn

You won't find a trace of trans fats or saturated fats in this bowl.

Per 3½ cups popped: 110 calories, 1.5 g fat (0 g saturated), 20 g carbs, 4 g fiber, 250 mg sodium, 3 g protein

Snyder's of Hanover Organic Whole Wheat & Oat Pretzel Sticks

These sticks are made exclusively with whole grains and are delightfully low in sodium, while still offering the salty crunch you crave.

Per ounce: 110 calories, 1.5 g fat (0 g saturated), 21 g carbs, 3 g fiber, 100 mg sodium, 4 g protein

Sugar

Ciao Bella Ecuadorian Passion Fruit Sorbet

This exotic fruit frozen treat is the perfect way to indulge your sweet tooth without blowing your diet.

Per ½ cup: 92 calories, 0 g fat, 22 g carbs, 0 g fiber, 4 mg sodium, 1 g protein

Popcorn, Indiana All-Natural Cinnamon Sugar Kettlecorn

All the hot-buttered satisfaction of carnival kettle corn in five simple ingredients, with no preservatives and only 7 grams of sugars.

Per 2½ cups: 130 calories, 4.5 g fat (0 g saturated), 21 g carbs, 2 g fiber, 115 mg sodium, 1 g protein

Breyers Pure Fruit Berry Swirls Bar

With only about as many calories as a small piece of fruit and 9 grams of sugars, you can truly enjoy this sweet treat guilt free.

Per bar: 40 calories, 0 g fat, 10 g carbs, 0 g fiber, 0 mg sodium, 0 g protein

Not only do these picks contain satisfying fiber, but they're also injected with air to fill your belly for fewer calories. If you nosh on air-puffed snacks, you'll be able to eat more without your gut suffering the consequences. The exception? Rice cakes. They're a poor source of fiber, vitamins, and minerals, so you should avoid them.

■ **TAKE SNACKS TO GO** Whenever you climb into your car, you're taking a chance. You'll likely pass dozens of convenience stores and fast-food joints, tempting you to fill your belly with unhealthy, grab-and-go fare. To avoid caving in a weak moment, stock your glove box with healthy, nonperishable snacks, such as 1-ounce portions of nuts, protein bars, or even beef jerky. That way, when hunger strikes on the go, you'll be prepared. Likewise, if you're headed to the mall, stow a smart snack in your purse (or pocket) so you don't have to hit up the food court.

■ **BROWN-BAG YOUR SNACKS** If you find yourself constantly battling 3:00 p.m. hunger pangs, plan ahead and keep healthy bites at your desk. This is the perfect opportunity to work in whole foods you can't easily eat on the go: instant oatmeal, canned tuna, fruit, or sliced veggies. Plan for drinks, too—sip on water all day, and if you need a flavor hit, work in healthy, low-calorie options, such as green tea or black coffee.

■ **CUT IT IN HALF** Cutting your snack in half can help you pare down your intake. In 2010, a study in the *Journal of the American*

Dietetic Association reported that people who were given the same snack, either whole or cut into halves, ate half as much when given the sliced version. It's a simple mind trick: When we're eating, we may feel satisfied based on the number of items (not the size of them) that we consume.

■ **SLURP A SMOOTHIE** When properly portioned, smoothies can be a perfect snack—they're quick, filled with fruit, and high in fat-blasting calcium. But, remember, a smoothie becomes a milkshake the instant you add ice cream. So base your shake around low-fat Greek yogurt or 1% milk. Try this tasty concoction: Blend ½ cup frozen berries with ½ cup yogurt or milk, plus ½ tablespoon of peanut butter. It's filled with fiber, protein, calcium, and healthy fats, all for fewer than 200 calories.

■ **CONTROL CRAVINGS WITH CHOCOLATE** Dark chocolate is usually reserved for dessert. But it can also be part of a sensible snack—and may even squash your cravings for junk. In a recent study from Denmark, researchers gave people either dark or milk chocolate, then 2 hours later offered them pizza. Those participants who downed the dark chocolate consumed fewer calories than the milk chocolate eaters and were also less interested in fatty, salty, and sugary foods. Try pairing a square or two of 70 percent cacao dark chocolate with fresh berries.

■ **RESIST THE SNACK-PACK TRAP** The pre-portioned snack industry is booming. In 2011,

Americans dropped more than $12 million on Snyder's 100 Calorie Pretzel Packs and $9.4 million on Cheetos 100 Calorie Packs. But be warned: These seemingly smart snacks are actually a weapon of waistline destruction. A recent study showed that people tend to eat more food and calories if the portions are presented in small sizes and packages. With smaller portions, you may not feel the need to regulate your intake, so you end up eating more than one serving. Besides, putting Cheetos into a tiny bag doesn't make them healthy. Create your own snack packs using nuts, seeds, and whole grain cereal instead.

■ **WORK FOR YOUR FOOD** If you struggle with portion control, choose snacks that require a little work: pistachios that have to be cracked, pumpkin or sunflower seeds still in their shells. You'll spend more time cracking and cleaning up than actually eating.

■ **PUT IT ON A PLATE** To avoid mindless munching, never eat from the bag or box—every snack belongs in a dish. This forces you to consider portion sizes and helps your brain register fullness.

■ **THINK BEFORE YOU EAT** A study in the *International Journal of Behavioral Nutrition and Physical Activity* showed that weighing the pros and cons of your next snack beforehand is strongly linked to weight-loss success. So rather than pressing that vending machine button without a second thought, pause and ask yourself, "Will eating this help me reach my weight-loss goals?" If the answer

is no, look for another option that you can truly feel good about.

■ **TURN OFF THE TUBE** It's *Modern Family* night. So what do you do? Grab your bag of chips and settle in for a half hour of entertainment. Be careful—you may eat more of those Lay's than you anticipated. A recent study found that TV watchers ate an average of 44 percent more potato chips while watching a program they considered entertaining. You're better off avoiding the snack/TV combination entirely; it's an invitation to eat mindlessly. But if you must, opt for a snack that won't cost you serious calories, such as plain popcorn.

■ **SNACK BEFORE YOU SWEAT** Exercising on an empty stomach lowers your blood sugar. This can switch your appetite into overdrive, so you end up gorging yourself afterward. Plus, eating the right snack before your workout can energize you and prepare your body for muscle building. Your preworkout prescription: About an hour before you hit the gym, grab a small snack that contains both carbs and protein, such as whole grain crackers and hummus or fruit and string cheese. In one study, exercisers who did this lost more than twice as much fat as those who ate nothing. Schedule your workout so it's time for a meal afterward, or grab a similar postworkout snack.

■ **SNACK CAREFULLY BEFORE BED** Before you hit up the pantry at 10:00 p.m., ask yourself: "Am I hungry or just bored?" If you are indeed hungry, go ahead and have a snack—you won't sleep well if your stomach is growling. Your go-to munchie: $\frac{1}{2}$ cup whole-grain cereal with 1% milk. In a Wayne State University study, people who snacked on cereal at least an hour and a half after dinner lost more weight in a month and ate a smaller percentage of their calories at night than non-cereal eaters. For an extra shot of fiber, top your bowl with sliced kiwifruit. In a recent Taiwanese study, insomniacs who ate two kiwis an hour before bed every night for a month conked out 35 percent faster. One explanation: Kiwis contain serotonin, a brain chemical that helps regulate your sleep cycle.

■ **LOG YOUR 8 HOURS** What could sleep possibly have to do with snacking? A lot, actually. In a University of Chicago study, people who lost 3 hours of sleep ate an extra 200 calories' worth of snacks the next day, compared to those who slept $8\frac{1}{2}$ hours. When you're short on shut-eye, you may experience a reduction in appetite-suppressing hormones and a spike in hunger-inducing ones. To ensure you snooze soundly, switch off the coffeepot at least 4 hours before bedtime and pair any late-day snacks with caffeine-free tea instead.

Soda

3 ways to kick your pop addiction

Simply put, soda is sugar water in a can—empty calories with zero redeeming nutritional value. And we're guzzling it by the gallon. A 2011 Emory University study found that the average American takes in 91 calories from added sugars in soda every day, and that sugary drinks now account for nearly 7 percent of our total calorie intake.

Unaccompanied by fiber, healthy fats, or protein, the sugar in soda spikes your blood glucose levels, triggering a flood of insulin, which tells your body to switch into fat-storing mode. That's not to mention the inevitable postsoda crash, which can leave you feeling sluggish and hungry. "People simply don't reduce their food intake when they drink their calories from soda and other beverages," says Barry Popkin, PhD, a professor of nutrition at the University of North Carolina at Chapel Hill. The upshot: Eliminating the empty calories in soda is the easiest way to instantly kick-start your weight loss. In a Johns Hopkins University study, dieters who cut liquid calories lost more weight—and kept it off longer—than those who cut food calories.

■ **DON'T BE FOOLED BY DIET SODA** Switching to diet soda *will* save you calories. But it won't necessarily help you lose weight. University of Texas researchers found that consuming as few as three diet sodas a week can raise your risk of obesity by more than 40 percent. One reason: The artificial sweeteners lurking in diet

(continued on page 248)

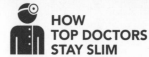

HOW TOP DOCTORS STAY SLIM

"I weigh and measure the food I eat, so I don't overpour the olive oil, salad dressing, or wine. When I go out to eat, my boyfriend and I split an entrée (unless we're in Paris—hey, sometimes prix fixe meals are too good to pass up!). I also exercise 6 days a week: I tend to do a 40-minute run and some sort of weight training at the gym four times a week, and a mind-body fitness class, such as yoga or Pilates, once or twice a week."

—**KARA MOHR, PhD,** co-owner of Mohr Results

POP STARS

Weaning yourself off of soda? You don't have to quit flavored beverages cold turkey. Simply switch to one of these fruity concoctions and gradually ease your way toward drinking mostly water.

CHERRY-VANILLA SODA

Makes 6 servings

3 cups 100% unsweetened black cherry juice

1 vanilla bean (about 6" long)

Seltzer or soda water

1. Place the juice and vanilla bean in a medium-size saucepan. Cover and bring to a gentle boil over medium-high heat, then reduce the heat to low and simmer uncovered for 35 to 40 minutes, until the liquid has reduced to 1 cup.

2. Remove from the heat and let cool until comfortable to handle.

3. Remove the vanilla bean and chill the syrup in a sealed glass jar in the fridge. It will stay fresh for up to 2 weeks.

4. To serve, pour $\frac{1}{4}$ cup syrup into a tall glass, top with 6 to 8 ounces chilled seltzer or soda water, and stir.

PER SERVING: 80 calories, 0 g fat, 18.5 g carbs, 0 g fiber, 5 mg sodium, 1 g protein

ORANGE-MANGO-STRAWBERRY SODA

Makes 6 servings

2 cups orange-mango juice, such as Santa Cruz Organic

1½ cups frozen strawberries, thawed

Seltzer or soda water

Orange slices for garnish (optional)

1. Pour the juice into a saucepan. Cover and bring to a simmer over medium-high heat, then reduce the heat to low and simmer uncovered for 20 minutes or until the liquid has reduced to $1\frac{1}{2}$ cups.

2. Put the strawberries and their juice in a blender and pulse to roughly chop. Pour through a strainer lined with a double layer of cheesecloth and squeeze to extract as much liquid as possible.

3. Mix both juices together and chill in a sealed glass jar in the fridge. The syrup will stay fresh for up to 3 days.

4. To serve, pour ⅓ cup syrup into a tall glass, top with 6 to 8 ounces chilled seltzer or soda water, and stir. Garnish with orange slice, if desired.

PER SERVING: 63 calories, 0 g fat, 16 g carbs, 1 g fiber, 8 mg sodium, 5 g protein

RED GRAPE AND THYME SODA

Makes 6 servings

5 branches fresh thyme	1½ tablespoons real maple syrup
2 cups red grapes	Seltzer or soda water

1. Use one of the sprigs of thyme to tie the rest of the thyme into a bundle.

2. Place the thyme, grapes, and maple syrup in a medium-size saucepan. Cover and bring to a gentle boil over medium-high heat, then reduce the heat to low and simmer uncovered for 10 minutes. Break up the grapes with a wooden spoon.

3. Remove from the heat and let cool for 15 minutes.

4. Remove the thyme bundle. Pour the liquid through a strainer lined with a double layer of cheesecloth and squeeze to extract as much liquid as possible.

5. Chill in a sealed glass jar in the fridge. The syrup will stay fresh up to 3 days.

6. To serve, pour ¼ cup syrup into a tall glass, top with 6 to 8 ounces of chilled seltzer or sparkling water, and stir.

PER SERVING: 50 calories, 0 g fat, 12 g carbs, 0 g fiber, 0 mg sodium, 0 g protein soda, which are significantly sweeter than sugar, may increase your taste for sweet things, says Popkin. In fact, in a University of North Carolina study, people who swapped their favorite sugary soft drink for the diet version ate more desserts and bread than those who swapped in water.

There's also the simple fact that the more flavored beverages you drink, the less water you're probably sipping. If you're a diet soda addict, slowly wean yourself off of the stuff by mixing it with an equal part of water or club soda. Gradually reduce the amount of soda in your drink, or replace it altogether with a jigger of juice.

■ **DRINK ICE-COLD WATER INSTEAD** Research shows that people who regularly drink water take in nearly 200 fewer calories a day than those who only sip on soda. The benefit is twofold: Choosing water not only slashes calories but it may also boost your metabolism. Research shows that when your cells are properly hydrated, you burn calories more efficiently. Even better, serve your water on the rocks. In a German study, people who drank six glasses of ice-cold water a day burned an extra 50 calories.

■ **EXPLORE FLAVOR ALTERNATIVES** Sometimes you crave flavor, fizz . . . or anything but water. That's okay—just don't heed the call of the Coke machine. Try sipping on unsweetened iced tea flavored with lemon, or indulge in a small glass of low-fat chocolate milk. One study found that people were significantly more satisfied half an hour after drinking low-fat chocolate moo juice than they were after sipping on soda. Dying for fizz? Mix seltzer and ice with a shot glass–full of juice. Just make sure to avoid clear sparkling beverages that look like seltzer but contain artificial sweeteners—they're no better than diet soda.

13 Ways to Stay Slim on the Road

Even when we travel for business, we tend to eat like it's a treat, a vacation, a special occasion—and we overindulge. The key to avoiding the extra baggage that travel can add to your body is to eat normally; that is, as closely to the way you eat at home as you can. That is assuming you eat right at home!

1 SKIP THE AIRPORT SALAD

Unfortunately, even the salads at airports are not to be trusted. Often loaded with more toppings than there are greens, prepackaged salads can be a sneaky source of big-time calories. Plus, the packets of dressing tend to be high in sodium, which can lead to bloat. That's bound to make you uncomfortable in an already-tight airline seat. You're better off with a deli sandwich that's as simple as possible: meat, veggies, and whole-grain bread.

2 STASH YOUR BAGS

If you have a long layover, stow your carry-on in a locker, then tour the airport. The time will pass faster, and, more important, you'll work in a little physical activity. Just make sure to stay off of the people movers.

3 PACK YOUR SNACKS

"There seems to be an assumption that when you travel, you can't eat healthfully, so you don't even make an attempt," says exercise physiologist Monika Woolsey, MS, RD, founder of CYST Institute for Hormone Health. Nice try. To avoid junky airport or gas station bites, pack a stash of portable snacks in your bag. A few good options: 1-ounce packets of nuts, protein-rich energy bars, puffed cereal, or low-fat string cheese. If you're on the road, you can even load up a cooler in your trunk with fruit and yogurt. Hint: Pack a stash of walnuts. A study in the *Journal of the American College of Nutrition* found that their polyunsaturated fats may dampen your body's natural stress reaction— perfect when you hit a traffic jam.

4 DRINK UP

The dry air in the airplane cabin or the recirculated air in your car will inevitably make you thirsty. Bad news: Your brain can misinterpret thirst as hunger, tempting you to snack when you're not actually hungry. Dehydration can also lead to fatigue, a known trigger of mindless eating. Drink 8 ounces of water before your flight, then down another 8 ounces for every hour you're in the air. If you're traveling by car, stock your backseat with plenty of fluids for the drive.

5 BE LEERY OF IN-FLIGHT MEALS

More often than not, airline food is little more than a glorified frozen meal. That means lots of sodium and empty carbs. It's okay to dine in the air—just follow these rules: Avoid any food with "pas" in its name, like pasta or pastries. Second, make sure to choose an entrée with lean protein, such as chicken breast, fish, or sirloin steak, and prioritize vegetable-based sides over bread (or pretzels). If you want a drink other than water, choose 1% milk. The protein will help keep you full for the duration of the flight.

6 SEEK FRESH FOOD

Yes, the gas station is only half a mile off the highway. But chances are, if you drive just a little farther, you'll encounter a grocery store. And there you'll find fresh, healthy foods, such as yogurt, fruit, and deli sandwiches. You don't have to eat Big Macs and Ho-Hos for every meal on the road.

7 BOOK THE TOP FLOOR

Ask for a room with a view. The higher up your hotel room, the more stairs you have to climb. That gives you the perfect opportunity to exercise each time you come and go from your room.

8 ELIMINATE TEMPTATION

Staying at a major hotel? Ask that your minifridge be stocked for a diabetic. This is a common request, and most hotels will oblige by swapping out sugary junk foods for milk, cheese, vegetables, and fruit, says Cynthia Finley, RD, a clinical dietician at the Johns Hopkins Weight Management Center. You can also create your own mini-bar. Ask the concierge for directions to the nearest supermarket, then stock up on healthy snacks. You'll spare your wallet and your waistline.

9 CONTROL YOUR CARBS

When you travel, you inevitably dine out. Too often, that means overfilled breadbaskets and other empty-carb fare. When whole grains and nonstarchy vegetables aren't an option, go ahead and eat the refined carbs; you can offset some of the damage by ordering a lean-meat entrée, such as chicken, fish, or steak with "loin" in the name. Just make up for your carbohydrate crime later: Each time you indulge in a carb-heavy meal, try to have a least three lower-carb meals or snacks before dipping into that well again.

10 DINE WITH A NEW CLIENT

If you're traveling on business, invite a new client to dinner with you. In a recent study, State University of New York at Buffalo researchers found that men consumed 35 percent fewer calories when eating with strangers than when breaking bread with friends.

11 SLOW YOUR SIPPING

When you're on vacation, it's easy to justify an extra margarita. But, remember, umbrella drinks are usually the most caloric, thanks to a heavy load of sugar. Enjoy your favorite fruity concoction as a treat after lunch or dinner, but rein in your intake the rest of the day. While you're lounging by the pool, for example, order water or seltzer with lime or a small all-fruit smoothie instead of another margarita.

12 SCHEDULE WORKOUTS

Pencil in your workout times, even when you're traveling. And refuse to fill that slot with another activity. If you treat exercise like an essential item on the itinerary, you're far more likely to stick to your fitness plan—which will also make it easier to jump back into your normal routine once you're home again.

13 TAKE ADVANTAGE OF THE SPA

If your hotel has a spa, book a massage during your stay. Studies have linked the occasional back rub to lower levels of cortisol, a hormone that can drive you to seek instant energy foods, such as empty carbs.

MAKE YOUR HOTEL ROOM YOUR GYM

There are millions of excuses for missing a workout—you're busy, the hotel gym is subpar, you're in meetings all day. None of them are valid: You can easily work in a few minutes of exercise in your hotel room, using only the resistance of your own body. "Your body weight is all you need to torch fat and build total-body muscle," says David Jack, director of Teamworks Fitness in Acton, Massachusetts. Start with these two moves (or try any of the body-weight exercises starting on page 306):

HUB SKATER HOP

Crouch over your right foot and lift your left leg off the floor behind you. Now bound to your left by pushing off with your right leg. Land on your left foot, lifting your right leg off the floor behind you. Continue hopping back and forth.

POWER SQUAT

Stand with your feet slightly beyond shoulder-width apart, toes forward, hands above your head. Simultaneously push your hips back and swing your arms down to your sides, lowering your body until your thighs are nearly parallel to the floor. Pause for 4 seconds, and then explode up to the starting position.

Sodium

12 tips to lick the salt

Your body needs sodium. It's an electrolyte, so it helps your muscles function and keeps your body hydrated. Besides, your body can't produce sodium on its own, making it an essential part of your diet. So why do we bother watching—even obsessing over—our intake? For the same reason sodium is beneficial: "Sodium acts like a sponge to help hold fluids in your blood," says Rikki Keen, RD, an adjunct instructor of dietetics and nutrition at the University of Alaska. In small doses, sodium helps your body rehydrate itself. But in large doses, sodium can cause your blood to hold too much water, forcing your heart to work harder and your blood pressure to rise. Plus, regularly overdoing it on sodium can increase your tolerance for salt, triggering cravings for it. And, unfortunately, salt-laden foods are rarely healthy—they may even cause you to retain water weight. That's a real motivation killer when you step on the scale.

The average person should consume no more than 2,300 milligrams of sodium per day, according to Institute of Medicine guidelines. That's about a teaspoon of salt. For middle-aged and older adults or people with hypertension or diabetes, the limit is even lower: 1,500 milligrams, or slightly more than ½ teaspoon per day. Most of us blow past our limit by leaps and bounds: The average American now takes in 3,400 milligrams of sodium every day! Try these strategies to tame your intake:

■ **WATCH YOUR SOUPS** Studies show that eating soup as an appetizer can help you lose weight. The heat slows you down, giving your brain more time to register fullness, and the liquid fills your belly for relatively few calories. The caveat: You should limit your slurping to low-sodium options—which can be tricky, since soups are one of the primary sources of sodium in the American diet. To be truly "low sodium," soups must contain no more than 140 milligrams of sodium per serving, according to USDA regulations. That's tough to find, although Campbell's does offer a few options. You can, however, easily find reduced-sodium soups, which have 25 percent less sodium than the original version. Look for a can with around 300 milligrams of sodium per serving, while still considering other factors, like calories and saturated fat.

■ **DON'T BE SUCKERED BY SEA SALT** Sixty-one percent of adults think sea salt is a low-sodium alternative to table salt, an American Heart Association survey found. (This may explain the roaring success of Wendy's sea-salt fries.) But, really, sea salt is no healthier than standard table salt—both are roughly 40 percent sodium, and any extra minerals that sea salt contains are in such trace amounts that the benefit is minimal (if it exists at all). One small advantage: Since sea salt's crystals are thick, you'll pick up and use less if you're sprinkling by hand.

■ **CHECK YOUR CEREALS** You probably don't expect breakfast cereals to be high in sodium. Outrageously sugary, yes. But loaded with sodium, no. You may be surprised: The sad truth is, even the healthiest-sounding cereals are often laden with ungodly amounts of salt. Wheat Chex, for example, contains an astounding 400 milligrams per cup! So before you toss that box into your cart, make sure the sodium level doesn't exceed 250 milligrams per serving.

■ **CHOOSE CANNED FOODS CAREFULLY** Processed vegetables are often canned just hours after harvest, so they tend to retain nutrients better than fresh produce. One problem: In order to keep canned goods fresh, food manufacturers have a habit of adding a heavy load of sodium to their produce. Your rule of thumb: If a canned good contains more sodium than calories, don't buy it. The same rule applies to frozen produce.

■ **OPT FOR UNSALTED NUTS** Healthy fats and protein make nuts naturally savory. That means you don't need a liberal coating of salt for them to satisfy your belly (or your cravings). Spare your arteries and stick to unsalted varieties. You can always add your own flavoring, whether it's garlic powder, cinnamon, or even cocoa powder.

■ **HIDE THE SALTSHAKER** It can be tough to gauge how much salt you're actually adding when you use a shaker. So use your fingers to add just a pinch. You'll never notice the difference in flavor, but your heart will thank you.

■ **FORGET PROCESSED FOODS** The more processed the food, the more sodium it usually contains. In fact, processed and restaurant foods account for 77 percent of the average person's sodium intake, according to Centers for Disease Control and Prevention data. Since sodium acts as both a flavor enhancer and a preservative, food scientists inject mass quantities of the stuff to make processed and restaurant foods taste better and last longer. Home-cooked meals, on the other hand, contribute only 5 percent of the sodium in the average person's diet. Your move: Stick with whole foods whenever possible, and prepare them in your own kitchen, using other flavor enhancers like pepper, herbs, lemon juice, garlic, ginger, or wine. If you do resort to packaged foods, scan labels for the phrases "low sodium" and "sodium free."

■ **FOCUS ON FRESH MEAT** Never confuse lunchmeats, hot dogs, and sausage with lean fresh meats. Since they're all highly processed, they tend to be packed with sodium, especially when canned, smoked, or cured. Opt for fresh

or frozen lean cuts that don't include sodium or salt in the ingredients list. Other signs of sodium-packed meat: labels that include the words "self-basting" or "broth." If you love lunchmeat, look for low- or no-sodium options.

■ **SAVE SALT FOR THE FINALE** You don't have to banish salt from your kitchen entirely. After all, without it, many foods would taste flat. Use this strategy to trim your intake: As you're cooking, skip the salt the recipe calls for (unless you're baking). Then if you want, add just a dash at the table, since you'll notice it more that way as opposed to adding the same

---

WHERE SODIUM HIDES

When you think of salty foods, pretzels and potato chips most likely come to mind. But have you considered that turkey on your deli sandwich? Or even the bread it's built on? In a 2012 CDC study, researchers analyzed the top sources of sodium in the average American's diet. Here's what they found:

1. Breads and rolls (7.5% of sodium intake)
2. Cold cuts/cured meats (5.3%)
3. Pizza (4.1%)
4. Poultry (4.2%)
5. Soups (4.4%)
6. Sandwiches (3.9%)
7. Cheese (3.8%)
8. Pasta dishes (3.1%)*
9. Meat dishes (3.5%)
10. Savory snacks (chips, popcorn, pretzels) (2.8%)

*Excluding macaroni and cheese

amount during cooking. Traditional baking soda and powder also contain sodium. Look for no-salt versions of these ingredients in your supermarket.

■ **PAIR SALT WITH GOOD FAT** If you're a sucker for salty snacks, it's okay to indulge every once in a while. When you do, just make sure to partner your pretzels or crackers with a little fat—a tablespoon of nut butter, a slice of avocado, a spoonful of hummus. The healthy fats slow digestion and, since they quickly fill you up, help you avoid downing the entire bag of pretzels.

■ **SCAN SALAD DRESSING LABELS** It's not just the fat in bottled salad dressings that you have to worry about. They're often loaded with sodium. As an alternative, you can use vinegar, lemon juice, or a small amount of olive oil, or simply hunt down bottled options that aren't laced with excessive amounts of salt, such as Annie's Naturals "lite" dressings.

■ **LOAD UP ON POTASSIUM** Packing in potassium may be as important as cutting back on sodium. The reason: Potassium blunts the negative effects of sodium on your blood pressure. Unfortunately, few of us consume the recommended 4,700 milligrams of potassium per day, possibly because levels in processed foods tend to be low. To work more of the mineral into your diet, load up on white beans, dates, baked potatoes, lima beans, and halibut. (For more smart sources, see page 11.)

Spices

4 ways to use flavor to fight fat

HOW TOP DOCTORS STAY SLIM

"I eat lots of protein, whole grains, produce, and heart-healthy fats like olive oil. I use spices like turmeric, ginger, and cinnamon often, and avoid processed foods and anything with added sugar. I also like Italian red wine—Montepulciano with dinner, Barolo for celebrations. This kind of diet has proven benefits for your heart and joint health."

—NICHOLAS DINUBILE, MD, an orthopedic surgeon and a clinical assistant professor of orthopedic surgery at the Hospital of the University of Pennsylvania

Jazzing up your food's flavor may lend your meal weight-loss powers. In a recent study in the *Journal of Nutrition*, people who ate dishes containing 2 tablespoons of spices—including black pepper, garlic powder, rosemary, paprika, cinnamon, and oregano—had 30 percent lower levels of triglycerides (a type of blood fat) afterward than those who skipped the seasonings. It's simple: Certain spices may slow the digestion of fat, says study author Sheila G. West, PhD. So start shaking!

■ **CAYENNE, CHILI POWDER, RED PEPPER** What makes these spices so hot? Capsaicin—an antioxidant that gives your tongue and your metabolism a jolt. One study found that spiking soup with red pepper helped people eat fewer calories at subsequent meals. There are a few factors at play: Not only does the heat force you to slow down, giving your brain time to recognize fullness, but it can also warm up your body, helping you burn a few extra calories as you eat. To maximize these spices' thermogenic effect, try to eat hot foods on a daily basis, says Jeya Henry, PhD, a professor of human nutrition at Oxford Brookes University.

Research suggests that capsaicin can also dampen your appetite and improve your body's ability to shuttle insulin out of your bloodstream after a meal. In fact, in a recent Australian study, overweight folks who added heat to their plates were more likely to burn fat afterward than those who didn't. The reason: Their levels of insulin, a hormone that signals your body to store fat, were 32 percent lower after the spicy meal. Harness some of the insulin-taming benefit by adding as much hot sauce to your dinner as you can handle. Another strategy: Sprinkle red-pepper flakes into omelets, stir-fries, hummus, and salads or on top of your pizza. (See "The Heat Index" on page 258 for the heat factor of various spices and peppers and suggestions for working them into meals.)

■ **CINNAMON** The ultimate cold-weather spice may help ward off the winter pounds. Cinnamon has been shown to help control people's blood sugar and insulin response to food; this can reduce your risk of storing fat, while also curbing your appetite. Sprinkle the warm spice onto your oatmeal, add it to frothy coffee drinks instead of sugar, or make it your go-to topping for frozen yogurt.

BONUS BENEFIT!

Cinnamon also does your heart a solid: A Pakistani study found that taking in ½ teaspoon of cinnamon per day could lower your cholesterol by 18 percent and triglycerides by 30 percent!

■ **GARLIC** Garlic doesn't contain the fiery capsaicin of chile peppers, but it's still considered a "warming spice." That means it may be able to rev up your body's fat burning (although not as much as peppers). You can add it to almost any savory entrée, side, or condiment: Try it in stir-fries, salsa, and hummus or as a veggie seasoning.

■ **TURMERIC** This woody, bitter-tasting spice is derived from the dried root of a tropical plant. What makes it an essential weapon in your weight-loss arsenal is curcumin, a compound thought to halt the growth of fat cells. Try adding a few dashes of turmeric to an omelet or scrambled eggs, or sprinkle it into your cooking water when making a pot of quinoa or brown rice.

THE HEAT INDEX

Want to fire up your metabolism with spicy foods? Scientists measure the level of capsaicin, the burn-boosting chemical in peppers, with Scoville heat units (SHU)—the higher the number, the more heat the pepper delivers.

Bhut jolokia

SHU: 1,000,000

This is the hottest pepper on the planet—it packs enough heat to send you to the ER.

Habanero peppers

SHU: 100,000+

To make a superspicy salsa, add a teaspoon of habanero to diced mangoes and onions. The hottest of the hot? Orange habaneros, which have an SHU of 210,000.

Thai bird peppers

SHU: 50,000+

Combine with coconut milk and lime juice for an instant Asian marinade.

Ground cayenne

SHU: 40,000

Mix garlic, cayenne, turmeric, and cumin with a little water. Add the resulting paste to sautéed onions and heat in a skillet for a quick, Indian-inspired sauce. You can also toss cayenne into homemade chocolate!

Crushed red pepper

SHU: 30,000

Stir it into hummus or sprinkle it on top of your pizza.

Serrano peppers

SHU: 25,000

Mince and mix with tomatoes, onions, and lime juice for a deliciously hot salsa.

Tabasco sauce

SHU: 15,000

You can add this to almost anything: steak, scrambled eggs, steamed veggies, even popcorn!

Chipotle peppers

SHU: 5,000–10,000

Chop up this smoky-flavored pepper and stir it into black bean dip.

Jalapeño peppers

SHU: 5,500

Dice up a couple and add 'em to your omelet, or top a bowl of chili with pickled jalapeños.

Bulgarian carrot

SHU: 5,000

The bright orange color lends itself nicely to fresh salsas and chutneys.

Poblano peppers

SHU: 1,000–2,000

Grill, peel off the skin, and slice. Add to tacos and quesadillas. They're also ideal for stuffing with brown rice and ground meat.

Chili powder

SHU: 1,000

Sauté leafy greens, such as kale, with chili powder, onion, ginger, and garlic for a spicy side. Or lightly spritz plain popcorn with olive oil, then sprinkle chili powder on top.

Anaheim chiles

SHU: 500–7,000

Redder means hotter. (Hint: Don't cut out the ribs, where much of the heat resides.) Stuff roasted Anaheims with diced veggies for an easy appetizer.

Canned green chiles

SHU: 500

Mix these guys into lean ground beef before throwing your burgers on the grill.

Senorita jalapeño peppers

SHU: 300–400

Far milder than standard jalapeños, senoritas are the perfect pepper to introduce sensitive taste buds to a little heat.

Sugar

9 simple sugar-cutting solutions

The average American eats about 20 teaspoons of added sugars every day. That translates to 317 empty calories from the sweet stuff on a daily basis! Your body wasn't built to handle all of that sugar. "Unlike fat, sugar is rapidly absorbed by the body, and the metabolic effects are immediate," warns Dianne Figlewicz Lattemann, PhD, a University of Washington professor who studies the effects of sugar in humans. "As a result, we seem to want more of it."

The sugar in our bodies, glucose, is a fundamental fuel for body and brain. The problem is, we're consuming gobs of it, and sweetened foods tend to make people overeat. A sudden influx of sugar forces your pancreas to crank out lots of glucose-clearing insulin—which also happens to signal your body to store fat. "The less sugar stress you put on your system, the longer it will function properly," says David Levitsky, PhD, a professor of psychology and nutritional sciences at Cornell University. Use the following strategies to control your intake:

■ **CUT SNEAKY SUGARS** Sugar can be tricky—detecting it in packaged foods is not always as simple as scanning for "sugar" in the ingredients panel. "Sugar hides in places you wouldn't expect because it's cheap to produce, tasty, and addictive," says Kristin

Kirkpatrick, RD, of the Cleveland Clinic Wellness Institute.

Learn to watch for—and avoid—sugar pseudonyms: barley-malt syrup, brown rice syrup, high-fructose corn syrup, dextrose, cane juice, fructose, galactose, glucose, maltodextrin, molasses, sorghum, sucrose, and turbinado. "This is the simplest way to clean up any diet," says nutritionist and weight-loss coach Jonny Bowden, PhD. Your rule of thumb: If any type of sugar is among the first four ingredients, leave that item behind.

■ **MAKE USE OF MANGO** A cup of mango contains about 22 grams of sugars. That sounds like a lot—but it's the natural stuff, unlike the sugar crammed into a Little Debbie. Add mango to your smoothie and you won't need to drop in a single teaspoon of sugar. Other perfect fruits for sweet sipping: apple and pineapple.

■ **SNACK WISELY** Simple-carb foods like bagels and pretzels are laden with starch, which your body quickly breaks down into sugar. Translation: These foods send your blood sugar soaring almost as quickly as desserts do—and they won't ward off hunger for long. Eat protein-packed fare, such as string cheese or hard-cooked eggs, as snacks instead.

■ **LAY OFF THE SODA** A study in the *Journal of the American Medical Association* found that the average man consumes nearly 46 percent of his added sugars from soft drinks and other sweetened beverages. That's especially dangerous, since soda has no nutrients to offset the effects on your blood sugar. Plus, soda doesn't make you feel full like water does—and that can make your appetite for it insatiable. To wean yourself off of the stuff, try writing down every soda you drink for a week, then work to cut your intake by 10 percent each week. Swap in nonsugary drinks, like unsweetened tea or black coffee.

■ **PREPARE MEALS AT HOME** Restaurant foods are notoriously high in sugar—and it's not just the desserts that are problematic. The oatmeal at IHOP, for example, packs 30 times more sugar than you'll find in Quaker Quick Oats! When you're behind the stove, you control the amount of sugar that makes its way into your meal. You can easily trim the sugar in a recipe without noticing a major difference.

■ **DRINK REAL JUICE** Before you guzzle that juice, check the label. Does it say "cocktail" or "juice drink"? If so, leave it on the shelf. These are euphemisms for "a little juice and a lot of added sugar." Stick to bottles that boast 100 percent juice, and even then, practice portion control, since juice lacks the sugar-balancing fiber of whole fruit.

■ **INDULGE THE RIGHT WAY** If you're dying for a treat, grab a sweet snack that has additional dietary benefits. For example, enjoy a sweet-tooth-satisfying handful of berries—the fiber will help slow the rush of sugar into your bloodstream. Or break off a couple of squares of 70 percent cacao dark chocolate, which is chock-full of antioxidants and healthy fats; these fats will reduce the rate at which you absorb sugar.

■ **TAKE A HARD LOOK AT YOUR YOGURT** In the hands of food scientists, a healthy snack can easily turn into a dessert. Case in point: yogurt, which is often "enhanced" with an outrageous amount of sugar. Every Yoplait Original flavor, for example, packs at least 26 grams of sugars! Switch to plain Greek yogurt and stir in fresh fruit. You not only up your protein intake by going Greek, but you reap the sugar-stopping benefit of the fiber in fruit.

■ **SAVORY FOODS ARE OFTEN SUGARY FOODS** Monitoring the sugar content of cookies, pies, and ice cream is a start. But, really, you need to diligently check the sugar content of every food you pick up. Even processed foods that you don't think of as sweet can contain a heavy load of added sugars; pay particular attention to pasta sauces, salad

dressings, breads, and crackers, which are often injected with sneakily high amounts of sugar. Look for varieties that don't have added sugars (often as high-fructose corn syrup) in the ingredient list.

HOW SUGARY IS YOUR DRINK?

A 2011 study in the journal *Obesity* found that some sweetened beverages pack significantly more sugar than listed on the label. Spot the offenders.

Drink	Percent Deviation from the Sugar Content on the Nutrition Label
Coke from McDonald's	+27
Sprite from McDonald's	+26
Sprite from Burger King	+22
Coke from Burger King	+18
Hawaiian Punch Fruit Juicy Red	+5
Tampico Citrus Punch	+4

Supplements

The truth about 16 weight-loss supplements

Weight loss doesn't come in a bottle. "You can take any combination of weight-loss supplements, but without diet and exercise, you won't manage your weight," says David Katz, MD, MPH, director of the Yale-Griffin Prevention Research Center. That's not to mention the safety concerns surrounding supplements like Hydroxycut and SlimQuick. They're not under the same FDA scrutiny that drugs are, so it's a bit of a mystery as to how their ingredients will behave inside your body. That said, there are some supplements that have stood the test of science and that, when combined with a sensible diet and exercise plan, may help you lose weight. Learn the truth about the most popular weight-loss aids below:

ALLI

The short answer: Leave it!

This FDA-approved pill is a reduced-strength version of orlistat, a prescription drug for weight loss. It works by disabling lipase, an enzyme that breaks down fat, so you absorb fewer calories and flush

HOW TOP DOCTORS STAY SLIM

"I drink a protein shake and a glass of milk for breakfast every day. For lunch, I usually have 2 cups of green vegetables, a fruit, and lean meat, like poultry or fish. In the afternoon, I have some cheese and fruit as a snack, and for dinner, I eat a salad, steak or fish, and fruit. I have a glass of wine occasionally."

–JOSE GARCIA, MD, PhD, an assistant professor in the department of diabetes, endocrinology, and metabolism at Baylor College of Medicine out much of the fat you consume. The downside is that Alli isn't selective about which fat it blocks, which means you may lose out on healthy monounsaturated and polyunsaturated fats. Plus, if you eat more than 15 grams of fat per meal (which you inevitably will), you may experience explosive diarrhea and gas that leave your underwear spotted with oil. Not worth it: Weight loss with Alli is generally minimal—an average 3 to 5 pounds per year, the Mayo Clinic reports.

BITTER ORANGE
The short answer: Leave it!

When the FDA banned ephedra, bitter orange swept onto the supplements scene, touted for its ability to elevate heart rate and boost weight loss. However, in one study, the supplement (paired with caffeine) led to only 2 pounds of weight loss over 6 weeks. And, scarily, it's been reported to spike blood pressure and cause heart attack and stroke in healthy people. In fact, a 2006 study review cautioned that bitter orange may raise the risk of "adverse cardiovascular events."

CAPSINOIDS
The short answer: Love them!

Capsinoids are compounds found in sweet peppers that may replicate the metabolism-boosting effects of the capsaicin in hot peppers. In fact, according to a study in the journal *Nutrition & Metabolism,* a supplement containing capsinoids can rev up your resting metabolism by 20 percent.

CALCIUM
The short answer: Drink milk instead.

You're better off relying on dairy. Calcium *has* been linked to weight loss—it may prevent some dietary fat from being absorbed. However, it works best when paired with the proteins in dairy products. In a University of Tennessee study, overweight people who took calcium supplements shed less belly fat than those who ate lots of calcium-rich dairy. Plus, recent studies suggest that supplemental calcium may raise your risk of heart attack.

CARB BLOCKERS
The short answer: Leave them!

These supplements contain a couple of compounds: chromium picolinate and/or vanadium. According to their makers, these minerals make it harder for your body to store carbs as fat. Not true. While your body does need chromium picolinate to regulate your blood sugar, you already have plenty in your system (unless you're diabetic). As for vanadium, you'd have to take it at dangerously high doses to see any effect.

CASEIN PROTEIN POWDER
The short answer: Drink milk instead.

Casein is a protein derived from milk. It's slower absorbing than whey, another milk protein, so it won't give you an instant shot of muscle-building amino acids. There is a bene-

THE ULTIMATE MEAL-REPLACEMENT SMOOTHIE

Makes 1 serving

A protein shake can be a sensible dinner—as long as you cover your nutritional bases the rest of the day. For the perfect balance of protein, carbs, and healthy fats, incorporate protein powder, frozen fruit, and a spoonful of peanut butter.

1 cup 1% milk

The calcium in milk may accelerate fat loss.

PLUS

2 tablespoons ground flaxseed

Flaxseed contributes a solid fiber punch, so you feel fuller longer.

PLUS

1 tablespoon natural peanut butter (such as Smucker's Natural)

Peanut butter has been shown to stave off hunger for 2 hours.

PLUS

½ cup frozen blueberries

The little blue guys sweeten your smoothie while adding antioxidants, fiber, and essential vitamins.

PLUS

1 scoop (32 grams) 100 percent whey protein powder (such as Optimum Nutrition Gold Standard 100% Whey)

The protein helps you build and maintain muscle and may rev up your calorie burn.

NUTRITION INFORMATION: 437 calories, 18 g fat (3 g saturated); 31 g carbs, 6 g fiber, 167 mg sodium, 39 g protein

---

fit, though: Because casein is digested slowly, it's better at delaying hunger than whey. Eighty percent of the protein in milk is casein, so there's no need to shell out cash for the powder.

FISH OIL
The short answer: Helps your heart.

What's the big deal with fish oil? Simple: The capsules contain the omega-3 fatty acids EPA and DHA, which have been linked to improved heart health, better brain function, and lower cholesterol. The downside: If you skip fish in favor of supplemental omega-3s, you miss out on the protein, vitamin D, and selenium found naturally in seafood. This may explain why fish oil supplements don't significantly speed fat loss, according to recent research out of the Cooper Institute in Texas. So go ahead and pop a pill for your heart—just don't expect it to help you drop weight. Choose a fish oil supplement that packs about 500 milligrams each of EPA and DHA.

GARCINIA CAMBOGIA
The short answer: Leave it!

This Asian plant extract is a natural source of hydroxycitric acid, purported to block fat production and suppress appetite. Not only is there no conclusive proof that garcinia aids weight loss—it may cause dangerous heart palpitations, stomach pain, dizziness, nausea, and headache.

GREEN TEA EXTRACT
The short answer: Love it!

Green tea is a bona fide fat burner. It contains epigallocatechin gallate, or EGCG, an antioxidant than can increase your resting metabolism and stimulate fat burning. One study found that exercisers who took green tea extract burned 17 percent more fat after a moderate-intensity workout than those who took a placebo. For maximum fat burning, make sure your supplement contains at least 200 milligrams of EGCG.

GUARANA
The short answer: Leave it!

This South American supplement is a sneaky way to pump up the caffeine content of diet pills. Although it may help you feel full longer, it's been linked to rapid heart rate, anxiety, and irritability.

HOODIA
The short answer: Leave it!

African tribesmen have eaten this bitter-tasting cactus for centuries to stave off hunger during long desert treks. However, there's no hard evidence that it works, and its health effects aren't known. Besides, the bottle on the shelf may not actually contain any of the cactus extract: In a study conducted by Alkemists Pharmaceuticals, scientists tested dozens of products listing hoodia as an ingredient and found that half of them didn't contain a trace of the plant.

PSYLLIUM HUSK
The short answer: Love it!

Taking this supplemental fiber can make it easier to reach your daily goal of 38 grams (men) and 25 grams (women). It's more than a colon clearer: In a recent Finnish study, the addition of psyllium to meals reduced participants' blood sugar and insulin response. Paired with protein, it was also shown to suppress ghrelin, a hormone that makes you hungry.

SOY PROTEIN POWDER
The short answer: Leave it!

Soy is safe when eaten as a whole or minimally processed food—for example, edamame (green soybeans), miso, or tofu. But processed soy, often found in protein powders, soy chips, and energy bars, can be dangerous. The reason: It's tough to determine the amount of phytoestrogens—plant chemicals that mimic the hormone estrogen—in supplemental soy. Exposure to high levels of these plant hormones may raise your risk of cancer and reduce men's sperm count.

VITAMIN D
The short answer: Love it!

It's true, sunlight triggers the production of vitamin D in your body. But you'd have to expose yourself to the sun's rays during peak hours—10:00 a.m. to 3:00 p.m.—without wearing sunscreen in order to meet your D needs. This is one area you don't want to risk deficiency: Low levels of vitamin D could cause your body to store fat instead of burning it. In fact, University of Minnesota scientists found that vitamin D deficiency makes it harder for people to lose weight. Insufficient D has also been linked to insulin resistance, which leads to hunger and overeating, says Liz Applegate, PhD, director of sports nutrition at the University of California, Davis. The recommended daily intake for adults is 600 IU; however, if you're obese, you may need up to five times that amount. To determine your D needs, ask your doctor to perform a simple blood test. Then select a supplement that contains vitamin D_3, the form that's absorbed most efficiently.

WHEY PROTEIN POWDER
The short answer: Love it!

Whey protein, derived from milk, leads the pack in the powder world. It's absorbed into your bloodstream very quickly—after only about 15 minutes, by some estimates—and is the best source of leucine. This amino acid activates protein synthesis in your body, which can help you build more fat-burning muscle. Plus, Swiss researchers recently found that whey protein provides a bigger calorie-burning boost than casein, while a study in the *Journal of Nutrition* showed that people who supplemented with whey protein for 23 weeks had less body fat and smaller waists than those who consumed soy protein.

YOHIMBE
The short answer: Leave it!

Weight-loss studies of yohimbe, an African bark extract, have been inconclusive. Its side effects, however, are clear: In a 1-year FDA study of poison control center calls, yohimbe products accounted for 18 percent of supplement-related inquiries. It's known to cause hypertension, anxiety, and agitation and may lead to headache, chest pain, and stroke.

Tea

8 ways to brew your belly off

One of nature's healthiest drinks may also help blast your belly. According to Japanese researchers, drinking a cup of tea—black, green, or oolong—can accelerate your calorie burning by an amazing 12 percent. A Taiwanese study showed that regular tea drinkers had 20 percent less body fat than nondrinkers.

It's not just the jolt of caffeine in tea that awakens your metabolism. In fact, a study in the *Journal of Nutrition* found that exercisers who drank four cups of green tea every day for 12 weeks lost more than eight times as much abdominal fat as those who drank an ordinary caffeinated beverage. The benefit of your brew lies primarily in its catechins, disease-fighting nutrients thought to accelerate the breakdown of fat. Maximize the waist-trimming potential of every cup with the tips below:

■ **OPT FOR LOOSE LEAF** Skip the ground stuff. For maximum flavor and metabolic benefit, you should buy loose-leaf teas. Loose-leaf tea releases more of its polyphenols than ground varieties do, allowing you to absorb more of the fat-burning compounds.

■ **GO GREEN** When you aren't drinking water, make green tea your go-to beverage. The catechins—specifically, EGCG—in this Asian brew can boost your body's fat-burning fire. A study in the *American Journal of Clinical Nutrition* found that people who downed 690 milligrams of green tea catechins daily had smaller waists than nondrinkers did. Plus, pairing green tea with meals can help you feel full 90 minutes longer, according to a study in *Nutrition Journal*. Try swapping in green tea for your morning coffee, sip on it when you hit the three o'clock wall, or drink it with your dinner. Make sure to steep your green tea as long as possible—at least 4 minutes—since darker-hued tea packs more catechins. Add a squeeze of lemon to boost your body's absorption of the fat-melting antioxidants.

■ **EXPERIMENT WITH OOLONG** Green tea is the brew best known for enhancing your burn. But there are other sippable solutions for a sluggish metabolism. Japanese researchers found that oolong tea can increase calorie burning by up to 10 percent for 90 minutes. To prepare it, pour 185°F water over oolong leaves and let them steep for 10 seconds. Then remove the leaves, discard the water, and put the leaves back into your cup. Pour hot water over them a second time. Steep this cup for at least 30 seconds. (This is the traditional preparation technique.) Too slow for your taste? Try ITO En Oolong Shots (www.itoen.com).

■ **SIP ON BLACK TEA** When it's a caffeine fix you're after, black tea is your best bet, since it has more caffeine than either green or oolong. Research shows that a shot of caffeine may accelerate your weight loss. In fact, USDA scientists found that people who drank black tea burned more calories than those who didn't. Beyond drinking the dark brew, you can use it as a marinade for your meats: Try warming a teaspoon of black tea leaves with a cup of fresh-squeezed orange juice. Remove the mixture from the heat and let it steep for 5 minutes, then strain and discard leaves.

■ **GO WILD WITH MATE** Mate tea comes from a tropical tree called yerba mate—the leaves of which are loaded with caffeine, other stimulants, and antioxidants. Together, these compounds are thought to give your metabolism a lift and suppress your appetite. To prepare your cup, steep dried mate leaves in hot (but not boiling) water for 5 to 8 minutes.

■ **TRAVEL THE ROAD LESS SWEETENED** Tea is calorie free—as long as you stick with unsweetened varieties. Before you sip, check the label to ensure your bagged or bottled brew contains zero grams of sugars. If you can't tolerate plain tea, look for a lightly sweetened option, such as those by Honest Tea. No nutrition info? That's a good sign—it means that the calorie content is negligible.

■ **SKIP THE ADD-INS** Don't let your afternoon pick-me-up morph into a 3:00 p.m. carb fest. Adding a glut of honey, sugar, or flavored syrups to your tea can quickly negate any nutritional benefits of your brew. If you need a little punch of sweetness, limit yourself to a light drizzling of honey. A squeeze of lemon is another ideal flavor enhancer.

■ **DRINK TEA FOR DESSERT** Not all teas will boost your metabolism. But that doesn't mean they don't belong in your cabinet. Caffeine-free dessert teas, such as Mighty Leaf's Chocolate Mint Truffle, make the perfect after-dinner treat—they taste wonderfully decadent but contain very few calories. Another good evening option: peppermint tea. Often used to aid digestion, this minty brew may also suppress your appetite, preventing late-night, postmeal munchies.

Vegetables

14 ways to pummel belly flab with plants

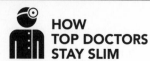
The golden rule of weight loss is simple: Eat more vegetables. In a study of 2,000 carb-conscious dieters, the biggest losers ate four servings of non-starchy vegetables every day. Another study conducted by the Centers for Disease Control and Prevention found that 71 percent of people who successfully shed their excess weight folded more produce into their diet.

The belly-slimming effect of vegetables starts with fiber—the more produce you consume, the more fiber rich your diet will be. The benefit starts before you even swallow: Research suggests that the act of chewing fibrous veggies can bump up your calorie burn by 30 percent! Once the rough stuff reaches your stomach, it occupies lots of space and can slow digestion, leaving less room for other, more-caloric foods. Insoluble fiber, which is found in vegetables, can even block the absorption of other calories! The high water content of veggies further enhances their fullness factor—without adding any calories. Grab a fork and dig in with the strategies below:

■ **EAT MORE** Only 11 percent of Americans consume the recommended servings of fruits and vegetables a day. You can—and should—do better. Even when you're dieting, never restrict your produce intake. Rather, make plants the center of your diet. Not only are vegetables packed with nutrients, but they're also filled with water. That makes them extremely satis-fying for relatively few calories. In fact, non-starchy vegetables are the fastest, healthiest way to bulk up any meal, whether you fold diced veggies into an omelet, top your salad with baby carrots or bell pepper strips, or replace half of your rice or pasta with steamed veggies. Ideally, the heft of the carbs in your diet will come from produce, so vegetables should occupy about a third of your plate.

GO CRAZY: NONSTARCHY VEGETABLES

- Artichokes
- Arugula
- Asparagus
- Bamboo shoots
- Bean sprouts
- Beets
- Broccoli
- Broccoli rabe
- Brussels sprouts
- Cabbage
- Carrots
- Cauliflower
- Celery
- Collard greens
- Cucumber
- Eggplant
- Green onions or scallions
- Green beans
- Jicama
- Kale
- Leeks
- Lettuce
- Mushrooms
- Mustard greens
- Okra
- Onions
- Pea pods
- Peppers
- Radishes
- Rutabaga
- Spinach
- Sugar snap peas
- Summer squash
- Swiss chard
- Turnip greens
- Turnips
- Zucchini

CONTROL YOUR PORTIONS: STARCHY VEGETABLES (One portion = a tight fist or half of a baseball)

- Corn
- Green lima beans
- Green peas
- Parsnips
- Potatoes
- Pumpkin
- Sweet potatoes
- Winter squash (acorn, butternut)
- Yams

BONUS BENEFIT!

Research shows that every daily serving of fruits or vegetables you add to your diet may decrease your risk of heart disease by 4 percent!

■ **TASTE THE RAINBOW** If you adore broccoli, eat it at every meal. Or if spinach is your thing, play Popeye and make it a staple in your diet. But don't let yourself fall into a veggie rut. Eating a range of vegetables ensures that you hit your nutrient quota—the more colorful the produce on your plate, the broader the spectrum of nutrients you're taking in. Aim to keep six or seven different kinds of veggies on hand rather than three or four. You don't have to go wild all at once, though: "Even though you may want to buy a bunch of interesting new veggies to kick off a diet, they can be so overwhelming that you don't eat any," says Lisa Dorfman, MS, RD, a sports nutritionist at the University of Miami. "Stick to one new vegetable at a time and buy others you know you like and will eat."

■ **START IN PRODUCE** As soon as you grab a cart at the supermarket, make a beeline for the produce section. This helps guarantee that vegetables will actually make their way into your cart. Even better, head to your local farmers' market. You'll find fresh, peak-season produce—the average supermarket apple travels 1,726 miles, compared to 61 miles for local apples—and avoid the temptation of processed foods. Find one near you at http://search.ams.usda.gov/farmersmarkets.

■ **EXPLORE THE FROZEN AISLE** Despite the ghastly reputation of the frozen aisle, it actually houses some of the healthiest foods in the supermarket. And, no, we're not talking about the Lean Cuisine frozen meals. Since produce is flash-frozen within hours of being harvested, frozen vegetables are often higher in essential nutrients than their fresh counterparts. Frozen spinach, for example, contains more vitamin A, vitamin K, and folate than fresh—and a study in the *British Journal of Nutrition* found that folks who took in the most folate were eight and a half times more likely to lose a significant amount of weight in a year than those who ate the least. A word of caution: Don't boil your frozen veggies, since a large portion of their nutrients will be leached into the water. Steam, roast, sauté, or microwave them instead.

■ **DON'T CAN CANS ENTIRELY** Like frozen veggies, canned produce is often richer in nutrients than fresh varieties. However, you're also at risk of consuming added sugars or excess sodium. Always check the label—the only ingredients should be the vegetable, water, and perhaps a little salt. (Make sure the amount of sodium is lower than the number of calories.) To maximize your nutritional payoff, warm canned vegetables in their liquid, which typically contains about a third of the nutrients. If you're concerned about BPA, choose canned goods from Eden Foods, Native Forest, and Trader Joe's.

■ **MOW THROUGH A SALAD** Noshing on vegetables before your main course can help you eat less, according to Penn State scientists. A salad built primarily on produce should be your appetizer of choice. You can also bulk up your greens with lean protein—beans, grilled chicken, sirloin steak—and eat salad as a low-carb entrée. Although romaine lettuce, green leaf lettuce, and spinach are the salad bar superstars, don't be afraid to use iceberg as your base. "Any lettuce that keeps you eating salads is a great vehicle for getting more produce into your day," says Dawn Jackson Blatner, RD, a nutrition consultant for the Chicago Cubs. The most nutrient-rich lettuce does you no good if it ends up in the trash.

BONUS BENEFIT!

Leafy greens—kale, collard greens, Swiss chard, mustard greens, spinach—are loaded with bone-protecting vitamin K. In a Harvard University analysis of 72,000 women dieters, those who ate at least one serving of lettuce per day had the lowest rates of hip fracture.

■ **HEAT 'EM UP** Raw fresh veggies are the perfect, portable snack. But when you're at home, consider heating up your produce; research suggests that some vegetables are more nutritious when they're cooked. Steam these guys: asparagus, broccoli, cabbage, carrots, cauliflower, kale, mushrooms, spinach, and zucchini. The cooking process can help unlock the disease-fighting power of their antioxidants.

■ **BULK UP GRAINS WITH PRODUCE** Rather than eat a heaping plate of pasta or rice, swap out half of the grain for nonstarchy vegetables. In a recent Penn State study, people who replaced half of the roast beef and rice on their plates with lightly buttered broccoli consumed 86 fewer calories—and felt just as full. "Vegetables are satiating because they contain water, which bulks food up," says

study author Jennifer Meengs, RD. Heat up 1 or 2 cups of chopped onions, peppers, broccoli florets, green beans, or spinach, and mix them into your cooked rice or pasta.

■ **LIGHTLY OIL YOUR VEGGIES** You shouldn't smother your vegetables in butter (or cheese). However, adding a pat to your produce won't do you in. In fact, studies show that the fat in butter improves your body's ability to absorb vitamins A, E, D, and K, which are abundant in vegetables. If you tend to go wild with butter, try pouring olive oil into a mister, such as the Misto Olive Oil Sprayer. It allows you to add a little flavor and fat to your food but keeps you from overdoing it.

■ **ADD VEGETABLES TO SOUP** Consider no soup complete until it contains a healthy portion of veggies. It's a painless way to work in more vegetables, plus the liquid will fill you up, so you eat less later. You can buy premade vegetable soup, or you can chop up and sauté your own vegetables, then stir them into a bowl of broth-based soup. Or, if you (or your kids) hate the taste of vegetables, puree them beforehand—you'll forget they're even there. Another perfect vessel for veggies: chili.

■ **DISPLAY YOUR PRODUCE** The crisper drawer is great in theory. But here's the problem: Tucked inside the bottom drawer of your fridge, veggies tend to be forgotten. To boost your intake, you should store your produce on an eye-level shelf—just seeing food makes you more likely to eat it, so your vegetables won't have time to go bad. Make a habit of prepping produce—washing, drying, and dicing or slicing—as soon as you buy it. This will encourage you to actually eat the vegetables you purchase, since you won't need as much time to whip them up for dinner.

■ **CHUG VEGETABLE JUICE** Fruit juice won't do much for you nutritionally. Low in calories and high in nutrients, vegetable juice is another story entirely. If you struggle to work produce into your diet, sip on a glass of low-sodium vegetable juice, such as V8, with lunch or dinner. In a Penn State study, people who downed a glass of vegetable juice before a meal ate 135 fewer calories later in the day.

■ **DON'T BE FOOLED BY IMPOSTERS** Frying vegetables negates their benefit. Period.

6 VEGETABLE MYTHS, BUSTED

1. Carrots are superhigh in sugar.

Only half of the 12 grams of carbs in carrots come from natural sugars—less than you'll find in the average piece of fruit. The remainder of carrots' carbohydrates comes from filling fiber and healthy complex carbohydrates. That's not to mention the wealth of vitamins and minerals, including vision-protecting beta-carotene and vitamin A, that accompanies the natural sugars in the orange veggie. So go ahead, eat the little guys. Try tossing grated carrots into marinara sauce, shredding them into tuna salad, or piling roast carrot slices onto your sandwich.

2. Celery is nothing more than water.

Yes, a stalk of celery is 95 percent water. But the other 5 percent consists of disease-fighting vitamins, minerals, and phytochemicals, including vitamin K, vitamin A, folate, and phthalides, compounds that may lower your blood pressure. The benefit doesn't stop there: Celery sticks can satisfy your urge to snack for virtually no calories—one large rib contains just 10 calories and offers 1 gram of belly-filling fiber. Ants on a log are, of course, the obvious way to enjoy celery, but you can also chop it up and add it to soups or stir-fries.

3. Corn is a carbohydrate nightmare.

Corn is classified as a starchy vegetable. That does mean it contains more carbs than most other veggies, but they're the best kind: high-quality, complex carbs, like those in whole grains. Plus, corn is loaded with fiber, as well as folate, thiamin, and lutein. For a simple corn salsa, toss fresh kernels with chopped jalapeño chile pepper, fresh cilantro, tomato, and onion.

That means french fries, chips, and onion rings don't count as a serving of vegetables. If you're craving something crispy, try this: Thinly slice root vegetables—parsnips, carrots, sweet potatoes, white potatoes—and toss them with a little olive oil, salt, and pepper. Roast them at 400°F until they're lightly browned and sufficiently crispy.

■ SWAP IN HEARTY VEGGIES FOR MEAT
You don't have to go vegetarian to lose weight. However, scaling back your meat intake *is* an easy way to cut calories. Don't make the classic mistake of swapping in carbs for meats, though. Instead, fill the void with hearty veggies, like portobello mushrooms and eggplant, both of which can be grilled like meat.

4. Organic vegetables are always better.

Not all organic produce is worth your dime. Produce that requires peeling—for example, avocados and onions—won't expose you to a heavy load of pesticides. According to the Environmental Working Group, it's not worth going organic when buying onions, sweet corn, avocados, asparagus, sweet peas, eggplants, cabbage, sweet potatoes, and mushrooms. Save your money for the veggies with the highest pesticide load: celery, spinach, sweet bell peppers, potatoes, lettuce, kale, and collard greens.

5. Sweet potatoes are healthier than white.

It's easy to assume that orange spuds rule over white. But that's only because we typically consume white potatoes in their most unflattering form: fried. The truth is, both sweet and white potatoes are good for you—just in different ways. While sweet potatoes are high in fiber and vitamin A, white potatoes are rich in iron, magnesium, and potassium. The bottom line: The form in which you consume your spuds—for instance, baked versus fried—is more important than the type.

6. Spinach wraps are healthier than regular tortillas.

The final word: Spinach wraps are not a source of vegetables! In fact, they're no better for you than run-of-the-mill flour tortillas. Consider Mission Garden Spinach Herb Wraps: The first ingredient is enriched flour (not whole grain), and the closest thing to a vegetable in this wrap is spinach powder. Stick with whole-grain tortillas and load them with real vegetables.

12 Restaurant Survival Tactics

The more often you dine out, the larger your waistline will likely be. On average, people consume 36 percent more calories at restaurants than when eating at home. And if you dine out as often as the average American does—about five times a week—those extra calories can add up. The smart solution is to cook and eat more meals at home, and when you do treat yourself to a restaurant meal, make the right choices. Before your next meal out, arm yourself with these calorie-saving, slim-eating strategies:

1 CONTROL YOUR IMBIBING

Don't assume one drink equals one serving. Alcoholic drinks at restaurants are often significantly larger than a standard drink, according to a Public Health Institute study of 337 drinks from 80 establishments. The scientists found that the average draft beer was 22 percent larger, spirit-based drinks were 42 percent larger, and glasses of wine were 43 percent larger than suggested serving sizes. Not only are you downing more calories than you bargained for, but being tipsy could also lower your inhibitions. And when your inhibitions drop, you're more likely to overeat. Limit yourself to a single 12-ounce bottle of beer, or ask your bartender to pour no more than 5 ounces of wine or 1½ ounces of spirits (a shot-glass size).

2 DOWNSIZE YOUR DINNER

Make an appetizer your entrée. In one Penn State study, people ate 30 percent more food when presented with bigger portions, but they didn't feel any fuller than when they ate smaller plates. You still need to use your discretion when perusing the starters: Avoid anything that's fried, covered in cheese, or includes the word "sampler."

3 DON'T FAST BEFOREHAND

If you prep for a big meal by avoiding food all day, you'll eat with fervor and without restraint. A better strategy: Eat a light lunch, then have a protein- and fiber-rich snack, such as an apple and string cheese, a few hours before your meal. That way, you won't be famished and will find it easier to make healthy choices.

4 FORGET ABOUT THE MENU

Before you leave the house, review the restaurant's menu and nutritional facts online. Ideally, you'll do this shortly after you've eaten, so you're not hungry when you're planning your next meal. If you wait to decide until you're at the restaurant, you're more likely to choose with your eyes and not with your head.

5 CONSULT AN EXPERT

Forgot to check the nutritional facts before you left home? Diet.com offers a cell phone service that will send you calorie counts when you text a restaurant name, a menu item, and the portion size to DIET1 (34381). The feedback is instant, and the service offers nutrition data for more than 36,000 menu items from over 1,700 restaurants.

6 DITCH THE BREADBASKET

Those breadsticks may be "complimentary," but they're far from free. Consider this: A single Olive Garden breadstick costs you 150 calories, as does a Cheddar biscuit from Red Lobster. And who eats just one? Rather than relying on your own willpower, ask the waiter not to bring the basket at all. If the bread isn't in front of you, you can't eat it.

7 AVOID THE DRIVE-THRU

The mere sight of a fast-food sign can make you feel rushed, causing you to make impulsive, unhealthy choices, according to a study in the journal *Psychological Science*. The effect will only be compounded if you have a line of cars on your tail. So, if fast food is truly your only option, find a parking spot and head inside. Standing at the counter will give you a few extra minutes to study the menu and choose the lesser of two evils.

8 FEAR THE DESSERT MENU

Not only are restaurant desserts outrageously high in calories, but they're served in enormous portions. If you must end with something sweet, split a dessert among your tablemates—and try to stop after a couple of bites. Savoring your sweets, even in small portions, can be just as satisfying as scarfing an entire brownie double fudge sundae on your own. Another strategy: Have a glass of wine for dessert. It's easier to estimate calories in wine than in a sundae.

9 PLAY RESTAURANT CRITIC

Imagine you're a restaurant reviewer: Critically examine the flavor and texture of whatever you eat. If the food is great and you're not full yet, have some more. But if the food is disappointing, push back the plate.

10 LOSE THE BUN

Many burger joints will wrap your meat patty in lettuce instead of a bun if you ask. At In-N-Out Burger, for example, ditching the bun is referred to as "protein style." Similarly, at some burrito joints, you can go naked and lose the carb-packed tortilla.

11 SKIP THE SAUCE

Sure, those little packets of special sauce seem benign. But, in reality, many of them are secret fat traps. A tiny cup of Chick-fil-A Sauce? 140 calories and 13 grams of fat. Papa John's Special Garlic Dipping Sauce? 150 calories and 17 grams of fat. If you need a shot of flavor, stick to ketchup and mustard, or leave the special sauce or dressing on the side and dip conservatively.

12 TAKE HALF TO GO

Consider your restaurant entrée two meals, not one. So before you dive in, divide your meal in half (or thirds, if it's huge). Leave one portion on your plate and stow the rest in a to-go box for later. Chances are, you won't even miss the packed-away portion.

Vitamin D

7 ways to use the weight-loss vitamin

Vitamin D does more than fortify your muscles and bones. It's also an essential nutrient for healthy weight loss. When your body has the vitamin D it needs, it releases more leptin, a fullness hormone that tells you it's time to stop eating. In an Australian study, people who loaded up on D and calcium at breakfast experienced a reduction in appetite over the next 24 hours. Sufficient D levels also make your body less likely to store fat, particularly around your middle, according to studies from the University of Minnesota and Laval University. One reason: Vitamin D may partner with calcium to tackle cortisol, a stress hormone that causes you to store belly fat.

Conversely, when your body is D-ficient, you may notice that the pounds start creeping in. Low levels of vitamin D have been linked to insulin resistance, which can cause you to overeat and gain weight, explains Liz Applegate, PhD, director of sports nutrition at the University of California, Davis. Vitamin D deficiency may also trigger the release of high amounts of parathyroid hormone and calcitrol, both of which tell your body to hang on to fat instead of burning it.

HOW TOP DOCTORS STAY SLIM

"My recipe for a quick and healthy meal: I use any brand of high-fiber/low-carb tortilla, and stuff it with organic arugula, shaved Parmesan cheese (optional), and smoked sliced salmon. I then add balsamic vinegar and black pepper."

—JOSE GARCIA, MD, PhD, assistant professor in the department of diabetes, endocrinology, and metabolism at Baylor College of Medicine

■ **CHECK YOUR INTAKE** If you're struggling to lose weight, it may be because you're vitamin D deficient. In a University of Minnesota study, people who were low on D had trouble shedding excess weight. Although adults need a daily 600 IU of vitamin D, according to National Institutes of Health guidelines, obese people may require two to five times that amount. Body fat prevents D from being used in your body—it essentially becomes trapped in your fat, unable to circulate through your bloodstream. (Turn to page 13 for instructions on calculating your BMI. Thirty or above is considered obese.) Ask your doctor to perform a blood test to determine whether you're deficient and how much you should aim to take in every day.

■ **POP A SUPPLEMENT** Your body produces its own vitamin D when your skin is exposed to sunlight. However, it's not always as easy as stepping outside for a few minutes to soak up some sun. The darker your skin or the deeper your tan, the higher your natural SPF and the more sunlight your skin requires to make D. Plus, if you wear sunscreen (which you should), you stifle your natural production of the nutrient; you'd have to sun yourself from 10:00 a.m. to 3:00 p.m., skin unprotected, in order to manufacture the vitamin D your body requires. Your solution? First, load up on vitamin D-rich foods (see "Foods That Deliver D"), but consider taking a supplement, too. Choose a pill that contains vitamin D_3, the most absorbable form. See "Check Your Intake," for dosing guidelines.

■ **POUR A BOWL OF D** Fortification is different from enhancement. Enhancement replaces ingredients lost during processing— think enriched white flour—but fortification simply tacks on extra nutrients that are often lacking in our diets. One biggie: vitamin D. When choosing your cereal, look for one that has added vitamin D while still observing the cardinal rules of cereal: 100 percent whole grain, no more than 120 calories per cup, lots of fiber, and a minimal amount of sugar. Try Wheaties or Multi Grain Cheerios.

■ **LOAD UP ON FORTIFIED DAIRY** Calcium isn't the only thing dairy products have to offer. Fortified milk, kefir, cheese, cottage cheese, and yogurt are all rich in vitamin D—a good thing, since there are few natural food sources of the nutrient. Vitamin D not only helps your body absorb the calcium in dairy, but the two nutrients may also team up to help you blast fat. A recent study found that people who ate a diet high in calcium and D from dairy lost 70 percent more weight than those who ate the same number of calories but without high levels of the nutrients. A cup of fortified low-fat yogurt offers 127 IU of vitamin D, while a cup of fortified 1% milk contributes 98 IU.

■ **SAVE THE YOLKS** Eating only the egg white has been a trendy way to cut calories for years. But when you lose the yellow stuff, you also lose the heft of the egg's nutrients, including 218 IU of vitamin D. Breakfast is the ideal time to work in eggs, whether in the form of an omelet, scrambled eggs, or even an Egg McMuffin, but don't confine your intake to the a.m. Whip up a batch of hard-cooked eggs to eat as midmorning or afternoon snacks.

■ **EAT MORE MUSHROOMS** All varieties of mushrooms have some vitamin D, but growers have raised levels in cremini, portobello, and white button mushrooms by exposing them to UV light. Mushrooms make the perfect meat substitute: Try grilling a portobello in place of a beef patty, or slice up button mushrooms and toss them with your greens.

■ **GO FISH** Seafood is an excellent source of vitamin D. Fatty fish can pack upwards of 800 IU per serving! Which fish top the list? Half of a sockeye salmon fillet contains 815 IU, 3 ounces of farmed rainbow trout has 645 IU,

and a serving of swordfish offers 566 IU. Canned pink salmon, halibut, flounder, tuna, and sardines are also great sources of the nutrient. Aim to eat fatty fish at least three times per week.

FOODS THAT DELIVER D

Fish and eggs are perhaps the easiest ways to load up on vitamin D, but there *are* other smart ways to bolster your intake.

Wild oysters (6 medium) = 269 IU
Fortified orange juice (1 cup) = 142 IU
Shrimp (3 oz) = 129 IU
1% milk (1 cup) = 127 IU
Canned mushrooms (1 cup) = 33 IU
Swiss cheese (1 oz) = 12 IU

Water

11 ways to liquidate your assets

You know that water is essential for life. But what about weight loss? First, consider what happens if you're not chugging enough: According to University of Utah scientists, dehydrated people experience up to a 2 percent decline in metabolic rate. And people who drink eight glasses of water a day have faster metabolisms than those who drink four. That's because every chemical reaction in your body, including your metabolism, depends on water. So, when your cells are well hydrated, you burn calories more efficiently. (And remember, your muscles are almost 80 percent water. You need water to keep them functioning properly, too.)

The best part? Guzzling a glass when you're dehydrated doesn't just bump your metabolism back up to its normal resting rate. Research in the *Journal of Endocrinology & Metabolism* showed that people experienced a 24 percent boost in calorie burn an hour after drinking two glasses of water. Another study found that women who increased their water intake without otherwise changing their diet or activity level dropped significant weight over the course of a year. Credit the metabolic boost water provides—but also another simpler factor. Water fills you up, helping to crowd out calorie-containing foods and beverages.

■ **CHECK THE BOWL** Worried you're not drinking enough? Peek in the toilet after you pee. Dark yellow- or amber-colored urine is a sign that you're not downing enough fluid. If you're drinking enough water, you will urinate every 2 to 3 hours.

■ **WAKE UP WITH WATER** After a full night's sleep, you haven't had water for 8 hours. Which means you should start rehydrating as soon as you roll out of bed. This will help your metabolism kick into gear for the day. Don't stop there, though. Set a water schedule: Have a glass when you wake up, one midmorning, one before lunch, one with lunch, and so on.

■ **DRINK BEFORE YOU EAT** Make it a policy to down a big glass of water 30 minutes before each meal and snack. In a study from Virginia Polytechnic Institute, overweight folks who drank 17 ounces of water before breakfast consumed 9 percent fewer calories than when they didn't start with agua. Another study in the journal *Obesity* found that folks who guzzled two glasses of water before each meal lost an extra 4½ pounds in 12 weeks. If you chug enough of the stuff, your stomach will think it's full, your hunger will switch off, and you'll eat less.

■ **HAVE ANOTHER GLASS WITH YOUR MEAL** Don't limit yourself to a predinner drink. During your meal, take a sip of water between every bite—it will slow your pace, giv-

ing your brain the time it needs to register fullness. Plus, drinking plenty of water will help prevent stomach irritation from the high amounts of fiber and protein in your new diet.

■ **SERVE IT ON THE ROCKS** Pour your bottled water over a cup of ice. In a German study, people who drank six glasses of cold water per day burned an extra 50 calories per day. One explanation: It requires calories to heat icy water to body temperature, says Madelyn Fernstrom, PhD, founding director of the University of Pittsburgh Medical Center Weight Management Center. Although the extra calories you burn drinking one glass won't amount to much, making it a habit can add up to pounds lost for essentially zero effort.

■ **KILL CRAVINGS WITH WATER** Thirst often masquerades as hunger, since both sensations are controlled by your brain's hypothalamus. So before you dive into those Twinkies, grab a glass of water. You may feel surprisingly satiated by the time you finish it.

■ **ADD LEMON** If the waiter offers lemon with your water, take him up on it. Fresh lemon can help suppress your appetite; plus, it acts as a natural diuretic, so you urinate more often. And urinating more often means you need to drink more often!

■ **USE A SMALL CUP** You want to drink as much water as possible—but skip the giant-size bottle, at least while you're at work. When you're sipping at your desk, using a small cup will force you to make repeated trips to the water fountain for refills. And that boosts your daily step count! To work in even more activity, stake out a fountain a couple of floors up.

■ **TRACK YOUR INTAKE** For on-the-go sipping, carry an Intak Hydration Bottle ($11, shopthermos.com). This BPA-free bottle is equipped with a handy meter that helps you gauge how much you're chugging. Bored at the doctor's office? Take a swig. Waiting in line? Have some water. You get the idea.

■ **AVOID FLAVORED WATERS** Just because a drink's name includes the word "water" doesn't mean it's healthy. Flavored waters often include sugar substitutes, such as acesulfame potassium and sucralose (Splenda), which are significantly sweeter than sugar. Research suggests that this can actually increase your overall liking for sweet things, causing you to crave sugar even more! That's

not to mention the load of artificial colors, flavors, and preservatives these waters contain. If you want something besides plain water, stick with seltzer water and a shot of juice.

■ **EAT MORE FRUITS AND VEGGIES** Taking frequent trips to the fountain isn't the only way to work more water into your day. Water in your glass is good, but water in your food can also have serious slimming power. In a study in the *American Journal of Clinical Nutrition*, dieters who added more water-rich foods to their diet while cutting back their fat intake lost more weight than those who only trimmed the fat. Fruits and veggies are 80 to 95 percent water, so adding more produce to your diet can also help you lose weight and satisfy your body's liquid requirements. It's a win-win: You stay hydrated, while taking in essential nutrients for very few calories.

Whole Grains

How to eat better-for-you carbs

Chances are, you weren't raised eating whole-grain bread. The majority of Americans grow up scarfing the white stuff—which may explain why so few adults willingly embrace the good-for-you grains. But consider this: Refined carbohydrates—the kind you find in white bread, pasta, and rice—lead to major spikes in your blood sugar. And when your blood sugar rises rapidly, your body releases a flood of insulin. This hormone helps shuttle the sugar out of your blood, but it also signals your body to store fat, especially around your midsection. Even exercise can't offset the negative effects of white bread. A study in the *American Journal of Clinical Nutrition* found that exercisers who ate refined grains every day had 12 percent more visceral fat—the most dangerous kind—than those who consumed the least amount of the processed stuff.

Convinced refined grains are bad? Here's the good news: In the same *American Journal of Clinical Nutrition* study, people who consumed the most whole grains had 17 percent less belly flab than those who consumed the least. Unlike processed carbs, whole grains include the entire plant seed: the germ, bran, the endosperm. That means all

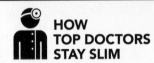

HOW TOP DOCTORS STAY SLIM

"I eat whole grains, especially whole-wheat pasta. If I haven't had an active day, I cut back on the pasta and add extra vegetables. If my day has been active and I need more fuel, I increase the ratio of pasta to vegetables."

—**TRAVIS STORK, MD,** author of *The Lean Belly Prescription* and host of TV's *The Doctors* of their natural fiber is intact, including a significant amount of insoluble fiber, which can block the absorption of other calories. Fiber also slows your body's breakdown of carbohydrates, so you avoid the blood sugar spike that occurs when you eat refined grains and feel fuller longer. Use the following strategies to make the whole grain switch:

■ **CUT REFINED CARBS** What, exactly, makes a carb refined? Simple: They're created when whole grains go through the milling process, stripping them of their vitamins, minerals, and about three-quarters of their fiber. That's serious business, because whole grains are a source of essential nutrients, like thiamin, riboflavin, vitamin E, iron, magnesium, and potassium. And their fiber is what fills you up, keeps you regular, maintains your blood sugar, and even helps you lose weight. Always opt for the whole-grain versions of food— brown rice, whole-grain bread, whole-grain pasta—whenever possible. The payoff is big: Penn State researchers found that dieters who ate whole grains lost twice as much abdominal fat as those who ate refined carbs.

■ **PRIORITIZE TRUE WHOLE GRAINS** One hundred percent whole-grain bread is undoubtedly good for you. However, the whole grains in it are paired with a host of other ingredients, including preservatives, oils, and sweeteners. You're better off eating pure whole grains: amaranth, barley, brown rice, buckwheat, bulgur, corn (including popcorn), millet, oats, quinoa, spelt, teff, and wild rice. (For a primer, see "Your Main Grains," opposite.)

■ **SELECT YOUR CEREAL CAREFULLY**
Pouring yourself a bowl of cereal is a fast way to fuel up in the morning—and research shows that people who do so tend to eat more whole grains throughout the day. But don't let whole grain frauds in the cereal aisle derail your breakfast. The makers of junky cereals have realized that whole grain claims sell, so even cereals like Cookie Crisp and Reese's Puffs boast about their whole grain content on the front of the box. Here's the thing: They may contain *some* of the good-for-you grains, but they're not built entirely on them. These sugary cereals are still loaded with the enriched flour you want to avoid. Flip the box over and check the ingredients list. Every grain or flour in your cereal should include the word "whole" in its name—whole-wheat flour, whole oats, whole corn, etc. A few smart picks: Fiber One Original, Post Shredded Wheat Spoon Size Wheat'n Bran, and Kashi 7 Whole Grain Puffs.

■ **GET MUSHY** Oatmeal is one of the easiest ways to eat more whole grains, since even the instant kind is chock-full of fiber and nutrients. Zap a packet of instant oatmeal and mix it with fresh berries and cinnamon for a quick and easy breakfast (or even a late-afternoon snack). Try Quaker Weight Control Maple & Brown Sugar—it tastes amazing and has more fiber, protein, and whole grains than the regular version. Of course, your best bet is to whip up a batch of steel-cut oats, which has more fiber than other oatmeal varieties. Try preparing a big batch at the beginning of the week, then reheat a bowl each morning.

(continued on page 290)

YOUR MAIN GRAINS

Ban white rice from your kitchen and your menu and expand your grain repertoire with these healthier (and tastier) alternatives.

Amaranth

Taste: Slightly sweet, yet peppery

Nutrition: 125 calories, 23 g carbs, 3 g fiber, 5 g protein*

Benefit: This gluten-free grain is approximately 14 percent protein (and it's the "complete" kind, like you'll find in animal products), making it one of the most filling grains. It's also one of few grains that contains vitamin C.

Whole-grain guarantee: If you see "amaranth" on the ingredients list, it's almost always whole amaranth.

Perfect it: Simply boil it for 15 to 20 minutes, being sure not to skimp on the water. For every cup of amaranth, use about 6 cups of water, the Whole Grain Council recommends.

Barley

Taste: Slightly nutty

Nutrition: 135 calories, 30 g carbs, 7 g fiber, 4 g protein

Benefit: Barley contains more fiber than any other whole grain. It's especially high in cholesterol-lowering beta-glucan, a type of fiber also found in oats.

Whole-grain guarantee: Although it's still high in fiber, lightly pearled barley isn't a whole grain. Look for whole barley, hulled barley, or hull-less barley.

Perfect it: Since barley can take up to an hour to cook, try whipping up a big batch and eating it throughout the week.

Nutrition information is per ½ cup cooked.

Brown rice

Taste: Hearty

Nutrition: 108 calories, 22 g carbs, 2 g fiber, 2.5 g protein

Benefit: Although lower in fiber than most whole grains, brown rice is rich in manganese, which helps your body break down fats and make use of the protein and carbs you eat. Plus, it's very easily digested (which is why it's often recommended for babies).

Whole-grain guarantee: Brown rice—as well as black and red rice—is always whole grain.

Perfect it: Unless you like sticky rice, don't stir it while cooking. The motion causes the grain to release extra starch, which acts like glue.

Buckwheat

Taste: Robust, nutty

Nutrition: 77 calories, 17 g carbs, 2 g fiber, 3 g protein

Benefit: Although not technically a grain— buckwheat is a cousin of rhubarb—its flavor and grainlike appearance allow it to be grouped with grains. Buckwheat is rich in rutin, a flavonoid that has potent antioxidant properties, and heart-healthy magnesium. Plus, it's gluten free.

Whole-grain guarantee: If you spot "buckwheat" on the ingredients list, it's almost always whole buckwheat.

Perfect it: Make sure to follow the package instructions to coat buckwheat with egg, and then heat it in a skillet until it's dry. Otherwise, it may swell up and turn into a thick, unsavory mass.

(continued)

YOUR MAIN GRAINS—Cont.

Bulgur

Taste: Mild, nutty

Nutrition: 76 calories, 17 g carbs, 4 g fiber, 3 g protein

Benefit: Like buckwheat, bulgur is loaded with the mineral magnesium. It cooks quickly, making it a nutritious fast food.

Whole-grain guarantee: According to the FDA, all bulgur is considered a whole grain.

Perfect it: It's already precooked, so just heat it up in boiling water for 20 to 25 minutes. Use about 2 cups of water per cup of bulgur.

Corn

Taste: Sweet, hearty

Nutrition: Yellow: 62 calories, 14 g carbs, 1 g fiber, 2 g protein; white: 66 calories, 15 g carbs, 2 g fiber, 2 g protein

Benefit: Corn does double duty as a vegetable and a whole grain. It contains a healthy shot of fiber, folate, and potassium.

Whole-grain guarantee: Look for "whole corn," whether you're buying cornmeal, corn flour, grits, or polenta. Avoid corn products that include the word "degermed." Or simply stick with fresh corn on the cob or popcorn!

Perfect it: Before you cook fresh corn, remove the silky fibers by rubbing a damp paper towel up and down the cob. According to the Whole Grain Council, you should avoid adding salt to the water when cooking sweet corn, since it can cause it to toughen up. Cook fresh corn no longer than 3 minutes.

Farro

Taste: Warm, nutty, slightly sweet

Nutrition: 100 calories, 26 g carbs, 3.5 g fiber, 4 g protein

Benefit: A staple for ancient Egyptians and modern-day Italians alike, farro has more fiber and protein than brown rice, along with calcium and iron.

Whole-grain guarantee: Make sure the ingredient list says "whole farro," and steer clear of pearled varieties.

Perfect it: Check the package: Some farros require presoaking. When ready to boil, use about 2 quarts of water per cup of farro. Expect it to double in volume during cooking.

Kamut

Taste: Rich, buttery

Nutrition: 126 calories, 26 g carbs, 3 g fiber, 5.5 g protein

Benefit: This heirloom grain has more protein and vitamin E than wheat.

Whole-grain guarantee: Shop exclusively for "whole Kamut."

Perfect it: Soak Kamut overnight, then boil it, using about 3 cups of water per cup of the grain. Let it simmer for about 30 to 40 minutes.

Millet

Taste: Mildly sweet, delicately nutty

Nutrition: 104 calories, 21 g carbs, 1 g fiber, 3 g protein

Benefit: This tiny grain is rarely eaten in the United States (unless by birds), but it should be: Half a cup contains 38 milligrams of magnesium, plus 54 milligrams of potassium, a known hypertension fighter.

Whole-grain guarantee: If you see "millet" on the ingredients list, it's almost always whole millet.

Perfect it: Use about 2½ cups of water per cup of millet. Allow it to simmer for 13 to 18 minutes.

Oats

Taste: Hearty, sweet

Nutrition: 83 calories, 14 g carbs, 2 g fiber, 3 g protein

Benefit: Steel-cut oats are rich in cholesterol-lowering fiber—and in particular, a special type of fiber called beta-glucan.

Whole-grain guarantee: Unlike most grains, oats are rarely stripped of their fibrous bran and germ. If you see "oats" or "oat flour" on the ingredient list, you're most likely eating the whole-grain version.

Perfect it: The easiest way to cook oats? In the microwave, of course.

Quinoa

Taste: Similar to wheat

Nutrition: 111 calories, 20 g carbs, 3 g fiber, 4 g protein

Benefit: This round, gluten-free grain won't spike your blood sugar, and it's a "complete" protein, meaning it contains all nine essential amino acids. For an extra antioxidant boost, look for red quinoa.

Whole-grain guarantee: If you see "quinoa" on the ingredients list, it's almost always whole quinoa.

Perfect it: Simply boil it for 15 minutes, then fluff it up with a fork before serving.

Spelt

Taste: Nutty

Nutrition: 123 calories, 26 g carbs, 4 g fiber, 5 g protein

Benefit: It can easily stand in for wheat—a good thing, since spelt is higher in protein.

Whole-grain guarantee: Not all spelt is whole grain, so make sure the ingredients list says "whole spelt."

Perfect it: Use 3½ cups of water per cup of spelt. Bring to a boil, reduce heat, then simmer for about 90 minutes.

Teff

Taste: Sweet, molasses-like

Nutrition: 127 calories, 25 g carbs, 3.5 g fiber, 5 g protein

Benefit: Teff is loaded with iron and leads the whole grain pack in terms of calcium content.

Whole-grain guarantee: All teff is whole grain—it's too tiny to be processed.

Perfect it: For creamy teff, cook a cup of the grain in 3 cups of water for 20 minutes.

Wild rice

Taste: Strong, nutty

Nutrition: 83 calories, 17.5 g carbs, 1.5 g fiber, 3 g protein

Benefit: Wild rice isn't actually rice. Rather, it's an aquatic grass, with more protein and fiber than brown rice.

Whole-grain guarantee: If you see "wild rice" on the ingredients list, it's almost always whole wild rice.

Perfect it: Follow the suggestions for cooking brown rice.

■ **WATCH YOUR CRACKERS** Crackers are surrounded by a "health halo." Since they're small and light, we tend to assume they're good for us. But really, the vast majority of crackers are made with enriched flour, which consists of nothing more than hunger-stimulating empty carbs. If you need a cracker fix, look for 100 percent whole grain options that have at least 3 grams of fiber, such as Wasa Whole Grain Crispbread or Kashi Snack Crackers Original 7 Grain.

■ **PICK THE RIGHT WRAP** Wraps can be healthier than bread, but only if you know what to buy. Your tortilla should contain as few preservatives and artificial colors as possible and no hydrogenated oils—that way, you avoid consuming your whole grains with a side of chemicals. Skip the standard flour tortilla. Instead, look for wraps made with whole wheat, spelt, teff, brown rice, or corn, and check the ingredients list to make sure that no refined grains slip into the mix. Smaller wraps, such as La Tortilla White Whole Wheat Soft Wrap Minis, are better, since a plate-size wrap can easily contain two servings of carbs.

■ **BE A BREAD DETECTIVE** First off, ignore the advertising copy on the front. Flip around to the ingredients list. Is every grain a whole grain? Does each slice have 2 or more grams of fiber? Do "inulin" or "polydextrose" show up? The correct answers should be yes, yes, and no. "With whole grain, nothing is stripped away," says Jim White, RD, a spokeperson for the Academy of Nutrition and Dietetics. That means you're noshing on natural fiber, not inulin or polydex-

trose, two additives used to artificially boost fiber.

■ **CRACK THE WHOLE GRAIN CODE** The ingredients list isn't the only place to spot a true whole grain food. In 2005, the Whole Grain Council introduced a labeling system to help consumers easily spot whole grain products. Their square yellow stamp, which has a sheaf of grain on it, flags foods that are "100% Whole Grain," making it easier for you to find healthy options while shopping.

■ **SNACK ON POPCORN** A recent study in the *Journal of the American Dietetic Association* found that people who eat popcorn consume up to two and a half times more whole grains than those who don't eat the stuff. Just don't buy the bucket at the movie theater. In its unadulterated—i.e., butterless—form, popcorn is one of the healthiest snacks in the supermarket. As a whole grain, it's high in fiber, and since it's made with air, it will fill you up for few calories. Although you should prioritize popcorn made with healthy olive or canola oils, you can also choose plain, lightly salted popcorn, such as Orville Redenbacher's Natural Simply Salted. (For instructions on making your own, see "Pick Your Popcorn" on page 238.)

■ **DON'T BE FOOLED BY MULTIGRAIN** *Multigrain* doesn't necessarily mean whole grain. The term may indicate a blend of whole grains, which is good, but it could also refer to a mix of refined grains. You don't know until you check the ingredients list. Other misleading ingredients: wheat flour (without the word "whole"), stoneground, durum wheat, bran, and wheat germ. These aren't whole grains.

YOUR FAVORITE FOODS, WHOLE GRAIN EDITION

Asian noodles

Annie Chun's Pad Thai Brown Rice Noodles

Wrap your fork around this: rice noodles with the same texture as those in your favorite takeout, but with bonus fiber.

Nutrition info (per 2 ounces): 200 calories, 1 g fat (0.5 g saturated), 44 g carbs, 4 g fiber, 10 mg sodium, 4 g protein

Bagel

Rudi's Organic Bakery Honey Sweet Wheat Bagel

The touch of honey will make your taste buds forget that this bagel is 100 percent whole grain.

Nutrition info: 130 calories, 1.5 g fat (0 g saturated), 28 g carbs, 5 g fiber, 240 mg sodium, 6 g protein

Bread

Pepperidge Farm Whole Grain 15 Grain

There's not a trace of high-fructose corn syrup lurking in this fiber-packed bread.

Nutrition info (per slice): 100 calories, 2 g fat (0.5 g saturated), 20 g carbs, 4 g fiber, 115 mg sodium, 5 g protein

Burger bun

Martin's Whole Wheat Potato Roll

Hearty *and* fluffy, these buttery-tasting rolls are the perfect base for your burger.

Nutrition info: 100 calories, 1 g fat (0 g saturated), 18 g carbs, 5 g fiber, 160 mg sodium, 7 g protein

Cereal (Cold)

Post Original Shredded Wheat

The folks at Post weren't lying when they described this cereal as "100% whole-grain goodness." A serving boasts 47 grams of whole grains—nearly three servings' worth—and 6 grams of belly-filling fiber. Add some chopped fresh fruit such as blueberries or sliced strawberries to boost the flavor and fiber.

Nutrition info (per 2 biscuits): 156 calories, 1 g fat (0 g saturated), 38 g carbs, 5 g fiber, 3 mg sodium, 5 g protein

Cereal (Hot)

Arrowhead Mills Organic Steel Cut Hot Cereal

Whole-grain carbs, like steel-cut oatmeal, provide an easy-to-access source of glucose for your body and brain first thing in the morning. Whip up a bowl of Arrowhead oats, then add flavor and texture with one of the oatmeal upgrades on page 109.

Nutrition info (per ¼ cup): 160 calories, 3 g fat, 27 g carbs, 8 g fiber, 0 mg sodium, 6 g protein

Cereal (Hot, Instant)

Quaker High Fiber Cinnamon Swirl Instant Oatmeal

This Quaker creation cooks up quickly but tastes slow-simmered. The 10 grams of fiber will keep you full throughout the morning, and the cinnamon will help stabilize your blood sugar.

Nutrition info: 160 calories, 2 g fat (0.5 g saturated), 34 g carbs, 10 g fiber, 210 mg sodium, 4 g protein

(continued)

YOUR FAVORITE FOODS, WHOLE GRAIN EDITION—Cont.

Cookies

Kashi Oatmeal Raisin Flax Soft-Baked Cookies

This delightful treat is the perfect way to satisfy a cookie craving while also gaining whole grains.

Nutrition info (per cookie): 130 calories, 4.5 g fat (0 g saturated), 20 g carbs, 4 g fiber, 70 mg sodium, 2 g protein

Crackers

Kashi Snack Crackers Original 7 Grain

You won't find enriched flour, hydrogenated oils, or artificial colors in these crackers.

Nutrition info (per 15 crackers): 120 calories, 3.5 g fat (0 g saturated), 19 g carbs, 3 g fiber, 160 mg sodium, 4 g protein

English Muffin

Weight Watchers Wheat English Muffin

Forget nooks and crannies. The Weight Watchers' take on the English muffin costs you minimal calories and effortlessly adds whole grains to your day. Toast and top with an egg and cheese for a homemade version of the Egg McMuffin.

Nutrition info: 100 calories, 1 g fat (0 saturated), 21 g carbs, 6 g fiber, 230 mg sodium, 6 g protein

Flour

King Arthur Premium 100% Whole Wheat Flour

If you switch to whole-wheat bread, why not do the same with your flour? The red wheat in this bag is more nutrient dense and protein packed than regular white wheat.

Nutrition info (per ¼ cup): 110 calories, 1 g fat (0 g saturated), 21 g carbs, 4 g fiber, 0 mg sodium, 4 g protein

Frozen pizza

Kashi Thin Crust Mediterranean Pizza

Instead of refined-carb crust, this Kashi creation—topped with spinach, red onions, and red peppers—is built on a base of whole grains, flaxseed, and sesame seeds.

Nutrition info (per ⅓ pizza): 290 calories, 9 g fat (4 g saturated), 37 g carbs, 5 g fiber, 640 mg sodium, 15 g protein

Granola

Nature's Path Organic Ancient Grains Granola with Almonds

This granola is heavy on nuts, not excess sugar. The result: a dose of healthy fats, along with a sizeable shot of fiber from the medley of whole grains, which includes oats and amaranth.

Nutrition info (per 3/4 cup): 250 calories, 9 g fat (1.5 g saturated), 39 g carbs, 6 g fiber, 135 mg sodium, 5 g protein

Mac 'n' cheese

Annie's Organic Whole Wheat Shells & White Cheddar

Healthier comfort food? Yes, please! Mac 'n' cheese gets a fiber and protein punch from whole grain noodles and velvety white Cheddar sauce.

Nutrition info (per cup): 260 calories, 4.5 g fat (2 g saturated), 43 g carbs, 5 g fiber, 570 mg sodium, 9 g protein

Pancakes

Batter Blaster Organic Whole Wheat with Brown Sugar & Cinnamon Ready-to-Cook Pancake & Waffle Batter

Just point, squirt, and cook for perfect fluffy pancakes on demand.

Nutrition info (per ¼ cup): 90 calories, 1 g fat (0 g saturated), 17 g carbs, 2 g fiber, 280 mg sodium, 2 g protein

Pita

Weight Watchers 100% Whole Wheat Pita

You won't find 9 grams of belly-filling fiber for only 100 calories anywhere else.

Nutrition info: 100 calories; 1 g fat (0 saturated), 24 g carbs, 9 g fiber, 260 sodium, 7 g protein

Pizza Crust

Rustic Crust Organic Great Grains Originale

The first ingredient is organic whole-grain flour—and it only gets better: organic rye flour, organic crushed oats, barley, to name just a few of the grains packed into this crust.

Nutrition info (per ⅙ crust): 140 calories, 2 g fat (0 g saturated), 28 g carbs, 5 g fiber, 190 mg sodium, 5 g protein

Rice

Uncle Ben's Ready Rice Whole Grain Brown

Zap this microwave-safe pouch for an instant whole-grain base for steamed veggies.

Nutrition info (per 1 cup): 190 calories, 3 g fat (0 g saturated), 39 g carbs, 3 g fiber, 15 mg sodium, 5 g protein

Sandwich thin

Arnold Fill'ems 100% Whole Wheat Sandwich Thins

Use these rectangular rolls in place of standard hot dog buns.

Nutrition info: 100 calories, 1 g fat (0 g saturated), 21 g carbs, 5 g fiber, 170 mg sodium, 5 g protein

Snack bar

Kashi Ripe Strawberry Cereal Bar

You wouldn't guess it, but this bar's soft-baked shell is made with whole grains.

Nutrition info: 130 calories, 3 g fat (0 g saturated), 24 g carbs, 3 g fiber, 100 mg sodium, 2 g protein

Spaghetti

De Cecco Enriched Whole Wheat Spaghetti

Gritty whole-grain pasta? Not here. The nutty, full flavor of this spaghetti is sure to satisfy.

Nutrition info (per 2 ounces): 180 calories, 1.5 g fat (0 g saturated), 35 g carbs, 7 g fiber, 0 mg sodium, 8 g protein

Tortilla

La Tortilla Factory EVOO Multigrain Soft Wrap

With these substantial tortillas, multigrain means whole-wheat flour, whole-grain millet, and whole-grain brown rice. Plus, an extra shot of oat fiber makes them super filling. Try warming one in a skillet before assembling your burrito.

Nutrition info (per wrap): 100 calories, 4 g fat (0.5 g saturated), 18 g carbs, 12 g fiber, 290 mg sodium, 9 g protein

Waffles

Kashi 7 Grain Waffles

This multigrain blend includes oats, whole wheat, rye, brown rice, barley, and buckwheat—all whole grains.

Nutrition info (per 2 waffles): 150 calories, 5 g fat (0.5 g saturated), 25 g carbs, 7 g fiber, 340 mg sodium, 4 g protein

Part 4
YOUR FITNESS

Move your body, lose more weight

Certain things go better together: coffee and coffee cake; Fourth of July and fireworks; kites and windy days. Diet and exercise. There's a reason the two nouns are often found in the same phrase. "One healthy behavior without the other will not work," says John Jakicic, PhD, chair of the department of health and physical activity at the University of Pittsburgh. "You need to diet and exercise to maintain long-term weight loss."

Sure, you can lose weight by dieting. You can lose it by exercising more. But studies show that combining the two efforts helps you shed pounds quicker and keep them off longer.

For those of you who dislike exercise, we suggest redefining what exercise means to you. If when you think "exercise," you imagine sweat and pain, then you need to open yourself to the notion that not all exercise is uncomfortable drudgery. Exercise can be fun. Also, view exercise as not just a way to change your appearance but also as a way to change your life, says J. Graham Thomas, PhD, a researcher at Brown University's Weight Control and Diabetes Research Center. Shift your focus from the scale to the other benefits exercise will bring: increased energy, elevated mood, greater self-esteem, and better health. Make this mental shift, and you may find that you actually look forward to your workout—the secret to sticking with it. This chapter includes expert advice to help you do just that.

Aerobic Exercise

15 ways to boost your cardio workout

Aerobic exercise is physical movement done at a low to moderate intensity—like walking, running, cycling, and swimming—where your lungs and heart are bringing enough oxygen in to feed your working muscles. *Aerobic* literally means "living in air." The opposite of aerobic exercise is anaerobic, which refers to very short-duration bursts of intense physical activity, such as lifting heavy weights to build muscle. It's effort that can't be sustained for longer than a few minutes.

Both types of exercise are useful for weight loss; as we've learned, more muscle on your body boosts your metabolism and burns more calories. But aerobic exercise has earned a reputation as one of the best ways to lighten your load—and rightfully so. A study in the journal *Obesity* found that just 80 minutes of cardiovascular exercise per week can slow weight gain and accumulation of abdominal fat a year after weight loss, while research in the *American Journal of Physiology* showed that an hour of intense cardio may quash appetite for up to 2 hours. Aerobic exercise stamps out the hunger hormone ghrelin while increasing levels of an appetite-suppressing hormone, says study author David Stensel, PhD. However, stepping on the treadmill isn't a guarantee that you'll blast fat—there's a right

HOW TOP DOCTORS STAY SLIM

"With three young kids and full-time work, it's really hard to fit in going to the gym. So I take walks with the kids, I take the stairs to my sixth-floor office, and I have small weights and resistance bands at home."

—NAOMI STOTLAND, MD, a doctor at the Center for Obesity Assessment, Study, and Treatment at the University of California, San Francisco

way to perform your aerobic exercise. Here are some useful tips:

■ **EASE INTO EXERCISE** One of the biggest mistakes people make when jumping into an exercise program is, well, jumping into an exercise program—one that's too rigorous and physically demanding. That's often a recipe for disaster. If you haven't been very active in a long time, you can easily injure yourself by starting too aggressively or may burn out quickly. Rather than going gung-ho and then petering out, start with just 2 or 3 days of light exercise a week for 2 to 4 weeks (walking is a great way to start), then gradually add more workout days to your routine. You don't have to start with hourlong sweat sessions, either—even 15 to 20 minutes of exercise will make a difference. Once you build up to a more regular routine, alternate intense workouts with easier ones, and allow yourself 1 day of rest and recovery in between.

■ **RETHINK YOUR WARM UP** Touching your toes is *not* the right way to warm up. In fact, any static stretching—the kind you learned in high school gym class—can actually cause injury because it stretches muscles that are cold, which can cause painful strains, pulls, and tears. The best warm up mimics the exercise you're about to do—a cardio workout should be preceded by a cardio warm up. The idea is for your heart to send warming blood to your limbs. An ideal warm up: 20 jumping jacks. You'll raise your heart rate and activate both lower- and upper-body muscles. Another

reason to keep it brief: A study in the *Journal of Applied Physiology* found that lengthy warm ups may wear you out, compromising your workout.

■ **LOG 30 MINUTES A DAY** You don't have to run a marathon every week to enjoy the benefits of cardio exercise. Aim to log 30 minutes of moderate aerobic exercise at least 5 days a week, whether it's walking, jogging, swimming, intervals, or cycling. Your heart rate should hit between 50 and 70 percent of its maximum rate. (See page 4 for the maximum heart-rate formula.) And don't just crank out a couple of miles on the treadmill at the same speed every day. You need to mix things up and push yourself—changing the intensity and type of exercise trains your muscles differently, so you'll see improvements more quickly.

■ **EXPERIMENT WITH INTERVALS** You can breathe a sigh of relief: Logging mile after mile won't necessarily help you lose weight. In fact, if you're already dieting, studies show that distance running does little to enhance your fat loss. Your aerobic prescription: intervals. A growing body of research suggests that intervals—short bursts of intense exercise, separated by brief rest periods—can accelerate your fat loss and improve your fitness more quickly than long bouts of exercise. In a study in *Medicine & Science in Sports & Exercise*, women who alternated 2-minute bouts of high-intensity running with 3 minutes of low-intensity jogging torched more calories the

SPIN OFF THE POUNDS

Spin class can be intimidating, especially if you're new to group exercise. The serious-looking equipment, the hard-core exercisers wearing special shoes, the dim lights and loud music—it's a lot to take in. But don't let that deter you from taking a class. In a Harvard University study of more than 18,000 women over a period of 16 years, those who biked for as few as 5 minutes a day gained less weight than those who didn't pedal. Spinning is the perfect combination of cardio and muscle-toning exercise, and it's easier on your hips and knees than running. Ready to start Spinning? Use these pointers from Olympian Alison Dunlap, who runs bike skills clinics in Utah and Colorado, to increase your confidence in the saddle.

Achieve the perfect setup

Positioning your bike is half the battle in Spin class. Adjust your seat so your knees are bent slightly when your foot is at the bottom of a rotation. Sixty percent of your weight should be in the saddle (seat) and 40 percent on the handlebar.

Pedal smoothly

You don't need to forcefully stomp the pedals. Rather, you should create fluid circles with your feet. Try this technique: Place the ball of your foot on the pedal, push down, and pull your foot through the bottom of the stroke. Then pull up and back around. A faster cadence is better—it boosts your heart rate and actually wears out your muscles less than slower pedaling does.

Keep your head up

Even when you're feeling fatigued, don't put your head down. This can hinder your ability to take in oxygen, which will only make you wear out faster.

Stabilize your core

While your legs are pedaling, keep your upper body relaxed and still—don't rock side to side. Maintain a flat back and keep your elbows bent and relaxed, holding your arms in line with your body (not out to your sides).

next day than those who ran at a slow and steady pace.

What makes intervals so effective? Studies show that they trigger an afterburn effect similar to strength training, so your body churns through calories long after you've finished your workout. The key to raising your metabolism is making the intervals sufficiently intense, according to a study in the *Journal of Physiology*. You need to push yourself out of your comfort zone and apply intense effort to win big. Try these interval strategies:

1. Find a flat section of road, visit a running track, or hop on a treadmill. Speed up to a hard but sustainable effort—you should be huffing and puffing—for 15 seconds. Jog or walk for 60 seconds. Repeat six times.

2. Speed up to a hard but sustainable effort for 30 seconds. Jog or walk to recover for 60 seconds. Repeat four times.

3. Run ¼ mile—the equivalent of one loop around a track—on flat or slightly hilly terrain at a hard but sustainable effort. Then jog or walk for 2 minutes. Repeat four times.

4. Try interval training on your bicycle. Pedal hard and fast for 30 seconds, followed by 60 seconds at a moderate (recovery) pace. Another way is to switch gears—back and forth between your largest and smallest chainrings—to change up pedaling resistance on a flat road.

■ **BEAT BOREDOM** The key to success with aerobic exercise is to find an activity that you really enjoy. If you find the elliptical a bore, try a Spin class. Or if you despise the treadmill, run around a lake. It's about finding what excites you to exercise, says Kristen Dieffenbach, PhD, an assistant professor of athletic coaching education at West Virginia University. "Try as many classes, running paths, and exercise machines as you can. Somewhere between swimming and Spinning, you will click with an activity or two." Actually liking your workout makes it that much easier to invest time in it.

■ **START STRONG** In a recent study from the College of New Jersey, exercisers who pushed themselves during the first half of their workout, then eased up for the second half, burned 23 percent more fat than those who did the opposite. So jump on the treadmill or elliptical, crank as hard as you can, then wind down toward the end.

■ **DON'T FEAR THE DUMBBELLS** Many women avoid one of the best calorie-burning activities—weight lifting—because they are afraid of becoming muscle-bound. Don't worry. It's unlikely to happen. Weight lifting doesn't necessarily increase your size. (It takes a special kind of heavy-weight lifting to do that.) Think of it this way: Lifting makes you stronger from head to toe, so you can exercise harder during your cardio workouts.

And you don't even have to "lift weights" to enjoy the benefits. *Resistance training* is a catchall term for any kind of strength training where you work your muscles against resistance. That resistance can come from exercise rubber bands or tubes, a medicine ball, a sandbag, even jugs of water or cans of beans.

MAKE CARDIO MACHINE WORKOUTS BURN FAT FASTER

Avoid common mistakes that reduce the effectiveness of your exercise.

Rowing machine

Common mistake: You do the entire workout at the same slow pace.

Fast fix: Set the machine to a medium level of resistance. Then complete four to six 10-minute sets of higher intensity rowing, separated by 2 to 3 minutes of easy resting strokes.

Treadmill

Common mistake: You run on a flat (zero-incline) platform.

Fast fix: Elevating the treadmill to a 1 percent grade mimics the outdoor air resistance that you lose when you exercise inside on a treadmill. Whenever you hop on a treadmill, crank up the incline to 1 percent. Then increase the incline from there to 2 percent and work up to a 10 percent incline and back down over the course of your workout. By walking or running at a higher incline, you make your workout more intense, burning more calories in a shorter period of time.

Stationary bike

Common mistake: Cruising instead of charging.

Fast fix: Cycle at a high cadence for 2 to 3 minutes, then rest for 3 minutes. Repeat this interval cycle for 15 minutes, varying the intensity and standing occasionally.

Elliptical

Common mistake: You glide like a gazelle, using the momentum of the pedals to carry your feet and legs.

Fast fix: Crank up the resistance. When you make a revolution, it should feel like you're pushing the ramp down. Try doing 90-second blasts at a high level of resistance, then recover for 90 seconds.

Stairclimber

Common mistake: Leaning on the hand supports, which is cheating yourself out of a good workout.

Fast fix: Pump your arms as you climb; only touch the bar for balance. Climb more slowly, using a higher level of resistance.

Body-weight calisthenics is an excellent resistance workout.

Recent research from the College of New Jersey confirms that resistance training can make your cardio workout more effective. In the study, people who performed a strength-training workout before riding a stationary bike burned more fat during their cardio session than those who didn't do any resistance training. Another study found that people who incorporated aerobic exercise and weight training into their 3-day-a-week routine lost 5 more pounds of fat than those who only performed aerobic exercise. Stressing your muscles through resistance training may activate fat-burning hormones that cardio doesn't.

■ **SQUEEZE IN AN A.M. RUN** The morning is prime workout time. "You're burning a higher percentage of fat before eating breakfast," says Lonnie Lowery, PhD, RD, a professor of exercise and nutrition science at Winona State University in Minnesota. That's because, after 8 hours of rest, your body's available carbohydrate supply is sapped, and your balance of hormones in the a.m. makes body fat more accessible. You'll reap the rewards for hours: Running triggers the release of thyroid hormones, which keep your metabolism on high well after you've showered.

BONUS BENEFIT!

You may feel grumpy when the alarm clock goes off—but your funk won't last for long. An early cardio workout will boost your mood, says Cedric Bryant, PhD, chief science officer for the American Council on Exercise. Aerobic exercise increases your brain's release of serotonin (a hormone associated with happiness) and dopamine (a hormone closely linked to motivation).

■ **WORK IN CIRCUITS** Circuit workouts, where you complete at least three exercises in a row without resting, can enhance your fat burn for up to an hour after you're finished. Try combining cardio and strength training into a fat-blasting circuit: Alternate 2 minutes of walking, jogging, cycling, or stairclimbing with a minute of body-weight exercises, like pushups, squats, and lunges. (This is especially useful if you only have a short amount of time for your workout.) The quick bursts of effort keep your heart rate up, giving you that cardio buzz you crave. (For more on circuits, see page 315.)

■ **WATCH YOUR POSTURE** Research shows that slumping during your cardio workout can make your workout feel harder. When running or walking, pull back your shoulder blades to open your chest; this allows you to breathe in more oxygen, so intense effort will feel easier and you'll burn more calories.

■ **FIND YOUR GROOVE** Listening to the right music can help you exercise harder and longer. A 2007 British study found that treadmill runners were more productive when they matched their pace to music with a tempo of

120 to 140 beats per minute (bpm). Another study found that people are more likely to stick to an exercise program if they listen to music. Not only is music motivating, but it also provides a beat that helps you keep your intensity on target.

For medium-intensity exercise, select songs with a tempo of about 120 bpm, and for high-intensity exercise, work out to tunes that are at least 140 bpm. Designate one power song to play when you start slowing down; it should have both a fast pace and lyrics that fire you up. Not sure where to start? Create your own mix at JogTunes.com, or try these perfect workout songs:

> "Pump It" by the Black Eyed Peas (120 bpm)
>
> "Livin' on a Prayer" by Bon Jovi (120 bpm)
>
> "You Shook Me All Night Long" by ACDC (127 bpm)
>
> "Moves Like Jagger" by Maroon 5 featuring Christina Aguilera (128 bpm)
>
> "The Time (Dirty Bit)" by the Black Eyed Peas (128 bpm)
>
> "Where Are We Runnin'?" by Lenny Kravitz (130 bpm)
>
> "On the Floor" remix by Jennifer Lopez and Pitbull (137 bpm)
>
> "How Far We've Come" by Matchbox Twenty (166 bpm)
>
> "Are You Gonna Be My Girl" by Jet (209 bpm)

■ **DIVERSIFY YOUR CARDIO WORKOUT** When the scale stops budging, it's time to switch up your workout—the more comfortable you are with your routine, the less effective it becomes. If you normally run on the treadmill, try a Spin class instead. If you love walking, switch to slow jogging or swimming. Even altering your favorite exercise routine slightly will do the trick. If you enjoy intervals, try shortening them, or if you love road biking, try mountain biking on a hilly trail. Then find another activity that complements your everyday routine. For example, add yoga to your routine to loosen and lengthen your muscles, or swim laps to build greater endurance. Adding variety to your workouts busts boredom, helping to keep you motivated.

■ **DON'T TRUST THE CALORIE COUNTER** The "calories burned" display on most treadmills and elliptical machines is unfortunately inaccurate. Why? The number reflects both calories burned through exercise *and* the energy you'd normally burn at rest, says Alex Koch, PhD, an exercise scientist at Truman State University. That means it's inflated by as much as 30 percent! For a more accurate estimate, multiply the number of minutes you exercise by 1.2—approximately how many calories you'd burn at rest. Then subtract this from the number on the treadmill display.

■ **WALK OR RUN UPHILL** If you're a treadmill runner, don't keep the platform flat the entire time. The extra effort of running on an

FOOD THAT FUELS

The right foods can energize your cardio routine—without derailing your diet.

BEFORE CARDIO

If your sweat session is 45 minutes or shorter, you don't need to munch beforehand (unless it's been several hours since your last meal or snack). For longer cardio workouts, grab a protein/carb combo, such as whole grain crackers with hummus or an apple with string cheese.

AFTER CARDIO

If you spent at least 45 minutes in motion or it'll be a few hours until your next meal, eat another carb/protein snack afterward. A couple of options: apple slices with a thin smear of peanut butter or low-fat chocolate milk.

incline can help blast fat. In fact, for each degree of incline, you could boost your burn by as much as 10 percent, says Jana Klauer, MD, a New York City–based physician and metabolism expert. That means running at a 5 per-

cent grade—the equivalent of a gentle hill—could help you burn 50 percent more calories than running on a totally flat surface! The reason is simple: To run forward *and* uphill, you have to recruit more muscles to propel you. Start by setting your treadmill at a 5 percent incline, and run at a hard but sustainable speed for 10 seconds. Reset your incline to zero until you catch your breath, about 45 to 60 seconds. Repeat, while gradually increasing the incline.

■ **KEEP AN EXERCISE LOG** Monitoring your progress will help keep you motivated. Carry a workout log with you to the gym, and write down everything you do. Go into specifics—for example, "jogged at 6 mph for 20 minutes," "took half-hour Spin class," etc. As you accumulate entries, you'll be able to track your growth on paper, reminding you of how far you've come. This creates a cycle of positive reinforcement that keeps you going back to the gym.

Body-Weight Resistance Exercises

Use what God gave you for the best workout of your life

There are many benefits to doing body-weight-only resistance exercises:

• No storage issues. Your body is your equipment.

• You won't drop a barbell on your toes.

• You won't have to schlep across town during a snowstorm just to exercise.

• It's free.

• You won't have to share space with intimidating muscleheads wearing Kataklysm T-shirts.

• You can do them just about anywhere.

On the following pages are classic body-weight exercises. String together five or six exercises that work different muscle groups for a total-body, calorie-frying workout.

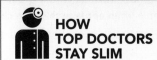

HOW TOP DOCTORS STAY SLIM

"I've got a pullup bar hanging above the door in my office. I don't do a lot of weights, but I do push-pull exercises—pushups, pullups, situps, using my own body weight—that I can do on the road when I travel. Strength training and isometrics seem to be particularly good for decreasing the body mass index."

—SANJAY GUPTA, MD, an assistant professor of neurosurgery at Emory University and CNN's chief medical correspondent

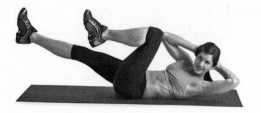

BICYCLE CURL

Firms the fronts and sides of your abs

Lie flat on your back, with your hands resting lightly behind your head and your feet flat. Then lift your head and upper back while extending your left leg off the floor and drawing your right knee toward your chest. Twist your torso to the right to bring your left elbow and right knee toward each other. Release and repeat, this time pulling your right elbow and left knee. Continue alternating sides.

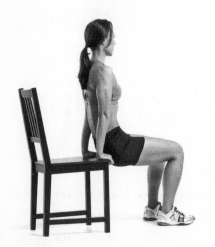

CHAIR DIP

Tones and tightens your shoulders and arms

Sit on the edge of a sturdy chair, with your knees bent and your feet flat on the floor. Your hands should be by your hips, grasping the seat. Press into your palms to lift your hips slightly in front of the seat. Bend your elbows back to almost 90 degrees, lowering your body toward the floor. Straighten your arms and repeat.

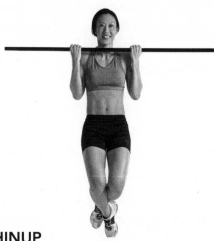

CHINUP

Works your biceps, back, shoulders, and core. Also strengthens the muscles that help you stand tall, so you look longer and leaner. Grab the chinup bar, using a shoulder-width, underhand grip. (Your palms should be facing your body.) Allow your body to hang so your arms are straight. Cross your ankles behind you, then pull yourself up until your chin is over the bar. Pause, then slowly lower your body back down to the hanging position. Don't get discouraged if you have trouble. This is a tough exercise, but it's worth working at. To improve, try the following beginner modifications.

Chinup beginner modification 1

Stand on a sturdy chair under the chinup bar. Use the chair to boost yourself into the up position. Now, lift your feet off the chair and bend them behind you. Very slowly lower yourself until your arms are straight. This is what's known a "doing a negative" in gym parlance, and it's very effective for building strength. Because the lowering phase of this move is easier than the lifting phase, doing negative chinups is a great way to work up to the full exercise.

Chinup beginner modification 2

This involves a partner. Ask a friend to grab your waist and push you up as you begin curling your body up to the bar from the down position. At the top, your friend will let go of you and you can perform a slow negative chinup until your arms are straight and you're ready for the next helper boost up. In time, you'll develop the strength to do chinups without help.

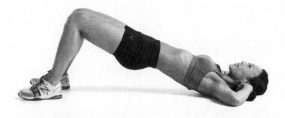

HIP RAISE

Exercises your glutes, the large muscles in your butt, and your hamstrings. Engages your core and lower-back muscles in order to keep your body stable.

Lie flat on your back with your knees bent at a 45-degree angle and your feet flat on the floor. Extend your arms at a 45-degree angle by your sides, with your palms facing up. Slowly raise your hips until your body forms a straight line from your shoulders to your knees. Pause for about 5 seconds, pushing your heels against the floor and squeezing your butt muscles. Lower your body to the starting position.

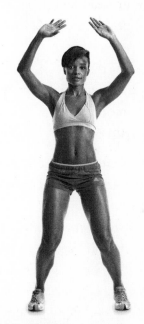

JUMPING JACK

A phys-ed classic that elevates your heart rate, primes your muscles for activity, and improves your flexibility

Stand with your feet together and your hands at your sides. Jump up just enough to spread your feet wide while simultaneously raising your arms overhead. Without pausing, jump back to the starting position.

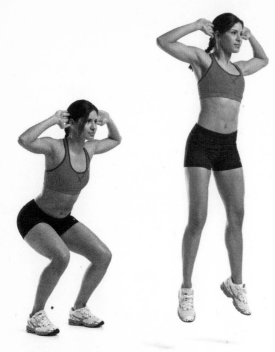

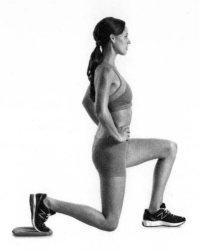

SQUAT JUMP

Activates the quadriceps, core, glutes, hamstrings, and calves and boosts your cardio endurance

Stand straight, with your feet hip-width apart. Position your fingers on the back of your head, pulling your elbows back so they're in line with your body. Bend your knees until your thighs are as close to parallel with the floor as possible. Now explosively jump as high as you can.

LUNGE

Works your quadriceps, as well as your glutes, hamstrings, and calves

Stand straight, with your feet hip-width apart. Place your hands on your hips or behind your ears. Step forward with your left leg, slowly lowering your body until your front knee is bent at a 90-degree angle. Your right knee should nearly touch the floor. Pause before pushing your body back to the starting position as quickly as possible. Repeat with the opposite leg.

MOUNTAIN CLIMBER

This is a great core exercise that also helps train you to keep your spine stable, which can help prevent lower-back trouble

Kneel on all fours and position your hands on the floor so they're slightly wider than shoulder-width apart. Draw your feet close together and straighten your arms and legs. Your body should form a straight line from

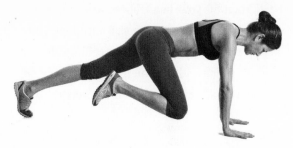

your head to your ankles. Lift your right foot, slowly drawing your knee as close to your chest as possible. Touch the floor with your right foot, then return to the starting position. Repeat with your left leg. Alternate back and forth for 30 seconds. Make sure to keep your core tight for the duration of the exercise.

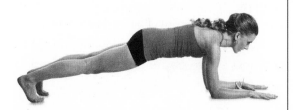

PLANK

Works your abs, glutes, thighs, and shoulders while stabilizing your spine

Lie facedown on the floor. Balance on your toes and prop up on your forearms. Your body should form a straight line from your ankles to your shoulders. Brace your abs and hold this position for 30 seconds, making sure to breathe deeply. If this is too difficult, try the following beginner modification.

Plank beginner modification

Lie facedown on the floor. Prop up on your forearms and knees. Bend your knees so they help support your body weight. Your body should form a straight line from your knees to your shoulders. Brace your abs and hold this position for 30 seconds. Make sure to breathe deeply. If you can't hold it for 30 seconds, try holding for 5 to 10 seconds, rest for 5 seconds, and repeat until you've completed 30 seconds in plank position.

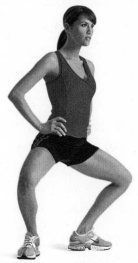

PLIÉ SQUAT

This ballet-inspired move works your inner thighs, glutes, and hips

Stand with your legs 2 to 3 feet apart, toes turned out. Place your hands on your hips. Push your hips back and lower your body until your thighs are parallel to the floor (or as close as possible). Pause, then slowly push yourself back to the starting position.

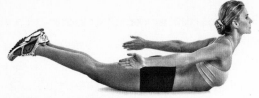

PRONE COBRA

Helps bolster weak muscles in your back while also strengthening your glutes and arms

Lie facedown on the floor with your legs straight and your arms by your sides, palms down. Tighten your butt muscles and your lower back, then lift your head, chest, arms, and legs off the floor. At the same time, rotate your arms so your thumbs point toward the ceiling. Ideally, only your hips and abdomen will be resting on the floor. Hold this position for 60 seconds.

PUSHUP

Works the large muscles of your chest (pectoralis major), shoulders (front deltoids), and triceps. Engages your core and hip muscles to keep your body stable.

BODY-WEIGHT WORKOUT UPGRADES

Whether you want to improve at golf or tennis, French cooking or organic gardening, technique is critical to getting the results you want. The same goes for fitness. Here are some tips that will help you get the most out of your body-weight workouts.

Stay off the ground

The fewer points of contact your body has with the floor, the more challenging the exercise. So lift one foot off the ground during your round of pushups, elevate an arm during the plank, or hold your foot in the air during squats. In these less stable positions, you'll be forced to engage more muscles to support yourself.

Add a mini-rep

Performing the toughest part of an exercise twice in 1 rep can boost your calorie burn—your body has to work harder to complete the extra movement with proper form. For example, when you're doing jump squats, drop into the squat position, rise up halfway, then lower back into the squat position before jumping up. As an extra challenge, try working in more than 1 mini-rep.

Lock it up

When performing lunges and squats, lace your fingers behind your head and pull your elbows back. This raises your body's center of gravity, forcing your core to work harder.

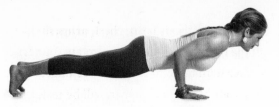

Kneel down on all fours and position your hands on the floor so they're slightly wider than shoulder-width apart. Draw your feet close together and straighten your arms and legs. Your body should form a straight line from your heels to your head. Keeping your elbows pulled in toward your sides, slowly lower your chest to an inch above the floor, then press back up. If this is too tough, try the exercise below.

Pushup beginner modification

Assume the modified pushup position—knees on the floor, forming a 45-degree angle with your torso. Make sure your back is straight from your butt to your head. Straighten your arms. Slowly lower your chest to the floor, keeping your core tight and your body in a straight line. Push back to the starting position.

Go doubles

Try combining two moves into one—you'll save time and work more of your muscles at once. For example, add a calf raise to plié squats.

Move the floor farther away

With many body-weight exercises—lunges and pushups, for example—your range of motion ends with the floor. Your solution: Place your front or back foot on a step when doing lunges, or your hands on books when doing pushups. This increases the distance your body has to travel from start to finish, so you do more work and spend more time in the most challenging part of the exercise.

Pause for 4 seconds

When you lower your body during an exercise, you accumulate "elastic energy," much like a coiled spring. This makes it easier to bounce back to the starting position. For an extra challenge, pause for 4 seconds in the down position of an exercise. This eliminates the elastic energy, so you have to work harder to return to the starting position.

Move in two directions

Add a rotational component to any exercise and you'll automatically work more muscles. Why? Rotating forces you to fully engage your core. For example, when you step back into a lunge, twist your torso in the opposite direction of your leading leg.

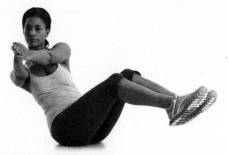

SEATED ROTATION

Targets your abs and obliques, helping you build a tighter midsection

Sit on the floor with your legs in front of you, your knees bent, and your heels lifted a few inches into the air. Lean back at a 45-degree angle and extend your arms straight in front of your chest, palms together. Slowly rotate your torso to the right, pause, then rotate to the left. Continue alternating.

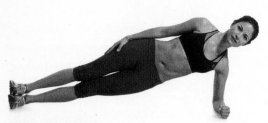

SIDE PLANK

Develops core strength and stability

Lie on your left side, with your knees straight. Prop your upper body up on your left elbow and forearm. Tighten your abs as forcefully as you can and raise your hips so your body forms a straight line from your ankles to your shoulders. Hold this position for 30 seconds, making sure to breathe deeply. Repeat on the opposite side. Too challenging? Try the move below.

Side plank beginner modification

Lie on your left side with your legs straight. Prop your upper body up on your left elbow and forearm, then bend and tuck your knees behind you at a 45-degree angle to reduce the amount of weight you have to lift. Now tighten your abs and raise your hips, forming a straight line from your knees to your shoulder. Hold this position for 30 seconds, then repeat on the opposite side. If you can't hold it for 30 seconds, try holding for 5 to 10 seconds, rest for 5 seconds, and repeat until you've completed 30 seconds in side-plank position.

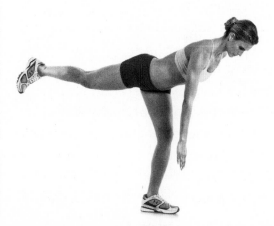

SINGLE-LEG DEADLIFT

Emphasizes your glutes and hamstrings but also targets your core and increases your lower-body flexibility

Balance on your right foot, with your knee soft and your hands on your hips, left leg lifted behind. With your abs tight and back straight, hinge forward from your hips, lowering your left hand toward your right foot. Pull through your right leg to return to standing. Switch sides.

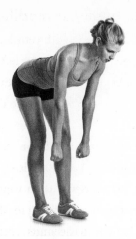

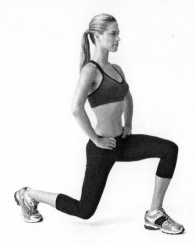

STRAIGHT-LEG DEADLIFT

Targets your glutes and hamstrings and strengthens lower back muscles

Stand with your feet hip-width apart, your knees slightly bent, and your hands held in front of your thighs. Without changing the bend in your knees, bend at your hips and lower your torso until it's almost parallel with the floor. Your back should stay naturally arched throughout the movement. Allow your hands to hang down by your shins. Pause, then raise your torso back to the starting position.

SPLIT SQUAT

Works the large muscles in your thighs, or quadriceps, as well as your hamstrings and glutes

Stand up straight, with your feet shoulder-width apart. Place your hands behind your ears or on your hips. Step forward about 3 feet with your left leg, then bend your knees and lower your back knee as close to the floor as

possible. Press through your left heel and return to standing. Switch legs and repeat.

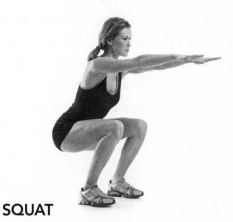

SQUAT

Targets your quadriceps, along with your glutes, hamstrings, and calves

Stand with your feet shoulder-width apart. Tighten your core and try to hold it that way for the entire exercise. Extend your arms straight out in front of your body at shoulder height, then lower your body by pushing your hips back and bending your knees. Your thighs should be parallel to the floor (or lower), and your weight should be on your heels. Pause, then slowly push back up to the starting position.

Y, T, I RAISES

Exercises your upper back, particularly your trapezius, the large muscles that run from your neck down to your shoulder blades

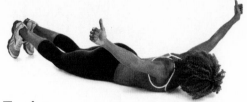

T raise

Lie facedown on the floor. Extend your arms straight out to your sides so your body forms a "T." Your thumbs should point up. Raise your arms as high as you can, pause, then slowly return to the starting position.

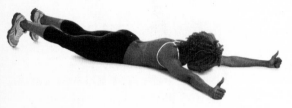

Y raise

Lie facedown on the floor with your arms at your sides. Lift your arms above your head, making a "Y" shape and allowing them to rest against the floor. Your palms should be facing each other. Now raise your arms as high as you comfortably can off the floor, pause, then lower them back to the starting position.

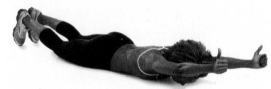

I raise

Lie facedown on the floor. Stick your arms straight out over your shoulders, so your body forms a straight line from toes to fingertips. Raise your arms as high as you can, pause, then slowly return to the starting position.

Circuit Training

6 fast-paced calorie-burning workouts

Circuit training has nothing to do with electricity. But you *can* expect it to spark your metabolic fire. This style of training involves short bursts of resistance training, one exercise after another, without rest, each move targeting a different muscle group. Since you emphasize different parts of your body with each exercise, you don't have to rest for long (or at all) in between sets, and you can maintain a higher intensity for a much longer time. This pumps up your heart rate, effectively adding an endurance component to strength training. To boost the cardio benefit, you can even work aerobic exercises into your routine, in what trainers call a "circuit plus."

Whatever your preferred circuit, one thing is certain: This style of training helps you burn fat fast. Research shows that circuit-style workouts can more than double your fat burn for an hour afterward. Circuits kick up the pace of your workout, increasing the challenge to your heart, lungs, and muscles, so you torch more calories. And the more muscles you work, the faster you'll lose your gut, since muscle is your body's primary fat burner. You can build your own circuits or try one of these sequences:

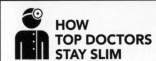

HOW TOP DOCTORS STAY SLIM

"Cities always have recreational sports leagues. I've played football through leagues like ZogSports. It's another way to keep active, but it's also a form of socializing. It's not just you and a treadmill in the gym."

—**THOMAS HILDEBRANT, PhD,** an assistant professor of psychiatry at the Mount Sinai School of Medicine who studies obesity

BODY-WEIGHT CIRCUIT

Take any four of the body-weight exercises found starting on page 305. Perform these four exercises one after another without resting in between. Complete 8 to 12 reps of each move, then repeat the entire sequence two more times, resting for a minute or two between circuits. Here's a good sample circuit:

1. Jumping jacks
2. Lunge
3. Pushup
4. Bicycle curl

SCULPTING DUMBBELL CIRCUIT

Grab a set of dumbbells heavy enough to lift just eight times. Complete two sets of 8 to 12 repetitions of the following four moves, resting 30 seconds between sets.

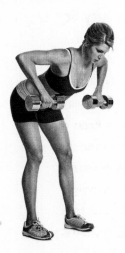

1. Row and Lift

Stand straight and hold your dumbbells in front of your thighs. Bend forward through your hips (45 to 90 degrees), keeping your weights close to your body. Let your arms hang below your shoulders, palms facing back. This is the starting position. Now bend your elbows and raise them toward the ceiling, pulling your dumbbells toward your chest. Lower the weights, then stand up, still keeping your dumbbells close to your body. That's 1 repetition.

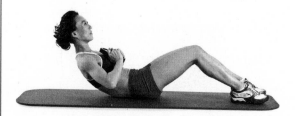

2. Curl and Press

Lie flat on your back with your legs bent. Hold your dumbbells (or a weight plate as shown) by your chest, elbows bent out to your sides. Tighten your abs as you lift your head and upper back off the floor. Press the dumbbells up, straightening your arms. Pause, then lower the weights and rest your head on the floor.

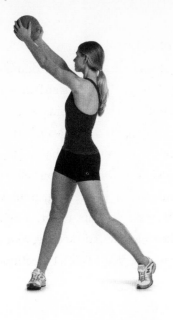

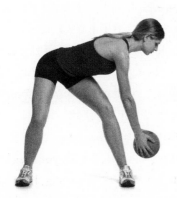

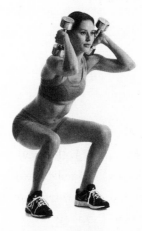

weight to the starting position. Repeat, doing half of your repetitions in this pattern, then lift the dumbbell above your left shoulder and do the exercise in the opposite direction, swinging the weight across your body to the right.

3. Cross Chop

Stand with your feet shoulder-width apart. Hold a lightweight dumbbell (or medicine ball as shown) with both hands. Lift the weight over your right shoulder, extending your arms straight. Now rotate your torso to the left and lower the dumbbell across your body and down toward your left shin in a chopping motion. As you swing the dumbbell, bend your knees and hips as if you were starting to sit back into a chair. Reverse the movement to return the

4. Double-Duty Squat

Stand with your feet shoulder-width apart, holding your dumbbells at your sides, your palms facing in. Bend your knees and hips, and lower your body as if sitting into a chair. Simultaneously bend your elbows to curl the weights up to your shoulders, palms facing your body. Keep your knees behind your toes by shifting your weight back into your heels and sticking your butt out. Press into your heels to stand up, and lower the weights.

RESISTANCE-CIRCUIT CHALLENGE

For this workout, you will need a pair of medium-weight dumbbells and a lat pulldown machine. Complete one set of 10 to 12 repetitions of each movement before resting for 60 seconds. Then repeat the entire sequence one or two times, for a total of two or three circuits. Every other workout, reverse the order in which you do the exercises. So in one session you'll start with the overhead squat, and the next you'll begin with the pushup.

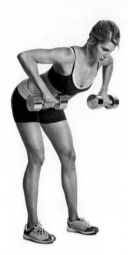

2. Dumbbell Row

Stand with your feet shoulder-width apart. Grab the dumbbells, bend at your hips and knees, and lean your torso forward until it's nearly parallel with the floor. Let the weights hang at arm's length, with your palms facing behind you. Bend your elbows and pull both dumbbells to the sides of your torso. Slowly return to the starting position.

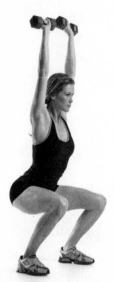

1. Overhead Dumbbell Squat

Stand with your feet slightly wider than hip-width apart. Hold a pair of dumbbells over your shoulders with your arms completely straight. Keeping your core tight, lower your body by sitting back with your hips until your thighs are as close to parallel with the floor as possible. Stand up, and lower the dumbbells to your sides. Repeat.

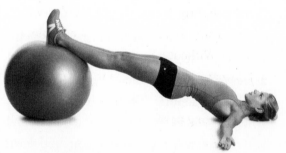

3. Lying Hip Extension

Lie flat on your back and place your heels on a bench or stability ball. Your hips should remain on the floor, and your legs can either be bent or straight. Extend your arms out to your sides for support, then raise your hips until your body forms a straight line from your shoulders to your knees. Pause, then lower yourself to the starting position.

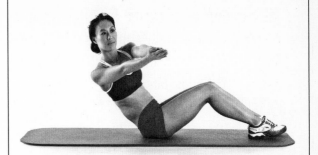

5. Russian Twist

Sit on the floor, knees bent and feet flat. Extend your arms straight out in front of your chest and hold your palms together. Lean back until your torso is at a 45-degree angle to the floor. Without raising or lowering your torso, rotate as far as you can to the right. Pause, then twist as far as you can to the left.

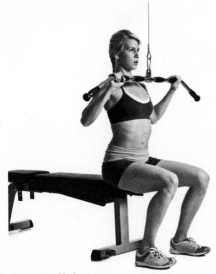

4. Lat Pulldown

Sit at a lat pulldown station. Grab the bar, using an overhand grip with your hands spaced slightly wider than shoulder-width apart. Your arms should be completely straight. Without moving your torso, pull the bar down to your chest, squeezing your shoulder blades together. Pause, then slowly return to the starting position.

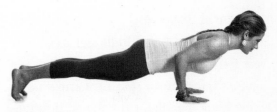

6. Pushup

Kneel down on all fours and position your hands on the floor so they're slightly wider than shoulder-width apart. Draw your feet close together and straighten your arms and legs. Your body should form a straight line from your heels to your head. Keeping your elbows pulled in toward your sides, slowly lower your chest to an inch above the floor, then press back up.

RESISTANCE + YOGA CIRCUIT

You will need a pair of lightweight dumbbells for this circuit. After completing each exercise, move immediately to the next without rest. Repeat the circuit two or three times.

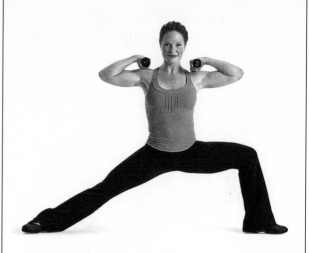

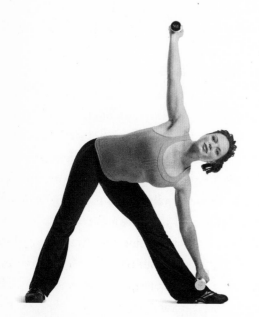

1. Lateral Bend and Dumbbell Reach

Grab a pair of dumbbells and stand with your feet about 4 feet apart. Turn your left foot out 90 degrees. Raise your right arm straight above your shoulder, palm facing in. Brace your abs and bend to the left, lowering the left dumbbell to your left ankle. Rise back up, keeping your right arm overhead. Do 12 to 15 reps, then repeat on the other side.

2. Biceps Warrior

Grab a pair of dumbbells and stand with your feet about 4 feet apart. Turn your left foot out 90 degrees and, hips and shoulders facing forward, bend your left knee 90 degrees. Extend your arms to shoulder height. With your upper arms parallel to the floor, do a biceps curl, bringing the dumbbells to your shoulders. Slowly extend your arms. Do 15 to 20 reps, then repeat on the other side.

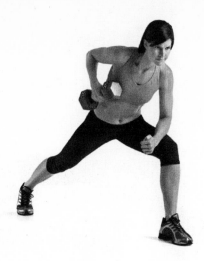

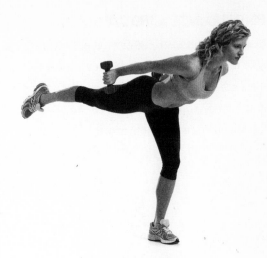

3. Warrior 1 Row

Hold a dumbbell in your right hand at your side and position yourself in a Warrior 1 yoga pose: Stand with your feet 3 to 4½ feet apart and turn your left foot and leg 90 degrees out to the left. Then turn your right foot inward, toward the left, until it achieves a 45-degree angle to your body. Next, rotate your hips and torso to face in the same direction as your left leg. Bend your left knee so its thigh and shin form a right angle. Keep your back foot pressed flat into the floor. Now, keeping your back flat and arms straight, bend your torso toward your front knee. Then bend your right elbow to lift the weight to the side of your chest. Slowly lower the weights back to the starting position. Complete 10 to 12 reps, then switch legs and repeat with the dumbbell in your left hand.

4. Warrior 3 Triceps Press

Starting in the Warrior 1 pose and holding a pair of dumbbells, lower your torso toward the floor, with your arms extended straight down from your shoulders. Straighten your front leg and lift your back leg off the ground as high as you can, keeping your core tight and back flat (Warrior 3 pose). Squeeze your shoulder blades and lift the weights to chest height, then extend your arms up and behind you. Slowly return to the starting position. Complete 10 to 12 reps, then switch legs and repeat.

ENDURANCE CIRCUIT

Perform each exercise for 30 seconds, then rest for 30 seconds before moving on to the next exercise in the circuit. Complete the circuit two or three times. Use 5- to 10-pound dumbbells or no weights at all.

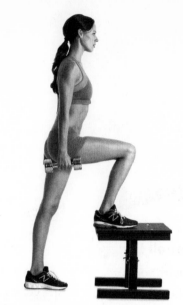

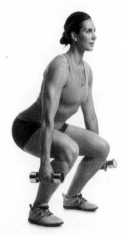

1. Dumbbell Squat

Stand with your feet shoulder-width apart. Hold the dumbbells at arm's length by your sides, with your palms facing your thighs. Tighten your core, then lower your body as far as you can by pushing your hips back and bending your knees. Pause, then slowly push back to the starting position.

2. Dumbbell Stepup

Hold the dumbbells at arm's length by your sides, with your palms facing your thighs. Standing in front of a bench or step, place your left foot firmly on the step. The step should be high enough that your knee bends at a 90-degree angle. Press your left heel into the step, and push your body up until your left leg is straight and you're standing on one foot on the bench, your right foot elevated. Step back down to the floor. Alternate legs.

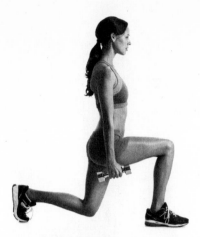

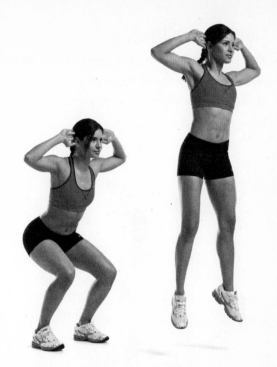

3. Dumbbell Lunge

Stand with your feet hip-width apart. Hold the dumbbells at arm's length by your sides, with your palms facing your thighs. Step back with your left foot, about 2 to 3 feet, and bend both knees until your front leg forms a 90-degree angle. Make sure your knee stays over your ankle. Return to the starting position as quickly as possible and repeat, alternating legs.

4. Body-Weight Jump Squat

Stand straight with your feet hip-width apart. Position your fingers on the back of your head, pulling your elbows back so they're in line with your body. Bend your knees until your thighs are as close to parallel with the floor as possible. Now explosively jump as high as you can.

CARDIO CIRCUIT

Perform these four cardio moves one after another, without resting in between. Repeat the circuit twice, with 1 minute of rest in between.

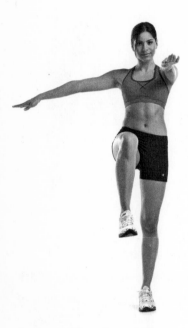

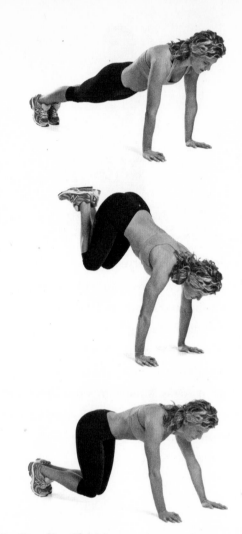

1. Standing Leg Lift

Stand with your feet shoulder-width apart, your arms at your sides. Lift your right knee as high as you can and swing your left arm forward until it's parallel to the floor. Return to the starting position, and repeat with your left knee and right arm. Continue alternating sides, completing as many reps as possible, for 1 minute.

2. Cardio Ski Hop

Start in the pushup position, with your arms completely straight. With your legs together, contract your abs and kick your legs to the right, bending them so your feet land just outside of your right shoulder. Hop back to the starting position and immediately repeat on the left side. Continue hopping side to side for 1 minute.

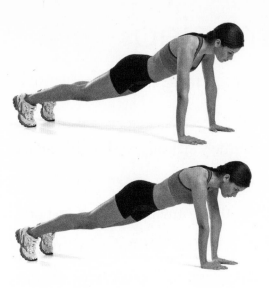

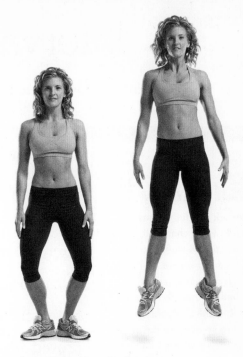

3. Hand Tap

Start in the pushup position, with your arms completely straight and your core tight. Lift your left hand, put it down next to your right hand, then return to the starting position. Repeat with your right hand and return to the starting position. Continue going back and forth for 1 minute, keeping your body in a straight line.

4. Plié Plyometric Jump

Stand with your legs together, your toes pointed out to form a V, and your arms at your sides. Tighten your abs, bend at the knees, and quickly jump up in the air, landing in the starting position. Repeat 20 times. Move your feet to wider than shoulder-width apart, your knees and toes still turned out. Jump in the air, keeping your legs wide. Repeat 20 times. Alternate between the first and second positions for 20 more reps.

Interval Training

5 ways to burn more calories during intervals

HOW TOP DOCTORS STAY SLIM

"I work out four times a week, and I change it up every 6 to 8 weeks to keep myself interested. I might run long distances for 8 weeks, then do intervals for 8 weeks. I'm always trying something different. The idea is never to commit to one approach."

—**THOMAS HILDEBRANT, PhD,** an assistant professor of psychiatry at the Mount Sinai School of Medicine who studies obesity

Our bodies are extremely efficient and highly adaptable machines. That actually makes weight loss more difficult: As you become more fit, your body's "exercise efficiency" improves—that is, your body learns to adapt to the exertion and conserve calories. Researchers at the University of California, Berkeley, proved this in a study monitoring runners who, despite their dedication to regular exercise, gained weight with each passing year. In order to avoid gaining weight, the researchers found, the runners had to boost their weekly mileage by 1.7 miles each year. They had to keep pushing their bodies with greater physical challenges in order to increase calorie burn. You can use this fact of life to your advantage and get the most effective workout for your time by regularly changing your exercise routine to keep your body from adapting and, well, getting lazy about calorie burning. One of the easiest ways to do that is interval training.

Intervals involve alternating between slow- to moderate-paced physical activity and short bursts of high-intensity effort. Studies have shown that this type of exercise forces your body to release fat-burning hormones that stoke your metabolism and keep it revving on high long after you've finished exercising. This is what sports scientists call the afterburn effect, the calories used while your body cools off and repairs muscles stressed by the exercise. Afterburn alone can torch an extra 100 to 200 calories, more than you'd burn off by running a mile.

You'll notice the difference on the scale quickly once you begin a program of regular interval training. In an Australian study, people who cranked out 20 minutes of high-intensity interval training 3 days a week dropped 10 percent of their body fat, while those who exercised longer but at a lower intensity didn't lose any. Another study showed that short, high-intensity workouts helped exercisers shed 20 percent of their visceral fat in just 3 months.

What makes intervals so effective? They mimic weight training. Running intervals forces you to crank out lots of power in a short amount of time, the same way that lunges, for example, intensely challenge your legs. Plus, intervals are thought to give your testosterone a boost, helping you build calorie-burning muscle and further elevating your metabolism.

The benefits of intervals aren't just metabolic. Since you're kicking up your intensity, you can shorten your gym sessions. You're enjoying the benefits of a 60-minute workout in half an hour. Some tips on getting the most from interval training:

■ **ESCAPE YOUR COMFORT ZONE** To really fire up your fat burners, don't just find an interval workout you like and stick with it forever. A study in the *Journal of Physiology* found that pushing out of your comfort zone can help you blast more fat. In fact, if you raise your level of effort, you could burn 10 percent of the total calories used during the workout shortly after exercising. It's all about keeping your muscles guessing with more effort and varied activity. If your normal interval effort is a 4 on an effort scale of 1 to 10, push your intensity up to a 7. You can increase the difficulty by adding more sets to your workout or by incorporating hills.

Need some inspiration? Rotate the following routines to constantly force your body through new challenges. Make sure to warm up and cool down with 5 to 10 minutes of slow jogging or fast walking.

1. Run at a hard but sustainable pace for 15 to 30 seconds and then jog or walk for 60 seconds.

2. Sprint all out for 30 seconds and then walk for 30 seconds or jog for 90 seconds.

3. Set the treadmill on an incline and run for 30 seconds. Then walk for 1 minute. Start with a 4 or 5 percent incline and work up to as much as 10 percent.

4. Jump rope doubles for a minute, then do 2 minutes of singles.

5. Alternately jog and walk in 1-minute intervals for 30 minutes. You can also alternate between speed walking and regular walking.

6. Run a quarter of a mile—the equivalent of one loop around a track—on flat or slightly hilly terrain at a hard but sustainable effort. Then jog or walk for 2 minutes.

7. Try a ladder drill: Run 1 minute hard, 2 minutes easy, 2 minutes hard, 3 minutes easy, 3 minutes hard, 4 minutes easy, and then work back down.

8. Whether running or cycling, speed up to a comfortably hard pace—where you can't say more than a few words at a time—and hold steady for 10 to 15 minutes. Then slow down and recover at a conversational pace for 5 minutes.

9. Find a hill in your neighborhood and run up it at a faster-than-average pace. At the top, turn around and slowly jog or walk back down, then power up and do it again.

10. On a stationary bike, sprint for 8 seconds, then slow to an easy pace for 12 seconds.

11. Set the treadmill incline to 10 percent and walk at a quick pace for a minute. Then lower the incline to zero and recover for a minute.

3 TYPES OF INTERVALS TO REV YOUR FAT BURNERS

TIME-SPECIFIC INTERVALS
Run, cycle, or swim hard for 20 seconds and then recover for 40 seconds. Ten minutes of these intervals—at the beginning or end of a regular workout or as a stand-alone training session—is plenty to start. Fifteen to 20 minutes is the max for anyone.

VOLUME-SPECIFIC INTERVALS
Rather than timing your exercise segments, log a specific distance, then recover for however long you need. You can easily train like this for a full 30- to 45-minute workout.

TIMED VOLUME-SPECIFIC INTERVALS
Try to hit a specific distance every minute. The faster you run, the more time you have to recover. With each set, your pace will slow down—but don't worry, that's a sign that you're working hard.

■ **CREATE AN INTERVALS PLAYLIST** For interval workouts, build a playlist that alternates fast songs with medium-tempo tunes. Then, as you're exercising, move faster during the high-tempo songs and take it down a notch during the slower ones.

■ **MAKE INTERVALS A WORKOUT STAPLE** It's okay to stick with steady-state cardio on occasion. Ideally, though, you'll work intervals into your routine at least 3 days a week—they more effectively blast fat than running at a consistent pace. Need some motivation to start moving? Consider the time you'll save by switching to intervals: In a study from Canada, exercisers who did 30-minute interval workouts shed three times as much fat in 15 weeks than those who performed 45-minute steady-state routines. That's an extra 15 minutes you could spend relaxing!

■ **STICK WITH IT** At first, interval training will leave you feeling sore and exhausted. But don't give up: The pain of interval training may subside after just six sessions. In a new study from California State University, cyclists produced more power and felt less leg pain by their sixth day of high-intensity intervals. Over time, interval training boosts your muscle stores of glycogen and phosphocreatine, two fuels for intense exercise. And as your body adapts, your perceived effort declines, says study author Todd A. Astorino, PhD.

■ **SHORTEN YOUR INTERVALS** The shorter your intervals, the more effective your workout may be. Researchers from the University of Nebraska at Omaha found that cyclists who performed 30-second intervals at 90 percent effort could exercise 20 percent longer than when they did 3-minute intervals—even though their heart rates were higher during the short sprints. Try doing 15 to 20 half-minute sprints at 90 percent of your heart rate max. Rest for 30 seconds in between.

Resistance Training

17 strategies to accelerate weight loss by building more muscle

HOW TOP DOCTORS STAY SLIM

"I work out at home for 45 to 60 minutes, alternating strength training one day with cardio the next. I use free weights and the Powertec system, which I like because it has no cables or pulleys. I also love dips. I do five sets of 10 dips, and every now and then I bang out 25 just to prove I can still match my old school record."

—JOHN ELEFTERIADES, MD, chief of cardiothoracic surgery at the Yale School of Medicine

New research has demonstrated how important resistance training is in the weight-loss game. Studies have shown that people who complete a strength-training workout experience a boost in metabolism for 16 hours afterward. One particular study at Skidmore College found that people who combined cardio with resistance training shed twice as much body fat—and more than four times as much abdominal fat—as people who did only aerobic exercise. Although cardio torches more calories minute for minute, weight training keeps your internal furnace going long after you put down the weights.

There are long-term benefits, too. By building muscle, you help ensure that you don't regain lost weight. "Whenever you lose weight, it typically comes from both fat tissue and muscle," says Michele Olson, PhD, an exercise researcher at Auburn University. In fact, for every pound of muscle you lose, your resting metabolism declines by about 2 to 10 calories per day. That's not to mention the muscle loss you inevitably experience as you age—starting around age 25, you lose about 1 percent of your muscle mass every year. (For most of us, this is replaced with fat.) "Resistance training helps maintain or even add muscle mass, which prevents a slowdown in metabolism," says Olson. For every 3 pounds of muscle you gain, you increase your calorie burn by about 6 to 8 percent.

Your strength-building, calorie-burning plan: Lift weights two or three times per week. Use a weight that challenges your muscles but that you can still lift 8 to 12 times.

■ **FOCUS ON LARGE MUSCLES** To make the most of your workout, focus on exercises that recruit your body's largest muscle groups: your back, legs, chest, and arms. Rather than isolating small muscles, you want to work the muscles that will help you build the most lean mass, since that's what helps you burn calories around the clock. Make sure to choose large-muscle moves that work more than one joint—for example, squats, pushups, and any exercise that combines upper- and lower-body movements. That way, you're working more than one muscle per exercise, maximizing your calorie burning.

■ **LOWER WEIGHTS SLOWLY** Take your time on the bench—remember, it's your goal to work your muscles as hard as possible with each repetition. If you slowly lower weights, you increase the challenge to your muscles and may give your metabolism a jolt for up to 3 days, according to recent research from Wayne State University. Conversely, when you perform an exercise too quickly—for example, bouncing up from a squat—you transfer stress from your muscle to your tendons, which reduces the metabolic benefit. Try to take 3 seconds to lower the weight, then pause for a second before lifting it back up.

BONUS BENEFIT!

Lifting weights can lower your blood pressure. In a recent Brazilian study, hypertensive men who lifted weights 3 days a week for 12 weeks experienced an 11.5 percent drop in their average blood pressure.

■ **EXPERIMENT WITH CIRCUITS** Circuits are the weight-lifting equivalent of sprints. How to do them: String together a series of exercises and perform one after another, with little (or no) rest in between. The key is choosing moves that work different muscles so you can maintain a high intensity throughout the entire circuit.

Completing a single circuit of eight exercises can expend up to 230 calories. That number is high, considering the time you save with circuits. In a Spanish study, people who performed circuit workouts achieved the same strength gains as those who lifted in a more traditional manner—yet their workouts were 42 percent shorter. The best part? The quick bursts of effort keep your heart rate up, adding a cardio component to your resistance workout. (For circuit workout ideas, see Circuit Training on page 315.)

■ **BUILD MUSCLE WITH BODY-WEIGHT MOVES** You don't have to hit the gym to make strength gains. You can do pushups, squats, and other body-weight exercises in your living room—and still tone and tighten as much as you would using machines. "Your muscles don't know the difference between working against your body's own resistance and on a fancy piece of equipment," says Wayne Westcott, PhD, fitness research director at Quincy College in Massachusetts. Try this mini-workout: Perform 10 reps each of push-ups, squats, mountain climbers, lunges, and chair dips. (For exercise descriptions, see Body-Weight Resistance Exercises on page 305.) If you can't complete all 10 reps, try cutting your repetitions in half and doubling the number of sets you do.

■ **HOLD WEIGHT OVERHEAD** You can work your abs while toning the rest of your body. While doing lunges and squats, hold a light weight overhead. "Your core is the main connection between your upper and lower body," explains sports nutritionist and exercise physiologist Christopher Mohr, PhD, RD. "By creating more length from your center to your fingertips, your abs have to work extrahard just to keep you upright." This helps tone up your midsection.

■ **PUMP UP WITH PROTEIN** What you eat before and after your workout can make a big difference in transforming your body. In a recent Syracuse University study, people who drank a combination of carbs and amino acids—the building blocks of protein—burned more calories the next day than those who only consumed carbs. Protein may dampen the effects of the stress hormone cortisol, and this could in turn enhance your postworkout

metabolic boost, says study author Kyle Hackney, PhD, CSCS. Aim to consume about 20 grams of protein with a shot of healthy carbs before and after intense exercise (of 45 minutes or longer).

■ **DO THE RIGHT NUMBER OF REPS** No matter the exercise, try to complete 8 to 15 repetitions per set. Research shows that this rep range stimulates the greatest increase in fat-burning hormones. The caveat: You have to use a weight that sufficiently challenges your muscles. Doing 8 reps when you could do 15 won't do much for your muscles. If you're struggling by your last repetition, you know you're in the right weight ballpark.

■ **. . . AND SETS** Perform two to four sets of each exercise. In a recent Ball State University study, scientists found that levels of fat-burning hormones spike after just one set of an exercise. Doing more sets will further raise your hormone levels, but there's a limit: Greek researchers recently determined that there's no difference between doing four sets and six. Two to four sets is the optimal number for fat loss. If you're just starting out, try two sets, then increase your number as you become better conditioned.

■ **HIT THE WEIGHTS FIRST** Resistance training burns through your body's carbohydrate stores. After about 20 minutes of lifting, once your carb supply is sapped, you begin to use fat as fuel. What that means: If you start your workout with strength training, you prime your body for fat burning during the cardio portion of your routine. Core exercises, such as planks and mountain climbers, should come first. By training your core when your muscles aren't weary, you'll achieve the fastest strength gains. That will boost the rest of your workout, since your core is involved in almost every exercise.

■ **USE THE RIGHT WEIGHT** If your weights are too heavy, you can easily injure yourself. But if they're too light, you won't reap the full benefit of your workout. If you haven't been lifting, start with 3- to 5-pound dumbbells or the lightest weights on the machines at the gym. Once you can crank out 12 to 15 repetitions at that weight with good form, add more weight.

■ **SHORTEN YOUR REST PERIODS** No need to dilly-dally around between sets. If you allow your muscles to fully recover between sets, you miss out on some of the fat-burning potential of weight lifting—it's tiring out your muscles that makes them grow. The perfect rest period: 60 to 75 seconds. This gives your body just enough time to regain strength for your next set, but it doesn't permit total recovery. Bonus: The shorter your rest periods, the shorter your workout can be.

■ **WATCH YOUR FORM** Using proper form while weight lifting helps you build stronger muscles, according to Brazilian scientists. In their study, they found that men who performed curls with a full range of motion were about 10 percent stronger than those who failed to bring the weight all the way down and back up. Use the following table as a guide to proper form for the exercises that people most commonly do incorrectly.

FIX YOUR FORM

THE EXERCISE	THE MISTAKE	THE FIX
Lunge	Leaning forward, so the heel of your leading leg lifts off the ground.	Focus on moving your torso only up and down, rather than pushing it forward. This helps keep your weight balanced, allowing you to press into the floor with your heel.
Squat	Beginning the exercise by bending your knees (putting unnecessary strain on your joints) and leaning forward on your toes.	Imagine you're sitting down into a chair—push your hips back and sit back into your heels. As you stand, think about pushing the floor away from your body, rather than lifting your body.
Deadlift	Rounding your lower back as you bend over, which can predispose you to back trouble.	Pretend you're holding a tray of drinks and have to close the door behind you with your backside. That way, you push your hips back and put less strain on your back. When standing up, squeeze your butt muscles.

■ **TRAIN YOUR WHOLE BODY** The more muscles you activate during a workout, the more calories you will burn. That's why it makes sense to build workouts around exercises that work your largest muscles and multiple muscle groups. University of Wisconsin researchers recently found that men who performed a total-body workout experienced an elevation in metabolism for 39 hours afterward, and they burned more calories from fat than those who didn't do a total-body routine. Besides, if you consistently favor a single muscle, you'll eventually create muscle imbalances that can lead to injury. If you frequently work your biceps, make sure to train your triceps, too. Or if you favor exercises that strengthen your quads, incorporate a few extra hamstring-boosting moves.

■ **LENGTHEN YOUR MUSCLES** Make sure to use your full range of motion with every exercise. What this means: Fully bend or extend your joints until they can't go any farther (without locking them). Not only will you make faster gains, but you may improve your flexibility, according to recent research. Each time you reach the "down" position of the lift (where you feel the stretch), pause for 2 or 3 seconds without relaxing your muscles.

■ **ALTERNATE BETWEEN TWO EXERCISES** Why spend more time in the gym than you have to? After completing one set of an exercise, rest briefly, then do an exercise that works muscles that weren't involved in the previous move, and rest again. For example, pair an upper-body move that works the muscles on your front side (say, bench press) with a lower-body exercise that emphasizes muscles on your back side (the deadlift, for example). By coupling noncompeting moves, you can cut your rest time in half—or eliminate it entirely—without fatiguing quickly.

■ **SWITCH IT UP** It can be tempting to stick with a lifting routine indefinitely—especially if it seems to be working. But here's the thing: As your body becomes familiar with an exercise, it stops responding to it. That's when your progress plateaus. "Even replacing one exercise can create enough of a surprise to keep results coming," says Michele Kettles, MD, head of the Cooper Clinic in Dallas. As a general rule, you should temporarily retire moves that work more than one joint—for example, squats and bench press—after 8 weeks, and single-joint moves, such as biceps curls and triceps pushdowns, after a month. The key: Replace them with exercises that work the same muscles, just in different ways. You don't have to give up your favorite exercises for good. You just need to give them time to become "new" again.

■ **FINISH WITH CARDIO** Add treadmill time to the end of your workout. "Resistance training is mostly a carb-burning activity," says Wayne Westcott, PhD, fitness research director at Quincy College in Massachusetts. "After about 20 minutes of strength training, you deplete your glycogen [carb] stores, so fat is readily available to burn." This is especially important if you're using the same muscles during weight training and cardio—say, you're doing both lower-body exercises and jogging.

Walking Workouts

12 strategies for shedding pounds one step at a time

Whatever keeps you moving can help you lose weight. And one of the easiest and most effective ways to shed pounds is simply to put one foot in front of the other. According to University of South Carolina scientists, the number of steps you take each day influences how much fat you store. In their study, people who logged at least 9,000 steps per day—that's about 4.5 miles—were more likely to be slim and fit than those who took fewer than 5,000 steps a day—or less than 2.5 miles.

Your goal should be at least 10,000 steps a day. That, of course, includes the nonexercise walking you do—but don't expect your regular steps to suffice. According to a recent Centers for Disease Control and Prevention study, fewer than 12 percent of women actually take 10,000 steps per day. Make a habit of walking around the block or stepping onto the treadmill, and use the following strategies to ensure you torch as many calories as possible.

■ **GAUGE YOUR EFFORT** How do you know when you're walking at the right pace? Listen to your body, using the chart on the following page to guide you.

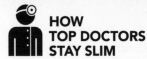

GAUGE YOUR EFFORT

EFFORT LEVEL	PHYSICAL RESPONSE
Light	Comfortable breathing
Moderate	Breathing hard
Brisk	Slightly breathless
Fast	Breathless

You can also gauge your speed by counting the number of steps you take per minute. (The formula is based on the average stride length of 2.5 feet.) Walk for 20 seconds and count your steps. If you take 40 steps, that's 120 steps per minutes, or about 3 miles per hour; 45 steps is 135 steps per minute, or about 3.5 to 4 miles per hour; and 50 steps is 150 steps per minute, or about 4.5 miles per hour.

■ **TRACK YOUR STEPS** The easiest way to track your steps is to strap on a pedometer. Wearing the device may even motivate you to get moving: Research suggests that sporting a pedometer can spur people to walk 2,000 more steps per day! Don't stop there: To maximize your results, set step-count goals and track your progress in an activity log. According to a recent study review in the *Journal of the American Medical Association*, setting a specific step goal can help you walk an extra mile every day. A good start: Measure your baseline steps, then shoot for an extra 2,000 steps per day. Work your way up to 10,000 steps. No pedometer? Use these references to estimate your steps:

Basic activity (taking out trash, cleaning house)	100 steps per minute (spm)
Walking casually but lively (like around the mall)	100 spm
Walking with purpose (about 3 mph)	120 spm
Walking briskly (about 3.5 to 4 mph)	135 spm
Power walking (about 4.5 mph)	150 spm

1 mile walked = ~ 2,000 steps

■ **WARM UP THE RIGHT WAY** Don't bother stretching before you embark on a walk. The best warm up is one that mimics the exercise you're about to do, so prepare your muscles by walking at a leisurely pace for 5 to 10 minutes. Then, wrap up your walking workout with 5 minutes of strolling to let your muscles cool down. Stretch at the very end.

■ **ADOPT A DOG** Walking your dog can help you stay lean. In a recent George Washington University study, people who walked their dogs were half as likely to be overweight as couch-bound dog owners. "You may feel guilty if your dog doesn't get a lot of activity," explains study author Cindy Lentino, MS. "That guilt could motivate you to walk your pet more and become more active." Of course, if you can't bring home Fido, you can volunteer at a local animal shelter or offer to dog-sit for a neighbor.

■ **PRACTICE SELF-AWARENESS** Walking can be relaxing—but don't let yourself feel too Zen or you might slow down. To maximize your workout, continually ask yourself: Do I have the energy to walk faster? Am I breathing quickly but evenly? By checking in with yourself, you ensure that you don't slack off.

■ **PUT THE TREADMILL IN AN INTEREST- ING ROOM** If you're a treadmill walker, don't make the mistake of setting up your machine in the basement. Think about it: How motivated can you possibly feel while staring at a cement wall? Research shows that if you enjoy a workout, you'll stick with it. So set up shop in a pleasant space with lots of light and easy access to a TV or radio.

■ **HIT THE TRAILS** Walking on uneven terrain, such as hiking trails or cobblestones, will force you to flex muscles you don't normally use—for example, your glutes (in your butt) and adductors (in your thighs). According to Oregon Research Institute scientists, it can also improve your balance.

■ **KICK IT UP A NOTCH** You've hit a weight-loss plateau. First off, be encouraged— plateaus are a sign you've lost weight, since a slimmer body burns fewer calories. To bust through, you need to take your activity to a higher level. If you're very overweight or just beginning to be active, "leisurely" walking several days a week may be enough to help you lose a few pounds. But once your body adjusts, you'll need to step it up. Try adding some hills to your walks (or set the treadmill on incline), combine walking and light jogging, or simply speed it up. Picking up your pace can help send your body into fat-burning mode.

■ **APPLY THE INTERVAL PRINCIPLE** Intervals aren't just for hard-core athletes. You can use the exercise method—short bursts of intense activity, followed by brief rest periods— to blast fat while you walk. Alternate 1-minute bursts of power walking with 1 minute of strolling. This not only helps you burn more calories while you exercise, but it can also increase your number of mitochondria, the powerhouses inside your cells. The result: You incinerate more calories even while you sleep!

■ **SQUEEZE IN WALKS** "No time" is no excuse to skip exercise. A 2005 National Institutes of Health study showed that short-but-frequent workouts—10 minutes, four times a day—produced the same health benefits as a daily 40-minute sweat session. So throughout the day, take a quick walk whenever you have a few spare minutes. Always keep it brisk: Walk at a pace where you are breathing hard but can still maintain a conversation. Try these short-walk suggestions:

WAKE-UP WALK

Start your day with 6 minutes of walking outside, then climb up and down your stairs for 4 minutes. (You can also step on and off a curb if you want to stay outside.)

PEP TALK WALK

Walk around your house or office for 5 to 10 minutes and mentally organize your to-do list to motivate you for the coming day. You can jot down your thoughts afterward.

CAFFEINE-FREE JOLT

Crank up the radio and step in place. Drop your chin toward your chest, then lift it with each step for 1 minute. Next, lift your knees high (as though you're marching) for 1 minute, do jumping jacks for 1 minute, and, finally, climb the stairs for 2 minutes.

ON-THE-GO MEETING

Propose a walking meeting to your coworkers. Share ideas and discuss upcoming projects over a couple of laps around your floor or head outside if the weather is nice.

LUNCHTIME BOOST

Rev up your metabolism before your afternoon meal. Warm up at an easy pace for 5 minutes, then kick it up to your "I'm late and in a hurry" pace for 10 minutes. Cool down for 5 minutes.

POWER WALK

Warm up at a casual pace for 5 minutes. Speed up to a hurried pace for 10 minutes, and then walk as fast as you can for 3 minutes. Bring it back down to a purposeful walk for 4 minutes. Finally, cool down for 5 minutes.

NOON TUNES

Pop in your earbuds (use only one if you're in a traffic-heavy area) and head outside during your lunch break. Warm up for 5 minutes, then cue up upbeat songs with fast-paced tempos, such as "California Gurls" by Katy Perry, "Brown Eyed Girl" by Van Morrison, or "Born in the USA" by Bruce Springsteen. Walk to the beat for 20 minutes, then round out your workout by strolling for 5 minutes to cool down.

WALK AND TALK

Grab your cell and cruise around the block at a lively pace, walking and talking for 10 minutes.

SHOPPING STROLL

Make a lap around the inside perimeter of your supermarket before you put any items into your basket.

ARE YOU WALKING FIT?

Take this simple test, designed by James Rippe, MD, a professor of biomedical sciences at the University of Central Florida, to assess your fitness.

The test: Find a flat 1-mile loop, and grab a stopwatch. Warm up for 5 minutes, then walk the mile as quickly as you can without stopping. Compare your time against the standard for your age group.

You're in great shape if you can walk a mile in . . .

Under age 30: 13 minutes

Ages 30–39: 14 minutes

Ages 40–49: 14 minutes, 42 seconds

Ages 50–69: 15 minutes

Ages 70+: 18 minutes, 18 seconds

If you exceed the ideal time for your age group by 3 to 6 minutes, you're not in the best aerobic shape. But don't worry: With consistent walking, you'll lower your time!

MEDITATION WALK

Choose a quiet place to walk. Start by standing tall with your feet together, close your eyes, and inhale deeply for three breaths. Open your eyes and stroll at a casual pace for 4 minutes, focusing on your breathing and posture.

AFTERNOON PICK-ME-UP

Walk up and down a flight of stairs for 2 minutes. Take another 2 minutes to walk around your office building. Repeat.

AFTER-DINNER TREAT

Before you eat dessert, go outside for a 15-minute walk around the block with your family. Stick to a pace that's slightly faster than a stroll, and you may find that your sugar cravings die down. There's another reason you don't want to skip this walk: A recent 12-week study showed that evening walkers dropped seven times more weight than morning walkers!

COMMERCIAL BREAKS

Don't park yourself on the couch for the duration of your favorite TV show. During commercials, get moving: Straighten your living room, take out the trash, or carry the laundry upstairs. The steps will add up!

■ **HEAD FOR THE HILLS** To kick up your cardio, hit as many hills during your walk as possible. (If you don't live in a hilly area, climb stairs or stadium bleachers.) Time how long it takes you to go up a hill, staircase, or set of bleachers, then recover by walking on level ground for about half that time. For instance, if you're climbing for 45 seconds, recover for 20 to 25 seconds.

■ **INCORPORATE STRENGTH TRAINING** Cardio exercise, walking included, is a great way to jumpstart your weight loss. But in the long term, you need to work in weight training so that you avoid shedding muscle as you drop pounds. An easy way to do it: cardio-strength circuits. Try alternating 2 minutes of walking or marching in place with 1 minute of toning moves, such as pushups, squats, and lunges. Research shows that circuit workouts can more than double your fat burn for an hour afterward!

Yoga

9 poses for slimming stress relief

HOW TOP DOCTORS STAY SLIM

"My morning stretch starts with my hips. If I can't touch my toes, I know I'm too stiff. Then I loosen up my neck, because that's where I store tension. A lot of times I'll think, I'm too tired to do my situps today. But after stretching for 15 seconds, I have the energy for them. I also do yoga in the morning. I try to feel enough discomfort in the poses so I can breathe through it and loosen up my body."

—**MEHMET OZ, MD,** host of TV's *The Dr. Oz Show*

Yoga's ability to calm mind and body is legendary. What's less understood is the practice's other benefits, namely toning muscles, reducing weight, and boosting self-esteem. Regular yoga practice activates the parasympathetic nervous system, which helps calm your body. A calm body is generally a slimmer one: One study found that women who practiced yoga for at least 4 years gained less weight over a decade than those who didn't. And a study in the *Journal of the American Dietetic Association* reported that yoga may help you become more mindful of what you eat.

There's even a connection between yoga poses and trimmer thighs. "Cellulite is a symptom of reduced lymph circulation," says Atma JoAnn Levitt, MA, RN, head of the integrative weight loss program at the Kripalu Center for Yoga and Health in Lenox, Massachusetts. Lymph is the bodily fluid that contains white blood cells; yoga helps it flow more freely through fatty areas, effectively reducing cellulite, says Levitt. Think of yoga as the perfect complement to traditional strength training. Roll out a mat and give these basic yoga poses a try:

BRIDGE

Stretches: *chest, neck, spine, hips*
Strengthens: *neck, back*

Lie flat on your back with your knees bent, your feet flat on the floor, and your palms facing down. Lift your hips and torso off of the floor, pressing into your palms and feet. Interlace your hands under your back and press your shoulders and upper arms into the floor. Lift your hips higher toward the ceiling and hold for five to seven breaths. Lower your butt back to the floor and separate your arms.

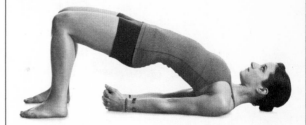

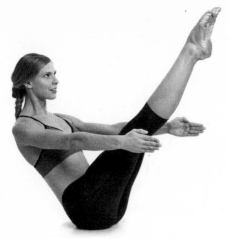

BOAT POSE

Stretches: *spine, lower back, hips*
Strengthens: *core, back, arms, hip flexors, thighs*

Sit with your knees bent and your feet flat on the floor. Grab your legs under your thighs, just above your knees, and lean back slightly. Lift your feet off of the floor, pressing your feet together, until your shins are parallel with the floor. Extend your arms straight out in front of you at shoulder height, palms up. Straighten and raise your legs toward the ceiling until your body forms a V shape. Hold for three to five breaths. Lower your shins until they are parallel with the floor, place your hands back under your thighs, lower your feet to the floor, and return to an upright position.

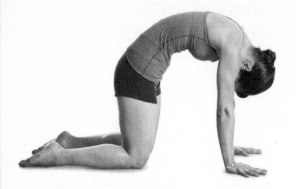

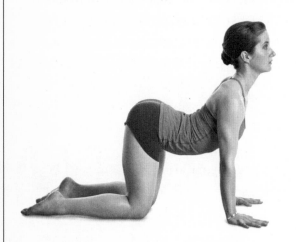

CHAIR

Stretches: *shoulders, chest*
Strengthens: *thighs, calves, spine, ankles, butt, back*

From a standing position with your feet hip-width apart, extend your arms over your head, keeping your shoulders relaxed. Exhale as you bend your legs until your thighs are nearly parallel to the floor. (Imagine yourself sitting in a chair.) Keep your heels flat on the floor.

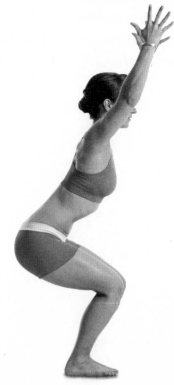

CAT COW

Stretches: *hips, lower back, spine*

Assume an on-all-fours position on the floor, with your shoulders directly over your wrists and your hips over your knees. Inhale and slowly arch your back, then exhale and reverse the motion, tucking your pelvis and looking up.

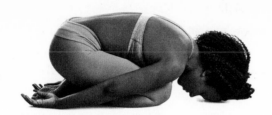

CHILD'S POSE

Stretches: *lower back, hips*

Sit on your heels, and place your hands on your thighs. Lower your chest and forehead until your chest rests on your thighs and your forehead touches the floor. Straighten your arms behind your body, with your palms faceup.

DOWNWARD-FACING DOG

Stretches: *feet, shoulders, hamstrings, calves, chest*
Strengthens: *arms, legs, core*

Start on all fours with your wrists about 6 to 12 inches in front of your shoulders. Position your knees so they are hip-width apart, then curl your toes under. Push evenly into your palms and lift your knees off of the floor. Lift your "sit" bones (those in your butt that you sit on) toward the ceiling and push the tops of your thighs back so your body forms an inverted V. At first, keep your knees bent and your heels lifted off the floor, then gradually straighten your knees (without locking them). Gently move your chest back toward your thighs until your ears are even with your upper arms; don't let your head dangle. Keep your hips lifting and push firmly into your hands.

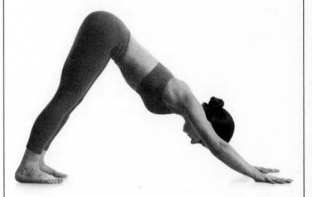

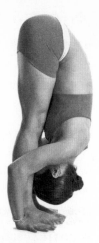

FORWARD FOLD

Stretches: *hamstrings, calves, hips*
Strengthens: *legs, knees, abs*

Stand up straight with your feet together. Bring your hands to prayer position in front of your chest, then place your fingertips where your thighs meet your hips. Lift your chest and gaze toward the ceiling. Then pour your torso forward, bending from your hips and keeping your spine straight. If you can, rest your palms on the floor, just outside your toes. Come to your fingertips, lift your chest, and gaze slightly forward. Rest your palms on the floor again, lower your chest toward your thighs, then lower your head toward your knees. Hold for three to five breaths. Come to your fingertips, lift your chest, and gaze slightly forward. Place your hands on your hips, then bring your torso upright while maintaining a straight spine. Bring your hands to prayer position.

HERO POSE

Stretches: *ankles, knees, thighs*

Kneel on the floor with your knees nearly together and your feet hip-width apart, toes pointing straight back. Exhale as you sit on the floor between your feet (if you can't, place a prop, such as a block, thick book, or folded blanket between your feet and sit on the prop). Place your hands on top of your thighs, palms facing down. Relax your shoulders and upper body, keeping your chest lifted. You should feel the stretch in your thighs.

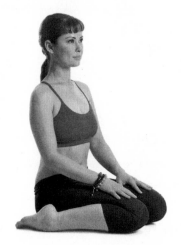

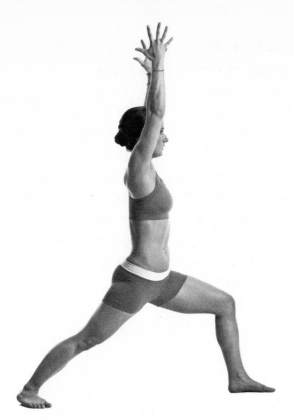

WARRIOR 1

Stretches: *shoulders, hips*
Strengthens: *legs, abs*

Stand tall with your feet together and your arms by your sides. Step out, so your feet are 4 to 4½ feet apart (and still parallel). Inhale and lift your arms up overhead, shoulder-width apart, palms facing each other. Exhale and turn your left foot and leg 90 degrees out to the left. Then turn your right foot in, toward the left, until it achieves a 45-degree angle. Rotate your hips and torso so they're facing the same direction as your left leg. Take a deep breath, and then as you exhale, bend your left

knee so your left thigh and shin form a right angle. Only bend your knee as far as you can while keeping the outer edges of your back foot pressed flat into the floor. To align your spine, imagine drawing your ribs in toward your body, pressing your tailbone toward the floor and elongating the back of your neck.

3 STICK-WITH-IT STRATEGIES FOR YOGA BEGINNERS

1. MOVE TO THE FRONT OF THE CLASS.
Even if it's your first time in yoga class, roll out your mat in the front of the room. Research shows that hiding out in the back of the studio, where you can't hear and see what's going on, prevents you from learning the practice and feeling competent. Plus, if you get to know your teacher, you're more likely to keep coming back.

2. CALL ON YOUR INNER CHEAPSKATE.
Find a yoga studio in your area and buy a package of classes. (Hint: Look on Web sites like Groupon for great deals.) You won't want to throw away workouts you've already paid for.

3. FIND THE RIGHT OM FOR YOU.
Pick a practice that you enjoy so much you'd do it even if it weren't good for you. If you're interested in what you're doing, your performance will improve—and that will feed your desire to go back for more. See "Choose the Right Yoga for You" on page 346 to find the style that suits your needs.

CHOOSE THE RIGHT YOGA FOR YOU

There's a yoga practice to fit almost any preference. Use this guide to demystify the most popular yoga styles, so you can find the right class for your health and fitness goals.

Ashtanga

What to expect: A fast-paced, athletic practice that links each movement to an inhale or exhale. In an authentic Ashtanga class (called "Mysore"), you memorize the series of moves and progress at your own pace.

Try it if: You're looking for a calorie-burning workout and enjoy exercising independently. This style appeals to type A personalities.

Avoid it if: You prefer an instructor.

Sweat factor: 7 out of 10

Bikram

What to expect: Twenty-six heart-rate-revving poses, each done twice, in nearly 105°F heat. (This isn't "hot yoga," which is Vinyasa in a hot room.)

Try it if: You like pushing your body to extremes, or you want to lose weight. You can burn up to 600 calories per class! Just make sure to pack water and a towel.

Avoid it if: You have heat sensitivity, high blood pressure or heart disease, or an injury.

Sweat factor: 10 out of 10

Iyengar

What to expect: A slow class that concentrates on the alignment of your body. Prepare to hold poses for several minutes and to focus on achieving proper form (great for injury prevention).

Try it if: You're a perfectionist—with this style, precision is key. It's also great for beginners, since it's less intense than many other common styles.

Avoid it if: You get antsy if you aren't always moving or you're uncomfortable partnering with strangers.

Sweat factor: 6 out of 10

Jivamukti

What to expect: A meditative but highly physical class involving spiritual elements, like chanting and scripture. Beginners' classes emphasize standing poses.

Try it if: You desire enlightenment and exercise.

Avoid it if: You don't relish discussing social and political activism during your workout.

Sweat factor: 7 out of 10

Kripalu

What to expect: A three-part practice that teaches you to know, accept, and learn from your body. You begin by doing different poses to show you how your body works, then move into longer postures and meditation, and wrap up with a series of linked poses.

Try it if: You want to prove to yourself that your body is powerful.

Avoid it if: You're not prepared to talk openly about self-discovery.

Sweat factor: 5 out of 10

Kundalini

What to expect: A focus on breathing, non-traditional movements, and Eastern philosophy. Instructors usually wear white apparel, use gongs, and emphasize balancing your body's energy.

Try it if: You want spiritual-based yoga.

Avoid it if: Chatting about chakras makes you roll your eyes.

Sweat factor: 5 out of 10

Power

What to expect: An active, aerobic style adapted from Ashtanga. (Some studios add a "hot" element.) Power yoga is great for toning and lean-muscle building.

Try it if: You are not afraid of challenging yourself and if you want to kick your metabolism into high gear.

Avoid it if: You're a routine person—power yoga classes rarely stick to the same sequences of poses each time.

Sweat factor: 8 out of 10

Restorative

What to expect: Relaxing poses, lying down with support from blankets, blocks, or bolsters. You'll rest in each pose for several minutes and may do guided meditation. Snoozing is completely acceptable.

Try it if: Stress is driving you insane.

Avoid it if: Your main goal is weight loss.

Sweat factor: 2 out of 10

Sivananda

What to expect: A sequence of 12 basic postures, paired with sun salutations and corpse pose (*savasana*). Each class opens and closes with chanting and meditation.

Try it if: You seek an intense spiritual experience.

Avoid it if: You're a meat lover—one of the central tenets of the Sivananda philosophy is vegetarianism.

Sweat factor: 5 out of 10

Viniyoga

What to expect: A highly individualized practice, where you're taught to adapt poses to your body. Teachers usually work one-on-one with students.

Try it if: You have specific injuries or pains you'd like to address.

Avoid it if: You're a back-of-the-class type of exerciser.

Sweat factor: 5 out of 10

Vinyasa

What to expect: A "flow" of continuous movements. Most classes keep a fast pace, but you can also find gentle "slow flow" classes. Unlike with most yoga styles, you can expect to move to music during this flab-melting workout.

Try it if: You enjoy dancing, want to challenge your muscles in new ways, and hope to drop a few pounds.

Avoid it if: You're a beginner—most instructors will expect you to know the poses.

Sweat factor: 8 out of 10

Part 5
YOUR PLAN

Putting *The Doctors Book of Weight-Loss Remedies* to work in your life

Every page of this book is loaded with useful tips to help you take the steps toward improving your body and your health. You can achieve successful weight loss simply by choosing a selection of strategies from the previous four parts and building them into your lifestyle. However, we recognize that some people prefer a prescriptive plan that walks and talks them through every step in the journey. That's what you'll get in this section—a well-designed prescription for weight loss that includes specific diet and lifestyle changes plus recommended cardio- and strength-exercise routines that will help you shed pounds and tone up flabby muscle.

Your job is to figure out what exactly you'd like to achieve. What's the point of your plan? "Specific goals help focus your attention and increase your effort, which helps you persist longer," says Gary Latham, PhD, a professor of organizational effectiveness at the University of Toronto. In other words, if you have a roadmap for weight loss, you're much more likely to stick with it—and reach your final destination faster. In the pages ahead, you'll find a simple plan built around the core strategies in this book. Remember, your journey is an individual one, so you can always work in additional strategies from previous chapters to help target your unique trouble spots. But start here: Take some time to reflect on what it is that you'd really like to accomplish.

Your Goals

To arrive at your destination, you first need to know where you're going

Your car's GPS is about as useful as a rock for finding your route unless you plug in where you want to go. Well, shaping up is similar. The more specific you are in pinpointing where you want to ultimately be, body-wise, the more likely you'll be to arrive there . . . without taking a detour through a rough neighborhood in Cleveland. A good doctor, nutritionist, or trainer will always ask you what your goals are before prescribing a course of action. So take a few moments to reflect on where you would like to take your body. These six steps will help you to map our your most direct route.

■ **STEP 1: BE SPECIFIC** "Losing weight" does not count as a goal! After all, dropping even half a pound is technically "losing weight." When setting goals, you need to be specific—for example, *I want to lose 20 pounds by March. I want to fit into my size 6 jeans again.* (Overwhelmed by your weight-loss goal? Tell yourself you're going to lose 10 pounds 10 times.) And don't just focus on your figure; you should also set health and fitness goals—*I want to be able to run a 10-K. I want to lower my blood pressure by 10 points.*

HOW TOP DOCTORS STAY SLIM

"I'm 5'11" and I cap my daily calories at 2,500 to stay in my target zone of 175 to 182 pounds. If I put on a few pounds, I reduce my intake for a few weeks and double my exercise. Before long, I'm back in my zone."

—**JOHN ELEFTERIADES, MD,** chief of cardiothoracic surgery at the Yale School of Medicine

■ **STEP 2: FIND A WAY TO TRACK YOUR PROGRESS** If you can quantify your progress, you'll be more motivated to keep going. Track your goals, whether by weighing yourself, regularly taking your blood pressure, testing your body fat, or timing your mile runs. Set micro (weekly) and macro (monthly) goals to keep yourself on track for your final goal. Log your progress in a journal.

■ **STEP 3: MAKE SURE YOUR GOALS ARE ATTAINABLE** You want to aim high—but not so high that you end up discouraged and unmotivated. If you can barely find 20 minutes of free time, don't set yourself up for failure by committing to hourlong workouts everyday. Likewise, be realistic. Losing 20 pounds by next week simply isn't healthy or reasonable. Set no more than three to five major but attainable goals at a time. "Any more and your eyes glaze over and you burn out," says Gary Latham, PhD, a professor of organizational effectiveness at the University of Toronto.

■ **STEP 4: SET A TIME LIMIT** Deadlines create a sense of urgency and help you prioritize your goals. Give yourself a year to drop 75 to 100 pounds, 4 to 6 months to train for a marathon (if you're a new runner), and 2 months to lose 10 to 12 percent of your body fat.

■ **STEP 5: PUT IT IN WRITING** Write down your goals and your deadline, and treat that paper like an unbreakable contract. You can also build in rewards and cheat days to help you stay motivated, and even schedule your workouts to ensure you actually complete them. "If you schedule them like business meetings or lunch dates, you'll be more likely to follow through," says Bonnie Pfiester, co-owner of Longevity Fitness Clubs in Vero Beach, Florida.

■ **STEP 6: REVIEW YOUR GOALS** Don't just write down your goals and never look back. Regularly check in with yourself and make sure you haven't let old habits creep back in. You can even find a friend or family member to help you power through your weak moments, says Kelly Webber, PhD, RD, an assistant professor of nutrition at the University of Kentucky. Once you've achieved a goal, maintain the lifestyle changes you made. Otherwise, you'll end up right back where you started.

Your Diet

A simple yet effective meal plan that controls calories and boosts nutrition without sacrificing the enjoyment of eating—and how to customize it to your body and your goals

There are hundreds of diets from which to choose; some are effective, others useless. Some are intricate and complicated. Others are overly simplistic to the point that they require virtually no behavioral change—those simply don't work. You've probably tried many of them. Doctors and nutritionists agree: The best diet is one that eases you into making simple healthy dietary changes that quickly start to feel very natural. In short, a style of healthy eating that you can stick to for life. That's what you'll discover here. You won't find an overly complicated list of instructions in this chapter. Your long-term weight-loss strategy should be flexible—after all, you won't always want broccoli or eggs or whatever foods other plans tell you to eat at specific times of day. Our approach is simple: Avoid processed foods and restaurant foods as much as possible, and fill your plate with mostly vegetables,

DECODE YOUR MEAL!

You'll find the following symbols below each recipe. Use them to track your intake of important food groups—and make sure you eat a balanced diet.

fruit

nonstarchy vegetable

starchy vegetable

legumes

whole grains

lean protein

dairy

healthy fats

some fruits, whole grains, healthy fats, and lean protein. Do that and you will likely reduce calories automatically, without thinking or counting.

But because calorie counting can be such an effective weight-loss tool for many, and some people prefer playing a more active and strategic role in their weight-loss effort, we recommend also monitoring the number of calories you take in every day. It's particularly helpful to understand the true number of calories in certain foods (because Americans chronically underestimate the total calories in foods) for those times when we are tempted by treats or are eating away from the control of our homes.

Determining your ideal daily calories to reach your goal weight will also be helpful in planning meals. To that end, later in this section, we provide delicious recipes that are relatively low in calories and high in nutrients that you can build into your weekly meal plan. Combined with a program of regular exercise—such as the one we describe beginning on page 422—you are guaranteed to lose weight and transform your body into a fitter, healthier one.

FIND YOUR DAILY CALORIE GOAL

Begin by calculating your ideal daily calorie intake. You will divide those calories among meals and snacks built around produce, legumes, lean protein, whole grains, low-fat dairy, and healthy fats.

CALCULATE YOUR CALORIES

If you exercise 1 hour or less per week...

Goal weight × 10 = calorie goal

Example: If your goal weight is 150 pounds, multiply 150 by 10 to yield 1,500 calories.

If you exercise more than 1 hour per week...

Target body weight × (10 + additional hours, beyond 1, of exercise) = calorie goal

Example: If your goal weight is 150 pounds and you exercise 3 hours per week, multiply 150 by 12 to yield 1,680 calories.

Now that you have your target daily calories, try to stay within 200 calories of that figure per day. (As a general rule, most people can lose weight easily by limiting their per-meal calories to around 400 to 500.) By being cognizant of a calorie goal, you can create a flexible meal plan that allows you to enjoy the foods you love while also practicing portion control. The result: You'll feel satisfied, you won't feel denied, you'll gain the confidence that comes with discipline and control, and the regular fuel-ups will keep your metabolism fired up all day.

To make your planning easier, we've included healthy recipes for every meal, as well as smoothies, side dishes, snacks, and desserts. Every recipe meets the following general guidelines—which you can also use to evaluate recipes of your own:

BREAKFAST, LUNCH, DINNER ENTRÉES

≤ 400 calories

≤ 5 grams of saturated fat

≥ 12 grams of protein

≥ 3 grams of fiber

SNACKS

≤ 200 calories

≥ 5 grams of protein and fiber combined

SIDES

≤ 150 calories

Contains a fruit, vegetable, or legume

DESSERTS

≤ 200 calories

≤ 10 grams of fat

Contains fruit, low-fat dairy, or nuts

You can divide your calories into as many meals and snacks as you like—as long as you don't exceed your calorie limit. The key is balancing your day. If your breakfast option is primarily whole grains and fruit, opt for a lunch that focuses on lean protein, healthy fats, and vegetables. Or if your midmorning snack revolves around dairy, select an afternoon snack that's focused on fruit.

To help you construct a well-balanced menu, you'll find symbols that tell you what—fruit, nonstarchy vegetables, starchy vegetables, legumes, whole grains, lean protein, dairy, healthy fats—you'll find in significant amounts in each meal, snack, side dish, des-

sert, or smoothie. (If a meal recipe doesn't include produce, feel free to round it out with a piece of whole fruit or a side of vegetables.) You should track your intake of each nutritional group in a food log (find a sample log on page 435), which will make it easier to spot your dietary deficits.

WEEKS 1–2 GUIDELINES:

■ Eliminate sugary beverages.

■ Work lean protein and fiber into every meal.

■ Eat fruits and vegetables with at least two meals per day.

■ Drink a full glass of water before and during every meal.

■ Cheat one time per week.

■ Add your own goal: _____

_____

WEEKS 3–4 GUIDELINES:

■ Replace all refined grains with whole grains.

■ Limit your alcohol intake to one or two beverages per week.

■ Eat fruits and vegetables with every meal. Choose nonstarchy vegetables whenever possible. (Find a list on page 271.)

■ Add your own goal: _____

_____

Breakfasts

Fruit Parfait

Makes 1 serving

½ cup low-fat Greek yogurt

¼ cup Kashi GoLean Crisp! Toasted Berry Crumble cereal

1 cup strawberries, sliced

½ cup blueberries

2 tablespoons chopped pecans

Spoon half of the yogurt into a bowl or glass and top with half of the cereal, fruit, and nuts. Repeat with the remaining ingredients.

PER SERVING: 374 calories, 15 g fat (2 g saturated), 53 g carbs, 12 g fiber, 118 mg sodium, 17 g protein

DECODE YOUR MEAL:

fruit | whole grains | lean protein | dairy | healthy fats

Eggs Benedict

Makes 1 serving

2 tablespoons low-fat Greek yogurt

¼ teaspoon dried dill

¼ teaspoon lemon juice

½ teaspoon lemon peel

2 eggs

1 whole-wheat English muffin

1. Mix the yogurt with the dill, lemon juice, and lemon peel.

2. Poach the eggs and place them on top of the English muffin. Drizzle the yogurt sauce on top.

PER SERVING: 293 calories, 12 g fat (4 g saturated), 29 g carbs, 4 g fiber, 614 mg sodium, 21 g protein

DECODE YOUR MEAL:

whole grains   lean protein   healthy fats

AVOID "HARMLESS HABITS" THAT PACK ON POUNDS

Use every tip in your arsenal to lose weight. Here are three sneaky, seemingly harmless habits that can add unwanted calories and pounds—and how to avoid them:

■ **Listening to music** Music may soothe the savage beast, but it also can cause you to eat like a lion. Soft, soothing music encourages you to dine longer and order more food, recent research reveals. Loud, up-tempo beats cause you to eat faster, scarfing whatever is on your plate before your body has had a chance to recognize its feelings of fullness.

Do this instead: Keep the music off while dining at home and focus on the flavor and texture of each bite to savor the enjoyment of eating. If you're out at a restaurant and can't turn off the music, fill up on good conversation instead of dessert.

■ **Eating while standing** Standing is better than sitting—for burning calories, that is. But when it comes to eating, take your seat. Studies show that people who eat out of food containers while standing at a kitchen counter consume up to 50 percent more the next time they eat than those who sit at a table and eat off a plate. Why? Researchers believe that standing during a meal makes the food feel more like a snack, which people consider to be less satisfying.

Do this instead: Even if you are only munching on hummus and carrot sticks, take a seat at a proper table place setting to make the experience feel more like a meal.

■ **Sampling a little bit of everything** Variety can be dangerous to someone trying to lose weight. We humans like to take a taste of everything we see. No wonder, then, that in an experiment where people were given either 24 or 6 different flavors of jelly beans, the people offered more variety ate twice as many, according to the *Journal of Consumer Research*.

Do this instead: Shop before you shovel. At a party or a buffet, survey the food offerings and decide on a few choice selections rather than filling a plate with a little bit of everything.

Baked Oatmeal with Apple and Pecans

Makes 1 serving

¼ cup steel-cut oats

1 teaspoon baking powder

¼ cup 1% milk

1 egg

3 tablespoons unsweetened applesauce

Pinch of salt

½ teaspoon cinnamon, divided

2 teaspoons chopped pecans

¾ cup chopped apples

1 teaspoon honey

1. Preheat the oven to 350°F. Spray a ramekin with fat-free cooking spray.

2. Combine the oats, baking powder, milk, egg, applesauce, salt, and ¼ teaspoon cinnamon in the ramekin and bake for 6 to 7 minutes.

3. Top with the pecans, apples, honey, and the remaining ¼ teaspoon cinnamon.

PER SERVING: 363 calories, 12 g fat (3 g saturated), 57 g carbs, 8 g fiber, 742 mg sodium, 15 g protein

DECODE YOUR MEAL:

fruit | whole grains | lean protein | dairy | healthy fats

Huevos Rancheros

Makes 4 servings

1 can (16 ounces) whole peeled tomatoes, with juice

½ small onion, chopped

1 canned chipotle chile pepper in adobo sauce, finely chopped (about 1 tablespoon)

Juice of 1 lime, divided

¼ cup fresh cilantro sprigs

1 clove garlic

1 can (15 ounces) low-sodium black beans, drained

Pinch of cumin

8 large eggs

8 soft corn tortillas

1. Prepare the salsa by combining the tomatoes, onion, chile pepper, half of the lime juice, the cilantro, and garlic in a food processor. Pulse until well blended but still slightly chunky. Season with salt and pepper to taste. Let the mixture sit while you make the rest of the meal so the flavors have time to meld.

2. In a small mixing bowl, combine the beans with the cumin and the remaining lime juice. Add salt and pepper to taste. Use the back of a fork to lightly mash the beans; add a splash of warm water if the mixture looks too dry.

3. Coat a nonstick skillet with cooking spray and warm the pan over medium heat. Crack the eggs into the skillet and cook until the whites have set but the yolks are still runny. Set another skillet over medium heat and toast the tortillas for about 1 minute on each side.

4. Spread the beans on the warmed tortillas and top with the eggs and salsa. Serve immediately.

PER SERVING (2 TORTILLAS): 390 calories, 13 g fat (3 g saturated), 52 g carbs, 10 g fiber, 573 mg sodium, 22 g protein

DECODE YOUR MEAL:

nonstarchy vegetable | legumes | whole grains | lean protein | healthy fats

Greek-Style Frittata

Makes 4 servings

2 cups baby spinach leaves

1 tablespoon olive oil

1½ cups frozen diced potatoes, onions, and peppers (found bagged together in the freezer section)

4 large eggs

¼ cup 1% milk

½ cup crumbled feta cheese

½ cup sliced grape tomatoes

1 teaspoon oregano

1. Preheat the broiler to low. Meanwhile, warm a medium-size skillet over low heat. Add the spinach and cover until the leaves have barely wilted (about 1 minute). Place in a small bowl and set aside. Wipe out the skillet.

2. Add the olive oil to the cleaned skillet and warm over medium heat. Add the potato-vegetable mixture, cover, and cook, turning occasionally, until the potatoes are tender but firm, 5 to 7 minutes. Set aside.

3. In a medium bowl, whisk together the eggs and milk. Add the spinach, cheese, tomatoes, oregano, and salt and pepper to taste.

4. Spray an 8- to 10-inch ovenproof skillet (not nonstick) with cooking spray and place over low heat. Cover the bottom evenly with the potato-vegetable mixture and pour the egg mixture over the top. Cook until the eggs set, about 10 minutes.

5. Place the skillet under the broiler for 1 to 2 minutes to finish cooking the top of the frittata.

PER SERVING: 207 calories, 12 g fat (4 g saturated), 13 g carbs, 3 g fiber, 344 mg sodium, 12 g protein

DECODE YOUR MEAL:

nonstarchy vegetable | starchy vegetable | lean protein | dairy | healthy fats

Grilled Almond Butter and Berry Sandwiches

Makes 4 sandwiches

1 package (6 ounces) fresh
  raspberries (1–1½ cups)

¼ cup all-fruit raspberry spread

8 slices whole-grain bread or whole-
  grain cinnamon swirl bread

½ cup creamy natural almond butter

1. In a small bowl, mash the fresh raspberries into the raspberry spread with a fork.

2. Spread 4 slices of the bread with 2 tablespoons each of the almond butter. Spread about 3 tablespoons each of the berry mixture over the almond butter and top with the remaining bread slices. Lightly coat the outsides of the bread with cooking spray.

3. Place the sandwiches on a large nonstick griddle or skillet over medium-low heat (in batches, if necessary). Cook for 5 to 7 minutes, turning halfway through, to brown both sides. Cut each in half and serve.

PER SERVING: 400 calories, 21 g fat (2 g saturated), 45 g carbs, 8 g fiber, 360 mg sodium, 12 g protein

DECODE YOUR MEAL:

| fruit | whole grains | lean protein | healthy fats |

Green Eggs and Ham

Makes 4 servings

1 tablespoon white vinegar

8 eggs

2 tablespoons prepared pesto

2 tablespoons plain low-fat Greek yogurt

4 100% whole-wheat English muffins, split

4 slices deli ham

¼ cup sliced jarred roasted red peppers

1. Bring 3" water to a boil in a large skillet or saucepan. Reduce to a simmer and add the vinegar. Working in 2 batches, poach the eggs until the whites are just firm, 3 to 5 minutes. Using a slotted spoon, remove the eggs to a plate.

2. In a small bowl, mix together the pesto and yogurt until they're smooth and combined.

3. Toast the English muffin halves until golden.

4. Dividing evenly, top 4 of the muffin halves with the ham, red peppers, and eggs. Season with salt and pepper to taste and add the pesto mixture. Top the eggs with the remaining muffin halves.

PER SERVING: 343 calories, 16 g fat (5 g saturated), 28 g carbs, 3 g fiber, 815 mg sodium, 23.5 g protein

DECODE YOUR MEAL:

nonstarchy vegetable | whole grains | lean protein | healthy fats

Breakfast Melon Bowl

Makes 4 servings

1 cup low-fat ricotta cheese

¾ cup low-fat Greek yogurt

1 small cantaloupe

2 peaches, pitted and thinly sliced

½ cup sliced strawberries

½ cup blueberries

2 tablespoons chopped walnuts

Sprigs of mint

1. In a food processor or blender, process the cheese until very smooth. Transfer to a small bowl. Mix in the yogurt.

2. Halve the cantaloupe and remove the seeds. Cut into wedges, remove the rind, and cut the flesh into bite-size chunks. Place in a medium bowl. Mix in the peaches and strawberries. Add the cheese mixture and gently fold together.

3. Divide among 4 cereal bowls. Sprinkle with the blueberries and walnuts. Garnish with the mint.

PER SERVING: 193 calories, 7 g fat (3 g saturated), 26 g carbs, 3 g fiber, 180 mg sodium, 12 g protein

DECODE YOUR MEAL:

fruit | lean protein | dairy | healthy fats

Vegetable Omelet

Makes 2 servings

5 large eggs

2 tablespoons chopped flat-leaf parsley

Dash of reduced-sodium soy sauce

½ cup spinach

2 tablespoons broccoli florets, chopped

5 spears asparagus, chopped

¼ cup halved green beans

1 clove garlic, minced

Dash of freshly ground black pepper

2 teaspoons olive oil

1. Beat the eggs, parsley, and soy sauce in a bowl.

2. Coat a large skillet with olive oil. Add the spinach, broccoli, asparagus, green beans, garlic, and pepper to the skillet and cook over medium heat for 5 minutes.

3. Pour the egg mixture over the vegetables. Stir for about 30 seconds, then let it sit for 1 minute. Stir again until the eggs firm up, and let it sit for another minute. Fold it and remove it from the pan onto a plate.

PER SERVING: 262 calories, 17 g fat (5 g saturated), 9 g carbs, 3 g fiber, 235 mg sodium, 19 g protein

DECODE YOUR MEAL:

nonstarchy vegetable | lean protein | healthy fats

Ham and Cheese Waffled Sandwich

Makes 4 servings

8 slices firm 100% whole-grain bread

2 ounces extralean honey ham, thinly sliced

½ cup reduced-fat cheese, grated (such as Cheddar or Monterey jack)

1. Preheat the waffle iron until it's hot.

2. Cut the crusts off the bread slices. Coat one side of each slice with cooking spray.

3. Lay the bread, coated sides down, on the bottom of the waffle iron. Top each slice with a quarter of the ham and cheese. Top with the remaining bread slices, placing the coated sides up.

4. Cook the sandwiches until the bread is golden and crisp, about 2 to 4 minutes. Cut the sandwiches into 2 triangles each and serve.

PER SERVING: 386 calories, 10 g fat (4 g saturated), 46 g carbs, 8 g fiber, 943 mg sodium, 27 g protein

DECODE YOUR MEAL:

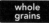 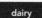 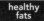

whole grains · lean protein · dairy · healthy fats

Lunches

Roasted Tomato-Basil Soup with Meatballs

Makes 4 servings

1 red onion, thickly sliced

1½ pounds plum tomatoes, halved lengthwise

2 red bell peppers, halved lengthwise and seeded

6 ounces lean ground turkey

¼ cup plain dried whole-wheat bread crumbs

¼ cup low-fat milk

⅛ teaspoon freshly ground black pepper

6 tablespoons chopped fresh basil, divided

2 cups chicken broth

1 tablespoon balsamic vinegar

1 clove garlic, minced

2 teaspoons paprika

½ teaspoon salt

1. Preheat the broiler.

2. Place the onion slices, tomatoes, and bell peppers, cut sides down, on a broiler pan. Broil 4" from the heat for 12 minutes, or until the pepper and tomato skins are blackened. When cool enough to handle, peel the tomatoes and peppers.

3. Meanwhile, in a medium bowl, combine the turkey, bread crumbs, milk, black pepper, and 2 tablespoons of the basil, stirring to thoroughly blend. Shape the turkey mixture into ¾" balls, using about 1 rounded teaspoon per ball.

4. Transfer the broiled vegetables to a food processor or blender and puree until smooth, about 1 minute. Pour the vegetable puree into a large saucepan along with the broth, vinegar, garlic, paprika, and salt. Bring to a simmer and cook for 3 minutes to blend the flavors.

5. Drop the meatballs into the soup, and simmer until cooked through, about 5 minutes. Stir in the remaining 4 tablespoons basil.

PER SERVING: 177 calories, 4.5 g fat (1 g saturated), 22 g carbs, 4.5 g fiber, 426 mg sodium, 15 g protein

DECODE YOUR MEAL:

nonstarchy vegetable | whole grains | lean protein

Grilled Chicken and Pineapple Sandwich

Makes 4 servings

4 boneless, skinless chicken breasts (4 ounces each)

4 teaspoons teriyaki sauce

4 thin slices Swiss cheese

4 pineapple slices (½" thick)

4 100% whole-wheat hamburger buns

½ medium red onion, thinly sliced

¼ cup pickled jalapeño chile pepper slices or 1 fresh jalapeño chile pepper, thinly sliced

1. Combine the chicken and enough teriyaki sauce to cover it in a resealable plastic bag. Marinate in the refrigerator for at least 30 minutes and up to 12 hours.

2. Heat a grill until hot (you shouldn't be able to hold your hand above the grates for more than 5 seconds). Remove the chicken from the marinade and place on the grill; discard any remaining marinade. Cook for 4 to 5 minutes, flip, and immediately add the cheese to each breast. Continue cooking until the cheese is melted and the chicken is lightly charred and firm to the touch. Remove from the grill; set aside. The chicken should reach an internal temperature of 165°F, as measured by a food thermometer.

3. While the chicken rests, add the pineapple and buns to the grill. Grill the rolls until they're lightly toasted and the pineapple slices until they're soft and caramelized, about 2 minutes per side.

4. Top each roll with chicken, pineapple, onion, and chile pepper slices. If you like, drizzle the chicken with a bit more teriyaki sauce.

PER SERVING: 355 calories, 10 g fat (4 g saturated), 32 g carbs, 4.5 g fiber, 703 mg sodium, 34 g protein

DECODE YOUR MEAL:

fruit | whole grains | lean protein | dairy | healthy fats

Asian Salmon Sliders with Citrus Yogurt Sauce

Makes 6 servings

½ cup low-fat Greek yogurt

Juice of ½ lime

Juice of ½ orange

1 teaspoon honey

1 pound skinless, boneless salmon, divided

1 tablespoon sesame oil

2 tablespoons low-sodium soy sauce

1 piece ginger (1"), chopped

2 cloves garlic, chopped

Juice of half a lemon

½ cup whole-wheat bread crumbs

½ cup cilantro, chopped

2 teaspoons canola oil

6 small 100% whole-grain pitas

1. In a small bowl, combine the yogurt, lime juice, orange juice, and honey; set aside.

2. Preheat a grill to medium. Wash the salmon and pat dry. Chop half of the salmon and place in a food processor along with the sesame oil, soy sauce, ginger, garlic, lemon juice, and salt and pepper to taste. Process into a pasty puree.

3. Chop the remaining salmon and add to the puree along with the bread crumbs and cilantro. Pulse until combined. Form into 12 small patties and brush with the oil.

4. Grill for 4 minutes per side, or until internal temperature is 145°F, as measured by a food thermometer. Stuff the pitas with the patties and yogurt sauce.

PER SERVING: 291 calories, 11 g fat (2 g saturated), 26 g carbs, 3 g fiber, 437 mg sodium, 23 g protein

DECODE YOUR MEAL:

whole grains | lean protein | healthy fats

Mediterranean Hummus Wrap

Makes 2 servings

¼ cup roasted red pepper hummus

1 100% whole-wheat wrap (9" diameter)

½ cup zucchini strips, sliced lengthwise

1 tablespoon sliced, pitted kalamata, black, or green olives

¼ cup shredded carrots

4 thin tomato slices

¼ cup shredded reduced-fat mild Cheddar cheese

½ cup shredded lettuce

1. Spread hummus on the lower third of the wrap.

2. Layer the zucchini, olives, carrots, tomatoes, cheese, and lettuce in the center of the wrap. Roll the wrap from the bottom toward the center. Fold the sides in, then roll the entire sandwich into a neat pocket.

3. Cut the wrap in half on an angle.

PER SERVING: 372 calories, 17 g fat (5 g saturated), 40 g carbs, 8 g fiber, 774 mg sodium, 17 g protein

DECODE YOUR MEAL:

nonstarchy vegetable | legumes | whole grains | lean protein | dairy | healthy fats

Thai Beef Salad Wraps

Makes 4 servings

12 ounces flank steak, trimmed

1½ teaspoons Asian chile sauce, divided

3 tablespoons lime juice

1 teaspoon fish sauce

2 teaspoons light brown sugar

1 cucumber, halved, seeded, and thinly sliced (1½ cups)

1 cup shredded carrots

2 cups Boston or Bibb lettuce, torn into bite-size pieces

¼ cup fresh mint leaves (packed), large leaves torn in half

4 100% whole-grain wraps (9" diameter)

¼ cup chopped unsalted peanuts

1. Preheat the broiler with the oven rack about 4" from the heat. Pat the steak dry and sprinkle each side with ½ teaspoon of the chile sauce. Place the steak on a baking sheet and broil for 4 minutes per side, or until internal temperature is 145°F, as measured by a food thermometer. Set aside.

2. In a large bowl, whisk together the lime juice, fish sauce, sugar, and remaining ½ teaspoon chile sauce. Add the cucumber, carrots, lettuce, and mint and toss well.

3. Slice the steak across the grain as thinly as possible, cutting the longer pieces in half as necessary, for 6 to 8 slices per wrap. Divide between the 4 wraps, placing the steak slices in the upper two-thirds of each wrap. Top with the salad mixture (about 1¼ cups each) and sprinkle with the peanuts. Fold up the bottom third and then roll in the sides, similar to a burrito with an open top.

PER SERVING: 340 calories, 11 g fat (3 g saturated), 44 g carbs, 5 g fiber, 488 mg sodium, 26 g protein

DECODE YOUR MEAL:

`nonstarchy vegetable` `whole grains` `lean protein` `healthy fats`

Tuna Salad Wrap

Makes 2 servings

2 scallions (white and green parts), cut into 1" pieces

1 rib celery, cut into 1" pieces

⅔ cup broccoli florets

½ cup packed flat-leaf parsley leaves

¼ Granny Smith apple with skin, cored and coarsely chopped

1 can (6.5 ounces) water-packed albacore tuna

2 tablespoons low-fat Greek yogurt

2 100% whole-wheat wraps (10" diameter)

2 large plum tomatoes, seeded and thinly sliced vertically

1. Place the scallions, celery, and broccoli into a food processor. Pulse 6 times to chop coarsely. Add the parsley and apple. Pulse 4 times to finely chop. The mixture should be moist but still crunchy. Scoop into a bowl. Wipe out the food processor bowl with a paper towel.

2. In the food processor, combine the tuna and yogurt. Process until the mixture is a spreadable pâté, about 45 seconds, scraping down the bowl as needed. Season to taste with salt and pepper.

3. Divide the tuna between the wraps, spreading firmly with a rubber spatula to cover all but ¾" along the outer edge of each wrap. Heap half of the chopped vegetables in the center of each wrap. Using your hand, spread them to cover the tuna, pressing lightly. Arrange the tomatoes evenly over the vegetables.

4. Roll the wraps from the bottom, pulling toward you slightly to make them tight. Trim off the ends, cutting them on a diagonal in the same direction. Cut each wrap diagonally in half. Wrap the pieces in plastic wrap and refrigerate 2 hours, or up to 24 hours, before serving.

PER SERVING: 248 calories, 2 g fat (0 g saturated), 37 g carbs, 6 g fiber, 671 mg sodium, 28 g protein

DECODE YOUR MEAL:

| fruit | nonstarchy vegetable | whole grains | lean protein | healthy fats |

Garden Vegetable Soup with Grilled Chicken

Makes 3 (24-ounce) servings

1⅓ cups whole-grain rotini pasta

1 teaspoon olive oil

¾ cup chunks (½") red onion

2 cloves garlic, quartered

1 teaspoon chopped fresh oregano or ¼ teaspoon dried

4 cups reduced-sodium chicken broth

1 can (14.5 ounces) reduced-sodium diced tomatoes, drained

½ cup chopped carrots

8 ounces grilled chicken breast, chopped

½ cup chopped fresh basil

1. Prepare the pasta according to the package directions.

2. Meanwhile, in a medium saucepan over medium heat, heat the oil, then add the onion, garlic, and oregano. Cook, stirring often, until the onion and garlic are tender, about 7 minutes.

3. Add the broth and bring the mixture to a boil.

4. Add the tomatoes and carrots. Lower the heat and simmer until the vegetables are tender, about 15 minutes.

5. Stir in the chicken and pasta. Simmer to heat the chicken through, about 2 minutes. Stir in the basil. Season with salt and pepper to taste. Serve hot or refrigerate in a plastic container and reheat before serving.

PER SERVING: 328 calories, 7 g fat (2 g saturated), 38 g carbs, 5 g fiber, 298 mg sodium, 28 g protein

DECODE YOUR MEAL:

| nonstarchy vegetable | whole grains | lean protein | healthy fats |

Italian Shrimp and Chickpea Salad

Makes 6 servings

2 cups rinsed and drained canned chickpeas

1 pound medium cooked, peeled, and deveined shrimp

2 medium tomatoes (about ½ pound), seeded and chopped

6 large leaves basil, chopped

¼ cup olive oil

4 cups arugula

1. In a large bowl, gently toss the chickpeas, shrimp, tomatoes, basil, and oil.

2. Season with salt and pepper to taste. Serve over the arugula.

PER SERVING: 270 calories, 12 g fat (1.5 g saturated), 21 g carbs, 6 g fiber, 180 mg sodium, 23 g protein

DECODE YOUR MEAL:

nonstarchy vegetable | legumes | lean protein | healthy fats

Turkey Tortilla Panini

Makes 2 servings

2 100% whole-wheat tortillas (9" diameter), toasted

2 tablespoons crumbled feta cheese, divided

4 ounces thinly sliced cooked turkey breast

4 thin slices red onion, separated

¼ cup jarred roasted red pepper strips

½ cup finely sliced kale leaves

1. Lay 1 tortilla in a dry, heavy skillet or griddle pan. Sprinkle evenly with 1 tablespoon cheese. Layer on the turkey, onion, red pepper, kale, remaining 1 tablespoon cheese, and remaining tortilla.

2. Place the skillet or griddle over medium-high heat. Cook, squeezing the sandwich with a panini press or other flat weight (like a heavy frying pan) until the tortilla is browned and the cheese melts, about 2 to 3 minutes per side. Reduce the heat slightly if the tortilla is browning too quickly. Remove and cut into 4 wedges.

PER SERVING (2 WEDGES): 231 calories, 6 g fat (2 g saturated), 26 g carbs, 4 g fiber, 478 mg sodium, 17 g protein

DECODE YOUR MEAL:

nonstarchy vegetable | whole grains | lean protein | dairy

Key West Chicken-Avocado Sandwiches

Makes 4 sandwiches

1 cup mashed avocado (about 1 medium)

1 tablespoon freshly squeezed lime juice (about ½ lime)

½ teaspoon green pepper sauce (such as Tabasco), optional

4 small whole-grain rolls (2 ounces each), split

1 cup baby spinach

10 ounces grilled or roasted chicken breast, sliced (about 2 cups)

1 mango, peeled, pitted, and sliced (about 1 cup)

1. In a small bowl, combine the avocado, lime juice, and green pepper sauce, if using. Spread the top and bottom halves of the rolls with 2 tablespoons each of the avocado-lime mixture.

2. Layer ¼ cup of the spinach, one-quarter of the chicken, and ¼ cup of the mango on the bottom halves of the rolls. Top with the other halves.

PER SERVING: 367 calories, 11 g fat (2.5 g saturated), 41 g carbs, 8 g fiber, 355 mg sodium, 29 g protein

DECODE YOUR MEAL:

| fruit | nonstarchy vegetable | whole grains | lean protein | healthy fats |

Dinners

Seared Scallops with White Beans and Bacon

Makes 4 servings

2 strips bacon, chopped into small pieces

½ cup finely chopped red onion

1 clove garlic, minced

1½ cans (15 ounces each) unsalted white beans, rinsed and drained

4 cups baby spinach

1 pound large sea scallops

1 tablespoon unsalted butter

Juice of 1 lemon

1. Heat a medium saucepan over low heat and cook the bacon until it begins to crisp. Pour off some of the fat and add the onion and garlic. Cook until the onion is soft and translucent, about 2 to 3 minutes. Add the beans and spinach and cook until the beans are hot and the spinach is wilted. Keep warm.

2. Put a large cast-iron skillet or sauté pan over medium-high heat. Blot the scallops dry with paper towels and season on both sides with salt and pepper to taste. Add the butter to the pan. After it melts, add the scallops. Sear 2 to 3 minutes on each side until they're deeply caramelized and the flesh is milky white or opaque and firm.

3. Before serving, add the lemon juice and salt and pepper to taste to the bean mixture. Divide the beans among 4 warm bowls or plates and top with the scallops.

PER SERVING: 283 calories, 7 g fat (2.5 g saturated), 28 g carbs, 7 g fiber, 361 mg sodium, 28 g protein

DECODE YOUR MEAL:

nonstarchy vegetable | legumes | lean protein | healthy fats

Tuscan Baked Zucchini

Makes 4 servings

4 medium zucchini

1 tablespoon olive oil, divided

1 jar (6 ounces) water-packed artichoke hearts, drained

2 cloves garlic, chopped

1 cup cooked whole-wheat orzo or couscous

3 tablespoons seasoned bread crumbs

¼ cup freshly grated Parmesan cheese

2 tablespoons toasted pine nuts

⅓ cup marinara sauce

½ cup shredded part-skim mozzarella cheese

1. Preheat the oven to 350°F. Spritz a 9" x 13" baking pan with cooking spray. Cut the zucchini in half lengthwise and use a spoon to scoop out the seeds and flesh, leaving a ¼"-thick shell. Discard the seeds and reserve the flesh. Brush the zucchini shells with ½ tablespoon of the olive oil and bake for 10 minutes. Remove the pan from the oven and set aside.

2. Place the pine nuts in an ungreased skillet over medium-low heat. Shake frequently as the nuts toast. Remove when lightly browned, after about 2 minutes.

3. While the zucchini is baking, chop the reserved zucchini flesh and the artichokes and place in a medium-size bowl. Add the garlic and combine. Heat the remaining ½ tablespoon oil in a nonstick skillet and cook the zucchini mixture for 3 to 5 minutes, until the zucchini is softened. Remove from the heat and add the cooked orzo or couscous, bread crumbs, Parmesan, pine nuts, and marinara sauce.

4. Fill each zucchini shell with about ⅓ cup of the filling and top each with 1 tablespoon mozzarella. Return the filled zucchini to the oven and bake for another 20 minutes, until the filling is heated through and the cheese is melted.

PER SERVING (2 HALVES): 300 calories, 13 g fat (3.5 g saturated), 34 g carbs, 8 g fiber, 630 mg sodium, 15 g protein

DECODE YOUR MEAL:

nonstarchy vegetable | whole grains | dairy | healthy fats

Honey-Mustard Salmon with Roasted Asparagus

Makes 4 servings

1 tablespoon unsalted butter

1 tablespoon brown sugar

2 tablespoons Dijon mustard

1 tablespoon low-sodium soy sauce

1 tablespoon honey

1½ pounds asparagus, trimmed

2 tablespoons olive oil, divided

¼ cup freshly grated Parmesan cheese

4 salmon fillets (6 ounces each)

1. Preheat the oven to 400°F. Combine the butter and brown sugar in a bowl and microwave on medium until they have melted together, about 30 seconds. Stir in the mustard, soy sauce, and honey.

2. Toss the asparagus with 1 tablespoon of the oil, the cheese, and salt and pepper to taste. Place the stalks in a baking dish and roast until they're al dente, about 10 to 12 minutes.

3. Meanwhile, heat the remaining 1 tablespooon oil in an ovenproof skillet over high heat. Season the salmon fillets with salt and pepper, then add to the skillet, flesh side down. Cook until browned on one side, 3 or 4 minutes. Flip the fillets, brush on half of the honey mustard, and place the pan in the oven. Bake until the fish is firm and flakes easily (but before white solids begin to form on the surface), about 5 minutes. (The internal temperature should be 145°F, as measured by a food thermometer.) Remove the fillets from the oven and brush with more honey mustard. Serve with the asparagus.

PER SERVING: 372 calories, 17 g fat (5 g saturated), 15 g carbs, 3.5 g fiber, 547 mg sodium, 40 g protein

DECODE YOUR MEAL:

nonstarchy vegetable   lean protein   dairy   healthy fats

Sweet-and-Sour Chicken Skewers

Makes 4 servings

1 pound boneless, skinless chicken breast, cut into bite-size chunks

2 medium zucchini, cut into large chunks

2 cups large pineapple chunks, drained

2 medium red onions, cut into large chunks

2 red bell peppers, cut into large chunks

1 tablespoon real maple syrup

3 tablespoons ketchup

½ tablespoon soy sauce

1 tablespoon vinegar (rice wine or cider)

1 teaspoon sriracha hot sauce

Fresh chopped cilantro (optional)

1. Preheat a grill or grill pan to medium-high. Soak 8 wooden skewers in cold water for 20 minutes. Thread the chicken, zucchini, pineapple, onions, and red peppers onto the skewers, alternating in the order listed. Season with salt and pepper to taste.

2. In a mixing bowl, stir together the maple syrup, ketchup, soy sauce, vinegar, and sriracha. Set aside half of the glaze in a separate container; brush the rest onto the skewered food.

3. Grill the skewers until lightly charred and the chicken is cooked through, about 4 minutes per side, or until the internal temperature reaches 165°F, as measured by a food thermometer. Then use a clean brush to coat with extra sauce. Top with the cilantro, if desired.

PER SERVING: 253 calories, 4 g fat (1 g saturated), 29 g carbs, 4 g fiber, 407 mg sodium, 27 g protein

DECODE YOUR MEAL:

fruit | nonstarchy vegetable | lean protein

Pizza Margherita

Makes 8 servings

1 tablespoon extra-virgin olive oil

1 teaspoon minced garlic

1 premade whole-wheat pizza crust

1½ cups shredded part-skim mozzarella cheese

1 pound tomatoes, sliced

½ cup fresh basil leaves

Freshly ground black pepper

1 tablespoon balsamic vinegar

1. Preheat the grill to medium-high.

2. Mix the olive oil and garlic. Brush half of the mixture onto the pizza crust.

3. Put the crust oil side down on the grill and heat until the bottom is golden brown, about 2 minutes.

4. Flip the crust, brush with the remaining garlic oil, and sprinkle the cheese evenly over it. Grill until the bottom is golden brown, about 2 minutes. Remove to a cutting board.

5. Scatter the tomatoes and basil evenly on the pizza. Sprinkle with pepper to taste and drizzle with the balsamic vinegar.

6. Cut into 8 slices.

PER SERVING: 374 calories, 12 g fat (5 g saturated), 56 g carbs, 10 g fiber, 146 mg sodium, 18 g protein

DECODE YOUR MEAL:

 fruit | whole grains | dairy | healthy fats

Mediterranean Pizza

Makes 8 servings

1 jar (3.5 ounces) roasted red peppers

¼ cup crumbled feta cheese

1 tablespoon red wine vinegar

1 cup marinated artichoke hearts

16 thin lemon slices

1 premade whole-wheat pizza crust

½ cup packed fresh baby spinach

8 kalamata olives, quartered and pitted

2 tablespoons extra-virgin olive oil

1. Preheat a grill to medium-high.

2. Rinse and drain the roasted peppers and puree in a blender with the cheese and vinegar.

3. Rinse, drain, and halve the artichoke hearts. Grill with the lemon slices, turning, until marked, for 2 minutes. Remove.

4. Lightly coat one side of the pizza crust with olive oil cooking spray. Put the crust oil side down on the grill and heat until the bottom is golden brown, about 2 minutes.

5. Flip the crust and spread evenly with the red pepper sauce. Sprinkle evenly with the spinach and olives. Scatter the artichokes and lemon over the top. Grill until the bottom is golden brown, about 2 minutes. Remove.

6. Top the pizza with the olive oil and freshly ground black pepper to taste.

7. Cut into 8 slices.

PER SERVING: 338 calories, 10 g fat (3 g saturated), 57 g carbs, 11 g fiber, 194 mg sodium, 13 g protein

DECODE YOUR MEAL:

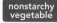

nonstarchy vegetable   whole grains   dairy   healthy fats

Raspberry-Pistachio Crusted Chicken

Makes 2 servings

½ cup raspberries

1 teaspoon Dijon mustard

1 tablespoon fresh lemon juice

¼ cup whole-grain bread crumbs

1 tablespoon coarsely ground pistachio nuts

1 tablespoon minced fresh parsley

Dash of white pepper

Pinch of sea salt

2 skinless, boneless chicken breast halves, pounded to ½" thickness

1 teaspoon olive oil

½ head kale, leaves trimmed and washed

1. In a food processor or blender, combine the berries, mustard, and lemon juice and process until smooth. Transfer to a shallow pan.

2. In another pan, combine the bread crumbs, pistachios, parsley, pepper, and salt.

3. Dip the chicken into the raspberry sauce, then into the bread crumb mixture to coat.

4. Heat the olive oil in a skillet and cook the chicken over medium heat, about 5 minutes per side, or until the internal temperature reaches 165°F, as measured by a food thermometer. Serve each chicken breast on a bed of kale.

PER SERVING: 243 calories, 8 g fat (1 g saturated), 9 g carbs, 3 g fiber, 450 mg sodium, 32 g protein

DECODE YOUR MEAL:

`fruit` `nonstarchy vegetable` `whole grains` `lean protein` `healthy fats`

Pesto Shrimp with Snow Peas over Quinoa

Makes 4 servings

¾ cup uncooked quinoa

1⅓ cups water

1 tablespoon olive oil

2 cloves garlic, minced

1 pound large peeled raw shrimp

3 cups snow peas (about 8 ounces)

¼ cup prepared basil pesto

2 tablespoons lemon juice

1. Put the quinoa in a fine mesh strainer and rinse well under cold water. Transfer to a medium saucepan and add the water. Bring to a boil. Reduce the heat to low, cover, and simmer until the water is absorbed and the quinoa is tender, 12 to 15 minutes. Fluff with a fork and cover until ready to serve.

2. Heat the oil in a large nonstick skillet over medium-high heat while the quinoa cooks. Add the garlic and cook, stirring, 30 seconds.

3. Add the shrimp and cook, stirring often, until just pink, about 3 minutes. Stir in the snow peas and cook, continuing to stir, 2 minutes longer.

4. Add the pesto and lemon juice and cook until warmed and the shrimp is done, about 1 minute. The flesh should be pearly and opaque. Serve over the quinoa.

PER SERVING: 372 calories, 14.5 g fat (3 g saturated), 28 g carbs, 4 g fiber, 293 mg sodium, 32 g protein

DECODE YOUR MEAL:

nonstarchy vegetable | whole grains | lean protein | healthy fats

Quick Pork Chops with Green Salsa

Makes 4 servings

1½ cups frozen shelled edamame

4 boneless pork chops (3 ounces each), trimmed of all visible fat

1 teaspoon ground cumin

¼ teaspoon salt

1 tablespoon canola oil

6 tomatillos, cut into wedges

4 scallions, cut into ½" pieces

1 clove garlic, minced

½ cup fat-free, reduced-sodium chicken broth

¼ cup chopped cilantro

1. Prepare the edamame according to the package directions. Drain.

2. Meanwhile, rub the chops with the cumin and salt. Coat a large nonstick skillet with cooking spray and heat over medium-high heat. Add the chops and cook for 4 minutes, turning once, or until a thermometer inserted in the center of a chop registers 160°F and the juices run clear. Remove to a plate and keep warm.

3. Heat the oil in the same skillet over medium-high heat. Cook the tomatillos, scallions, and garlic, stirring constantly, for 5 minutes, or until browned. Add the broth, cilantro, and edamame and cook for 3 minutes, or until the flavors meld. Serve with the chops.

PER SERVING: 239 calories, 10 g fat (1 g saturated), 11 g carbs, 5 g fiber, 278 mg sodium, 26 g protein

DECODE YOUR MEAL:

`nonstarchy vegetable` `legumes` `lean protein` `healthy fats`

Stir-Fried Beef and Broccoli

Makes 4 servings

1 pound top round steak, cut into ¼" strips

1 tablespoon reduced-sodium soy sauce

8 tablespoons orange juice, divided

3 tablespoons sherry, divided

2 teaspoons cornstarch, divided

⅓ cup hoisin sauce

⅛ teaspoon red-pepper flakes

1 tablespoon toasted sesame oil, divided

1 tablespoon grated fresh ginger

5 cups broccoli florets

2 carrots, sliced

3 tablespoons water

6 scallions, chopped

2 cups hot cooked brown rice

1. In a bowl, combine the beef, soy sauce, 2 tablespoons of the orange juice, 1 tablespoon of the sherry, and 1 teaspoon of the cornstarch. In a separate bowl, combine the hoisin sauce, red-pepper flakes, and remaining 6 tablespoons orange juice, 2 tablespoons sherry, and 1 teaspoon cornstarch.

2. Heat 1 teaspoon of the oil in a large nonstick skillet over medium-high heat. Add the beef, in batches if necessary so as not to overcrowd the skillet, and cook, stirring often, until lightly browned, about 2 minutes. Transfer to a plate and set aside.

3. Return the skillet to medium-high heat and pour in the remaining 2 teaspoons oil. Add the ginger and cook for 30 seconds, or until fragrant. Stir in the broccoli and cook for 1 minute. Add the carrots and water.

4. Cover and simmer for 2 to 3 minutes, or until tender-crisp. Uncover and stir in the beef and the orange juice mixture. Cook, stirring, until thick and bubbly, 1 to 2 minutes. Remove from the heat and stir in the scallions. Serve over the rice.

PER SERVING: 398 calories, 10 g fat (2 g saturated), 46 g carbs, 6 g fiber, 605 mg sodium, 31 g protein

DECODE YOUR MEAL:

nonstarchy vegetable | whole grains | lean protein | healthy fats

Turkey Gorgonzola Burgers

Makes 6 servings

1 pound lean ground turkey

3 ounces Gorgonzola cheese, chopped

½ cup sun-dried tomatoes, drained and chopped

2 cloves garlic, minced

2 teaspoons cumin powder

2 teaspoons canola oil

6 100% whole-grain buns

6 tablespoons barbecue sauce

Shredded cabbage (optional)

1. Preheat a grill to medium. In a bowl, combine the turkey, cheese, tomatoes, garlic, cumin, and salt and pepper to taste. Lightly mix together and form into 6 patties. Brush them with the oil.

2. Grill the burgers for 4 to 5 minutes per side, or until the internal temperature is 165°F. Toast the buns for 2 minutes. Serve the burgers on the buns; garnish with the barbecue sauce and cabbage, if desired.

PER SERVING: 293 calories, 11 g fat (4 g saturated), 27 g carbs, 4 g fiber, 545 mg sodium, 26 g protein

DECODE YOUR MEAL:

nonstarchy vegetable   whole grains   lean protein   dairy   healthy fats

Porchetta-Style Pork Loin with White Beans

Makes 6 servings

3 cloves garlic, minced

Peel of 2 oranges

1 tablespoon fennel seeds

1½ tablespoons chopped fresh rosemary, divided

1 tablespoon olive oil

1 pork loin (about 2 pounds), preferably with a thin layer of fat still attached

2 cans (15 ounces each) cannellini beans (white beans)

Juice of 1 lemon

1. Preheat the oven to 450°F.

2. On a cutting board, combine the garlic, orange peel, fennel seeds, and 1 tablespoon of the rosemary and chop until a paste forms. Scoop it into a small bowl and add the oil.

3. Season the pork with salt and pepper to taste, then rub it all over with the paste. (If you'd like, let it marinate up to 4 hours in the fridge before cooking.) Place the pork in a roasting pan and roast until a thermometer inserted into the middle reads 145°F, 25 to 30 minutes. Remove the pork from the oven and let it rest 10 minutes.

4. In a saucepan, heat the beans, lemon juice, and the remaining ½ tablespoon rosemary until warmed through. Season with salt and pepper. Slice the pork and serve with the beans.

PER SERVING: 313 calories, 8 g fat (2 g saturated), 21 g carbs, 6 g fiber, 216 mg sodium, 37 g protein

DECODE YOUR MEAL:

 legumes   lean protein   healthy fats

Sizzling Fajitas

Makes 4 servings

2 teaspoons olive oil

½ red or white onion, sliced

1 red, orange, or green bell pepper, sliced

2 cloves garlic, minced

2 whole chicken breasts, grilled and cut into strips, or ½ pound extralean (95%) ground beef

½ cup salsa

Chili powder

¼ cup low-fat sour cream

4 whole-wheat tortillas (7"–8" diameter)

1 cup shredded low-fat mozzarella cheese

1. Heat the oil in a medium skillet over medium-high. Add the onion, pepper, and garlic and cook briefly. Add the meat, reduce the heat to medium, and cook until no longer pink, about 10 minutes.

2. Stir in the salsa and chili powder to taste. Cook for 5 more minutes.

3. Spread 1 tablespoon of the sour cream in a thin layer on each tortilla. Divide the meat and vegetables on top of the tortillas, sprinkle each with the cheese, wrap, and serve.

PER SERVING: Chicken: 237 calories, 9 g fat (4.5 g saturated), 26 g carbs, 3 g fiber, 494 mg sodium, 15.5 g protein. Beef: 278 calories, 11.5 g fat (5 g saturated), 26 g carbs, 3 g fiber, 516 mg sodium, 22.5 g protein

DECODE YOUR MEAL:

nonstarchy vegetable | whole grains | lean protein | dairy | healthy fats

Quick Pad Thai

Makes 4 servings

6 ounces whole-wheat cappellini or angel-hair pasta (about ⅓ of a 16-ounce box)

2 teaspoons olive oil, divided

½ pound chicken breast, cut into bite-size pieces (about 1 cup precooked)

1 tablespoon fish sauce

1 tablespoon creamy natural peanut butter

1 tablespoon sugar

2 tablespoons red-pepper flakes

1 tablespoon water

3 eggs

⅓ cup chopped cilantro

Bean sprouts, crushed peanuts, or lime wedges (optional)

1. Cook the pasta according to the package directions. Drain and toss with 1 teaspoon of the oil.

2. Heat a wok or large skillet over medium-high heat and add the remaining 1 teaspoon oil. Add the chicken pieces and cook until just browned and no longer pink, about 4 minutes. Remove from the pan and set aside.

3. In a small bowl, whisk the fish sauce, peanut butter, sugar, red-pepper flakes, and water until smooth. Set aside.

4. Crack the eggs into a skillet and scramble until firm. Add the chicken and cook for another 2 minutes.

5. Add the cooked pasta and the peanut butter mixture to the skillet, tossing with the chicken and eggs. Add the cilantro. Garnish with the bean sprouts, peanuts, or a lime wedge, if desired.

PER SERVING: 326 calories, 9 g fat (2.2 g saturated), 38 g carbs, 3 g fiber, 464 mg sodium, 24 g protein

DECODE YOUR MEAL:

whole grains | lean protein | healthy fats

Pasta Primavera with Pine Nuts

Makes 4 servings

2 cups broccoli florets

3 cups dry whole-wheat pasta (a small style, such as rotini)

2 tablespoons olive oil, divided

1 large yellow bell pepper, sliced

3 tablespoons pine nuts

½ cup chopped oil-packed sun-dried tomatoes

1. Fill a large pot with water and bring to a rolling boil. Add the broccoli and cook until just tender and bright green, 2 to 3 minutes. With a slotted spoon, remove from the pot and place in a colander. Save the broccoli water. Run cold water over the broccoli for 1 minute, then place in a large bowl.

2. In the same pot, cook the pasta according to the package directions. Drain the pasta and add to the broccoli; toss with 1 tablespoon of the oil.

3. Add the remaining 1 tablespoon oil to a skillet and cook the pepper until soft, about 4 minutes. Remove from the pan and place in a pasta bowl.

4. Toast the pine nuts in a skillet until slightly browned, about 2 minutes, shaking the pan frequently to prevent burning. Add to the pasta bowl and toss with the other ingredients. Toss in the tomatoes and serve.

PER SERVING: 310 calories, 14.5 g fat (1.5 g saturated), 39 g carbs, 6 g fiber, 54 mg sodium, 8 g protein

DECODE YOUR MEAL:

nonstarchy vegetable | whole grains | healthy fats

Snacks

Edamame Hummus

Makes 4 servings

1 cup frozen shelled edamame

1 teaspoon chopped garlic

1 tablespoon tahini

1 tablespoon fresh lemon juice

3 tablespoons water

¼ teaspoon salt

½ teaspoon sriracha (optional)

1 tablespoon olive oil

1. Boil the frozen edamame for 4 to 6 minutes. Drain.

2. In a food processor, combine the edamame with the garlic, tahini, lemon juice, water, salt, and sriracha (if desired). Blend well. Drizzle in the olive oil. If the texture is too thick, add another tablespoon of water.

PER SERVING: 101 calories, 7 g fat (<1 g saturated), 5 g carbs, 2 g fiber, 152 mg sodium, 5 g protein

DECODE YOUR SNACK:

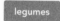 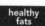

legumes | lean protein | healthy fats

Sweet-and-Spicy Yogurt Dip

Makes 4 servings

1 cup low-fat plain Greek yogurt

2 tablespoons finely chopped ripe peaches

1 teaspoon lemon juice

Dash of Worcestershire sauce

1½ teaspoons curry powder

¼ teaspoon cumin

¼ teaspoon salt

½ ring red bell pepper, chopped, for garnish

1 teaspoon chopped scallions, for garnish

1. In a bowl, stir together the yogurt, peaches, lemon juice, Worcestershire sauce, curry powder, cumin, and salt.

2. Chill for up to 2 hours to allow the flavors to develop. Top with the bell pepper and scallions before serving.

PER SERVING: 42 calories, 1 g fat (<1 g saturated), 3 g carbs, <1 g fiber, 165 mg sodium, 5 g protein

DECODE YOUR SNACK:

fruit | nonstarchy vegetable | lean protein | dairy

Tropical Guacamole

Makes 4 servings

½ avocado, pitted, peeled, and chopped

⅛ teaspoon salt

2 tablespoons chopped red onion

1½ tablespoons chopped fresh cilantro

2 teaspoons chopped jalapeño chile peppers

2 teaspoons fresh lime juice

¼ cup chopped pineapple

¼ cup chopped mango

¼ cup chopped cantaloupe

1. In a bowl, mash the avocado and salt together with a fork.

2. Gently stir in the onion, cilantro, peppers, and lime juice. Fold in the pineapple, mango, and cantaloupe.

PER SERVING: 107 calories, 4 g fat (<1 g saturated), 19 g carbs, 4 g fiber, 88 mg sodium, 2 g protein

DECODE YOUR SNACK:

fruit | nonstarchy vegetable | healthy fats

Green Goddess Dip with Vegetables & Homemade Pita Chips

Makes 20 servings

3 100% whole-wheat pitas (6" diameter)

2 teaspoons canola or olive oil

Ground cumin

Chili powder

Kosher salt

2 cups chopped avocado (about 2 whole)

1 cup low-fat plain Greek yogurt

¼ cup fresh lemon juice

¼ cup white wine vinegar

½ cup chopped fresh parsley

⅔ cup chopped fresh chives, divided

7 cups assorted fresh vegetables, raw or lightly steamed (e.g., beet slices, baby carrots, sliced fennel, julienned jicama, snow peas)

1. Preheat the oven to 350°F. Cut each pita into 8 wedges. Brush with the oil and sprinkle with cumin, chili powder, and salt—all to taste. Bake for 8 minutes, or until the edges begin to brown. Turn off the oven and let the chips stand for 15 minutes, or until crispy.

2. Meanwhile, put the avocado, yogurt, lemon juice, vinegar, parsley, ⅓ cup of the chives, and salt to taste in a small food processor or blender and puree until creamy. Stir in most of the remaining ⅓ cup chives, reserving some to garnish the dip.

3. To serve, spoon the dip into a small bowl and surround with the vegetables and pita chips on a platter.

PER SERVING: 78 calories, 3 g fat (1 g saturated), 11 g carbs, 3 g fiber, 95 mg sodium, 3 g protein

DECODE YOUR SNACK:

| fruit | nonstarchy vegetable | whole grains | dairy | healthy fats |

Maple Pepitas

Makes 8 servings

2 cups green pumpkin seeds	1½ teaspoons kosher salt
2 tablespoons pure maple syrup	½ teaspoon paprika or ground red pepper

1. Preheat the oven to 425°F.

2. In a bowl, toss together the seeds, maple syrup, salt, and paprika or red pepper and stir until the seeds are well coated. Transfer the seeds and any liquid to a parchment-lined baking sheet. Pat into a single layer.

3. Roast until the seeds are golden brown and aromatic, 10 to 15 minutes. Let cool. Pepitas will keep in an airtight container at room temperature for up to 5 days.

PER SERVING: 193 calories, 16 g fat (3 g saturated), 7 g carbs, 2 g fiber, 363 mg sodium, 10 g protein

DECODE YOUR SNACK:

lean protein   healthy fats

Spicy Roasted Chickpeas

Makes 7 servings

1 can (15 ounces) chickpeas, drained, rinsed, and patted dry

1 tablespoon olive oil

1 teaspoon smoked paprika

¼ teaspoon chipotle powder

¼ teaspoon sea salt

1. Preheat the oven to 400°F.

2. On a small baking sheet, toss the chickpeas with the oil, paprika, chipotle powder, and salt. Roast for 35 minutes, shaking the pan twice during cooking, until the chickpeas are crisp and dry.

3. Turn the oven off and leave the chickpeas inside to cool. Store in an airtight container.

PER SERVING: 91 calories, 3 g fat (0 g saturated), 14 g carbs, 3 g fiber, 250 mg sodium, 3 g protein

DECODE YOUR SNACK:

legumes | lean protein | healthy fats

Turkey Roll-Ups

Makes 2 servings

2 thick slices reduced-sodium, fat-free deli turkey breast

1 teaspoon honey mustard

2 thin slices reduced-fat cheese

½ red bell pepper, cut into thin strips

1. Lay the turkey slices on a flat work surface. Divide the mustard and spread evenly over each turkey slice. Top each with 1 slice of cheese.

2. Arrange half of the pepper strips on the center of each. Roll the turkey and cheese around the pepper strips.

PER SERVING: 102 calories, 4 g fat (2 g saturated), 5 g carbs, 1 g fiber, 228 mg sodium, 13 g protein

DECODE YOUR SNACK:

nonstarchy vegetable | lean protein | dairy | healthy fats

Side Dishes

Feta Quinoa Stuffed Tomatoes

Makes 4 servings

1 cup cooked quinoa, cooled

⅔ cup finely chopped bell peppers (orange, red, yellow)

½ cup reduced-fat feta cheese crumbles

¼ cup chopped fresh cilantro or parsley

¼ teaspoon finely grated lemon peel

1½ tablespoons extra-virgin olive oil

1½ tablespoons fresh lemon juice

¼ teaspoon salt

¼ teaspoon freshly ground black pepper

4 tomatoes

1. In a bowl, combine the quinoa, bell peppers, cheese, cilantro or parsley, lemon peel, oil, lemon juice, salt, and black pepper.

2. Cut the top off each tomato and scoop out the seeds and inner membranes. Stuff the tomatoes with the quinoa mixture and serve.

PER SERVING: 128 calories, 8 g fat (2 g saturated), 10 g carbs, 3 g fiber, 390 mg sodium, 5 g protein

DECODE YOUR SIDE:

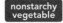

nonstarchy vegetable | whole grains | lean protein | dairy | healthy fats

Honey-Glazed Cashew Carrots

Makes 2 servings

2 cups baby carrots

4 teaspoons honey

Pinch of salt

2 tablespoons unsalted cashews, chopped

Fill a medium saucepan with 3" of water. Bring to a boil, then turn down the heat to low. Place the carrots in a steamer basket over the pot and cover, cooking until they're almost done, about 4 minutes. Remove from the heat, drain, then return to the pot along with the honey, salt, and cashews. Toss to coat.

PER SERVING: 143 calories, 4 g fat (1 g saturated), 26 g carbs, 3 g fiber, 139 mg sodium, 3 g protein

DECODE YOUR SIDE:

 nonstarchy vegetable lean protein healthy fats

Spicy Sweet Potato Sticks

Makes 2 servings

2 sweet potatoes, peeled

2 tablespoons olive oil

1 tablespoon paprika or chili powder

Pinch of salt and pepper

1. Preheat the oven to 400°F.

2. Cut the potatoes lengthwise into 3 or 4 pieces each, then cut each piece lengthwise into finger-size slices.

3. Toss the potatoes in the olive oil, then add the paprika or chili powder and salt and pepper to taste. Toss again to coat.

4. Spread the potatoes evenly on a baking sheet and cook for 30 minutes, turning them once halfway through.

PER SERVING: 148 calories, 7 g fat (1 g saturated), 20 g carbs, 4 g fiber, 324 mg sodium, 2 g protein

DECODE YOUR SIDE:

Spicy Black Beans

Makes 4 servings

1 tablespoon olive oil

½ cup chopped onion

1 teaspoon cumin seed or
½ teaspoon ground cumin

1 can (15.5 ounces) black beans,
rinsed and drained

½ cup water

1 teaspoon finely chopped
canned chipotle chile peppers
in adobo sauce

1. Heat the oil in a medium saucepan over medium heat. Cook the onion until tender, about 5 minutes. Stir in the cumin.

2. Add the beans and coarsely mash with a potato masher.

3. Add the water and peppers. Simmer over medium-low heat until the beans are creamy, about 5 minutes, adding more water if necessary to thin.

PER SERVING: 106 calories, 4 g fat (0.5 g saturated), 15 g carbs, 5 g fiber, 192 mg sodium, 5 g protein

DECODE YOUR SIDE:

nonstarchy vegetable   legumes   lean protein   healthy fats

Garlicky Asian Broccoli

Makes 2 servings

1 tablespoon finely chopped baby carrots

1 tablespoon finely chopped red onion

2 teaspoons canola oil

1 teaspoon minced garlic

1 teaspoon grated fresh ginger

8 ounces broccoli florets, cut into smaller chunks

1 tablespoon hot water

1. In a skillet over low heat, combine the carrots, onion, oil, garlic, and ginger. Add salt to taste. Cook, stirring, for 3 minutes.

2. Add the broccoli and stir to coat with the seasonings. Add the water and cover the pan. Cook, stirring occasionally, for 1 to 2 minutes.

PER SERVING: 86 calories, 5 g fat (0.5 g saturated), 7 g carbs, 3 g fiber, 106 mg sodium, 3 g protein

DECODE YOUR SIDE:

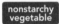 nonstarchy vegetable   healthy fats

Grilled Zucchini with Crispy Crumbs

Makes 4 servings

½ cup whole-wheat bread crumbs

2 tablespoons chopped pecans

1 teaspoon minced garlic

Pinch of salt

1 teaspoon olive oil

1 small zucchini

1. Mix the bread crumbs with the pecans, garlic, and salt. In a skillet over medium heat, heat the oil and toast the bread crumb mixture until golden brown, about 4 minutes.

2. Halve the zucchini lengthwise and grill over high heat until tender, about 8 minutes.

3. Top with the crumbs.

PER SERVING: 66 calories, 4 g fat (0.5 g saturated), 6 g carbs, 1.5 g fiber, 112 mg sodium, 2 g protein

DECODE YOUR SIDE:

nonstarchy vegetable   whole grains   healthy fats

Roasted Brussels Sprouts & Red Onions with Balsamic Vinegar

Makes 8 servings

1½ pounds Brussels sprouts, trimmed and quartered

1 tablespoon olive oil

1½ pounds red onions, thickly sliced

¼ cup balsamic vinegar

Sea salt

Freshly ground black pepper

1. Preheat the oven to 450°F. Line a large baking sheet with nonstick foil.

2. Spread the Brussels sprouts in a single layer on the prepared baking sheet and toss with the oil. Roast in the upper third of the oven, stirring occasionally, for 12 minutes.

3. Add the onions to the baking sheet, tossing to combine, and roast until the vegetables are tender and golden brown, about 10 minutes longer. Drizzle with the vinegar, tossing to combine, and roast for 2 minutes longer. Transfer to a serving bowl and season to taste with sea salt and black pepper.

PER SERVING: 85 calories, 2 g fat (0.5 g saturated), 15 g carbs, 4 g fiber, 24 mg sodium, 3 g protein

DECODE YOUR SIDE:

nonstarchy vegetable   healthy fats

Apple-Romaine Salad

Makes 4 servings

2 cups romaine lettuce, torn

1 cup chopped sweet red apples

⅓ cup shredded carrots

2 tablespoons honey

2 teaspoons olive oil

1 teaspoon poppy seeds

¼ cup lemon juice

1½ tablespoons low-fat plain Greek yogurt

Salt

Freshly ground black pepper

1. In a large salad bowl, toss together the lettuce, apples, and carrots.

2. In a small bowl, combine the honey, oil, poppy seeds, lemon juice, and yogurt. Add to the salad bowl and toss well. Season to taste with salt and pepper.

PER SERVING: 87 calories, 3 g fat (0 g saturated), 16 g carbs, 2 g fiber, 54 mg sodium, 1 g protein

DECODE YOUR SIDE:

`fruit`   `nonstarchy vegetable`   `healthy fats`

Desserts

Almond Chocolate Balls with Fleur de Sel

Makes 20 servings

1 cup natural almond butter	4 ounces dark chocolate
½ cup confectioners' sugar	Chopped fleur de sel
1 teaspoon vanilla extract	

1. In a bowl, combine the almond butter, sugar, and vanilla. Roll into 20 equal-size balls. Place on a baking sheet lined with waxed or parchment paper and freeze until firm, about 1 hour.

2. Stir the chocolate in a metal or glass bowl over a saucepan of simmering water until smooth. (Or microwave on medium power for 1 minute, stir, then continue microwaving on medium power, stirring every 20 seconds, until completely melted.)

3. Roll the almond balls in the melted chocolate, garnishing with the fleur de sel as you go. Refrigerate until the chocolate is set, about 30 minutes.

PER SERVING: 120 calories, 9 g fat (2 g saturated), 9 g carbs, 1 g fiber, 60 mg sodium, 2 g protein

DECODE YOUR DESSERT:

 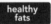

Honey Fruit Dip

Makes 4 servings

½ cup + 2 tablespoons frozen blueberries

4 ounces part-skim ricotta cheese

2 tablespoons orange juice

1 teaspoon vanilla extract

2 teaspoons honey

½ teaspoon cinnamon

1. Thaw the blueberries in the microwave on high until just warmed through, about 40 seconds.

2. In a food processor, combine the blueberries, cheese, orange juice, vanilla, honey, and cinnamon and blend until smooth. Chill in the refrigerator for at least 2 hours. Pair it with fresh-cut fruit or graham crackers.

PER SERVING (OF DIP): 68 calories, 2 g fat (1 g saturated), 9 g carbs, <1 g fiber, 35 mg sodium, 3 g protein

DECODE YOUR DESSERT:

fruit   dairy

Blueberry Cheesecake Parfait

Makes 4 servings

4 ounces Neufchâtel cheese, softened

½ cup reduced-fat sour cream

¼ cup confectioners' sugar

½ teaspoon vanilla extract

4 gingersnaps, crushed (2–3 tablespoons)

1½ cups fresh or frozen and thawed blueberries

1. Combine the cheese and sour cream in the bowl of an electric mixer and beat on high speed until smooth. Add the sugar and vanilla and beat until well combined. Reserve 4 teaspoons of the mixture and set aside. (You should have 1 cup for the parfaits.)

2. Fill each of 4 small parfait glasses or Champagne flutes with layers, starting with 2 tablespoons of the cheese mixture, then some cookie crumbs, and then a layer of blueberries. Repeat the pattern once more using the remaining cheese mixture, crumbs, and berries. Finish by dabbing 1 teaspoon of the reserved cheese mixture on top of each parfait. Use any extra berries and crumbs to garnish, if desired. Chill at least 30 minutes before serving.

PER SERVING: 200 calories, 10 g fat (6 g saturated), 24 g carbs, 1 g fiber, 190 mg sodium, 5 g protein

DECODE YOUR DESSERT:

fruit   dairy

Frozen Chocolate-Ricotta Sandwiches

Makes 16 servings

¾ cup part-skim ricotta cheese

1½ tablespoons all-fruit orange marmalade

1 tablespoon sugar

1 tablespoon mini dark chocolate chips

16 chocolate graham crackers

1. In a small bowl, stir together the cheese, marmalade, and sugar until combined. Fold in the chocolate chips. Place 8 graham cracker halves on a rimmed baking sheet.

2. Spoon a generous tablespoon of the cheese mixture onto each cracker half. Top with the remaining cracker halves and freeze until set, at least 1 hour. Once frozen, wrap separately. These will keep in the freezer for a week.

PER SERVING: 157 calories, 4 g fat (2 g saturated), 27 g carbs, 1 g fiber, 205 mg sodium, 3 g protein

DECODE YOUR DESSERT:

dairy

Crispy Rice Chocolate Pops

Makes 32 pops

3 tablespoons unsalted butter

1 package (10 ounces) marshmallows

2 teaspoons vanilla extract

6 cups organic puffed brown rice cereal

8 ounces bittersweet chocolate, melted

½ cup finely chopped pistachios

½ cup unsweetened coconut flakes, toasted

1. Melt the butter in a large pot over medium heat. Add the marshmallows and stir until melted, about 6 minutes. Remove the pot from the heat and stir in the vanilla and cereal until combined. Transfer the mixture to a baking sheet coated with cooking spray. Let stand until cool enough to handle, about 5 minutes.

2. With damp hands, form the mixture into 32 equal balls (about 2" diameter). Stick a small bamboo skewer into each ball, pressing gently to adhere.

3. Transfer the pops to a large sheet of greased foil and let stand about 15 minutes.

4. Dip each pop in the melted chocolate and return to the foil. Let stand about 10 minutes. Sprinkle half of the pops with the pistachios and the other half with the coconut.

PER SERVING: 161 calories, 6 g fat (3 g saturated), 16.5 g carbs, 1 g fiber, 33 mg sodium, 1.5 g protein

DECODE YOUR DESSERT:

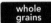

Caramel Corn

Makes 7 (1-cup) servings

2 tablespoons butter	1 tablespoon water
2 tablespoons brown sugar	7 cups air-popped popcorn
¼ teaspoon kosher salt	35 lightly salted peanuts

1. Melt the butter in a large stockpot over low heat. Whisk in the brown sugar, salt, and water.

2. Add the popcorn and peanuts. Toss until the mixture is evenly distributed. Let cool.

PER SERVING: 100 calories, 6 g fat (3 g saturated), 11 g carbs, 1 g fiber, 85 mg sodium, 2 g protein

DECODE YOUR DESSERT:

whole grains · lean protein · healthy fats

Grilled Tropical Fruit with Greek Yogurt

Makes 6 servings

½ pineapple	1¼ cups low-fat plain Greek yogurt
1 mango	2 tablespoons honey
Olive oil	1 teaspoon cinnamon
6 tablespoons toasted coconut	

1. Preheat a grill to high. Brush the pineapple and mango lightly with the oil.

2. Place the fruit on the grill grate, reduce the heat to medium-high, and cook until grill marks appear and the fruit is slightly tender, 2 to 3 minutes per side. Remove from the heat and let cool.

3. To toast the coconut, spread the shavings on a baking sheet and bake at 350°F for 5 to 10 minutes, until golden. Stir throughout.

4. In a bowl, mix together the yogurt and honey. Cut the fruit into small chunks and mix well in a large bowl. Serve the fruit salad topped with the yogurt dressing and sprinkled with cinnamon and coconut.

PER SERVING: 135 calories, 2.5 g fat (2 g saturated), 26 g carbs, 2 g fiber, 30 mg sodium, 4 g protein

DECODE YOUR DESSERT:

fruit | lean protein | dairy | healthy fats

Crunchy Peanut Squares

Makes 24 servings

1 tablespoon butter	3 cups plain air-popped popcorn
⅓ cup honey	2 cups crisp brown rice cereal
¼ cup packed brown sugar	2 cups oat circles cereal
⅓ cup natural peanut butter	⅓ cup unsalted peanuts, chopped
1 teaspoon vanilla extract	⅓ cup dark chocolate chips

1. Line a 13" × 9" baking dish with foil, extending the foil at the ends. Coat with cooking spray.

2. In a large nonstick saucepan, melt the butter, honey, and brown sugar over low heat, stirring frequently. Remove from the heat. Add the peanut butter and vanilla. Return to low heat and cook, stirring constantly, for 2 minutes, or until the mixture is well blended.

3. Remove the pan from the heat and add the popcorn, rice cereal, oat cereal, and peanuts. Stir until evenly coated with the peanut butter mixture. Turn into the prepared baking dish. Coat your hands with cooking spray and press the mixture firmly into the baking dish. Sprinkle with the chocolate chips. Cool completely on a rack. Lift from the baking dish using the foil. Cut into 24 squares to serve.

PER SERVING: 97 calories, 4 g fat (1 g saturated), 14 g carbs, 1 g fiber, 43 mg sodium, 2 g protein

DECODE YOUR DESSERT:

whole grains | lean protein | healthy fats

Raspberry Swirl Brownies

Makes 12 servings

- ½ cup + 2 tablespoons whole-grain pastry flour
- 1⅔ cups confectioners' sugar
- ¼ cup unsweetened cocoa powder
- ¾ teaspoon baking powder
- ⅛ teaspoon salt
- 1½ ounces unsweetened chocolate
- 2½ tablespoons canola oil
- 2 large egg whites
- 2 tablespoons raspberry all-fruit preserves
- 2 teaspoons vanilla extract
- 1 cup raspberries

1. Preheat the oven to 350°F. Line a 9" × 9" baking dish with foil, extending the foil at the ends. Coat with cooking spray.

2. In a medium bowl, mix the flour, sugar, cocoa, baking powder, and salt. In a large microwaveable bowl, combine the chocolate and oil and microwave on high power for 1 minute. Stir until the chocolate is completely melted. Stir in the egg whites, preserves, and vanilla. Stir in the flour mixture until just blended. Fold in the raspberries.

3. Pour the batter into the prepared baking dish and spread evenly. Bake for 24 to 26 minutes, or until the center is almost firm when tapped. Cool on a rack for 15 minutes. Lift the brownies from the pan using the foil. Cool completely on a rack. Cut into 12 squares to serve.

PER SERVING: 158 calories, 5 g fat (1.5 g saturated), 29 g carbs, 2 g fiber, 71 mg sodium, 2 g protein

DECODE YOUR DESSERT:

fruit | whole grains | healthy fats

Smoothies

Belly-Trimming Tropical Smoothie

Makes 2 servings

½ cup 1% milk

2 tablespoons low-fat vanilla yogurt

¼ cup frozen orange juice concentrate

½ banana

¼ cup whole strawberries

½ cup cubed mango

2 teaspoons vanilla whey protein powder

3 ice cubes

Toss everything into a blender and whip until smooth.

PER SERVING: 153 calories, 1 g fat (0.5 g saturated), 31 g carbs, 2 g fiber, 50 mg sodium, 7 g protein

DECODE YOUR SMOOTHIE:

fruit | lean protein | dairy

Awesome Almond Smoothie

Makes 2 servings

2 small frozen bananas, sliced

1½ cups kale, lightly packed, stems removed

1½ cups 1% milk

1½ tablespoons almond butter

¼ teaspoon cinnamon

¼ teaspoon nutmeg

¼ teaspoon ground ginger

Put all the ingredients in a blender and process until smooth.

PER SERVING: 269 calories, 10 g fat (2 g saturated), 40 g carbs, 4 g fiber, 156 mg sodium, 11 g protein

DECODE YOUR SMOOTHIE:

fruit | nonstarchy vegetable | lean protein | dairy | healthy fats

Red, White, and Blue Smoothie

Makes 2 servings

2 cups low-fat plain Greek yogurt

½ cup 1% milk

2 tablespoons sugar

1 teaspoon vanilla extract

1½ cups frozen blueberries

10 fresh raspberries

1. Blend the yogurt and milk with the sugar and vanilla. Pour half of the mixture into 2 glasses.

2. Add the blueberries to the remaining smoothie mixture in the blender and process. Pour over the vanilla smoothie in the glasses.

3. Top with the fresh raspberries.

PER SERVING: 279 calories, 5 g fat (3 g saturated), 41 g carbs, 3 g fiber, 93 mg sodium, 20 g protein

DECODE YOUR SMOOTHIE:

 fruit   lean protein   dairy

The Energy Booster

Makes 3 servings

2 frozen bananas, chopped

2 scoops chocolate protein powder

2 tablespoons peanut butter

2 tablespoons wheat germ

1 teaspoon cinnamon

1 tablespoon honey

¾ cup low-fat Greek yogurt

4 tablespoons nonfat dry milk

2 cups ice

Throw all of the ingredients into a blender and process until smooth.

PER SERVING: 294 calories, 7 g fat (2 g saturated), 38 g carbs, 4 g fiber, 102 mg sodium, 25 g protein

DECODE YOUR SMOOTHIE:

fruit | lean protein | dairy | healthy fats

Pumpkin Spice Smoothie

Makes 2 servings

1 cup canned pumpkin

1 cup 1% milk

2 teaspoons vanilla

1 cup crushed ice

2 tablespoons honey

2 teaspoons pumpkin pie spice

Toss all of the ingredients into a blender and process until smooth.

PER SERVING: 175 calories, 2 g fat (1 g saturated), 35 g carbs, 4 g fiber, 62 mg sodium, 6 g protein

DECODE YOUR SMOOTHIE:

starchy vegetable   dairy

Blueberry and Green Tea Smoothie

Makes 2 servings

¾ cup water

2 green tea bags

2 cups frozen blueberries

3 ice cubes

12 ounces low-fat vanilla yogurt

2 tablespoons whole dry-roasted, unsalted almonds

2 tablespoons ground flaxseed

1. Bring the water to a boil and pour over the tea bags. Steep for 4 minutes. Squeeze and remove the tea bags and discard. Chill the tea overnight.

2. Place the tea, blueberries, ice, yogurt, almonds, and flaxseed in a blender. Process until smooth.

PER SERVING: 369 calories, 12 g fat (3 g saturated) 57 g carbs, 7 g fiber, 105 mg sodium, 11 g protein

DECODE YOUR SMOOTHIE:

| fruit | lean protein | dairy | healthy fats |

Your Workout

The ultimate 4-week fat-burning exercise plan

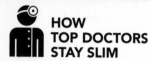

HOW TOP DOCTORS STAY SLIM

"The research is definitive: Staying lean isn't just about how many hours you spend in a gym, it's also about how many hours you're on your feet. I incorporate walking and standing into my day as much as possible. If I go to a coffee shop to work, I put my laptop up on the bar and do my work standing."

—TRAVIS STORK, MD, author of *The Lean Belly Prescription* and host of TV's *The Doctors*

Whether you've never walked into a gym or you took a 6-month exercise hiatus, this workout was created with you in mind. It's designed to be non-intimidating and easy enough for beginners yet effective enough to burn fat and tone muscle. Teamed with the eating strategy outlined earlier in this section, this exercise plan will deliver results you can see and feel within just 4 weeks. Do it as prescribed and we guarantee it will kick-start your new lifestyle of regular exercise and good eating habits. You'll feel and look so good, you won't want the benefits to ever end.

Now for some details. Each week, you'll complete six workouts: four walking workouts and two strength-training workouts. Initially, your aim is simply to get moving and perfect your exercise form. Then, as you advance, you'll shorten your rest periods between strength exercises and increase your cardio workout time to help you build endurance and blast fat. You will also build some lean muscle. Don't worry, those of you who fear becoming muscle-bound. It won't happen on this plan. You should, however, expect to build enough muscle to give your resting metabolic rate a nice boost and tone up your flabby parts.

WHAT YOU'LL DO:
6 workouts a week, divided into:
>   Fat-Torch Walk (2 days a week)
>   Calorie-Scorch Interval Walk
>   (2 days a week)
>   Belly-Blast Body-Weight Workout
>   (1 day a week)
>   Belly-Blast Dumbbell Workout
>   (1 day a week)

YOUR SCHEDULE
>   Day 1: Fat-Torch Walk
>   Day 2: Belly-Blast Body-Weight Workout
>   Day 3: Calorie-Scorch Interval Walk
>   Day 4: Rest
>   Day 5: Fat-Torch Walk
>   Day 6: Belly-Blast Dumbbell Workout
>   Day 7: Calorie-Scorch Interval Walk

FAT-TORCH WALK
Week 1

TIME	ACTIVITY	SPEED	INTENSITY
0:00	Warmup	3–3.5 mph	Light (You can sing.)
3:00	Brisk walk	3.5–4 mph	Moderate (You can chat with a friend.)
18:00	Cooldown	3–3.5 mph	Light
20:00	Finish		

Each week, for 4 weeks, increase the brisk walk by 5 minutes. By week 4, you should be able to turn the brisk walk into a light jog. (You can also do a walk/jog combination.)

CALORIE-SCORCH INTERVAL WALK
Week 1

TIME	ACTIVITY	SPEED	INTENSITY
0:00	Warmup	3–3.5 mph	Light (You can sing.)
3:00	Brisk walk	3.5–4 mph	Moderate (You can chat with a friend.)
4:00	Speed walk	Over 4 mph	Vigorous (You can barely talk.)
4:30	Alternate between 1-minute brisk walk and 30 seconds of speed walking 5 times		
12:00	Brisk walk	3.5–4 mph	Moderate
19:00	Cooldown	3–3.5 mph	Light
20:00	Finish		

Each week, for 4 weeks, increase the second brisk walk by 5 minutes. By week 4, you should be able to turn the brisk walk into a light jog. (You can also do a walk/jog combination.)

BELLY-BLAST BODY-WEIGHT WORKOUT

Perform these exercises as a circuit; in other words, do each exercise once in order. After completing one circuit, repeat the entire circuit once or twice more, depending upon how you feel. For the first 2 weeks, rest no more than 60 seconds between exercises. Then, for the second 2 weeks, shorten or eliminate your rest periods between exercises to increase your fat burning. Still, take a short rest in between individual circuits.

(Note: If you find any of these exercises too difficult, you may substitute a similar but easier body-weight exercise from the list of descriptions starting on page 306.)

Weeks 1–2

EXERCISE	REPS	REST
Forward lunge	10–12	45–60 seconds
Squat jump	10–12	45–60 seconds
Pushup	10–12	45–60 seconds
Bend and thrust	10–12	45–60 seconds
Plié squat	10–12	45–60 seconds
Jumping jack	As many as you can in 60 seconds	45–60 seconds
T-stabilization	10–12	45–60 seconds
Seated rotation	10–12	45–60 seconds

Weeks 3–4

EXERCISE	REPS	REST
Forward lunge	10–12	None
Squat jump	10–12	45 seconds
Pushup	10–12	None
Bend and thrust	10–12	45 seconds
Plié squat	10–12	None
Jumping jack	As many as you can in 60 seconds	45 seconds
T-stabilization	10–12	None
Seated rotation	10–12	45 seconds

SQUAT JUMP

Stand with your feet hip-width apart, your toes forward. Lightly touch your fingers behind your ears and extend your elbows to the sides. Bend your knees, then explosively jump as high as you can. Land softly on the balls of your feet and immediately lower into your next squat.

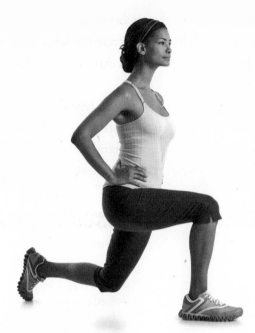

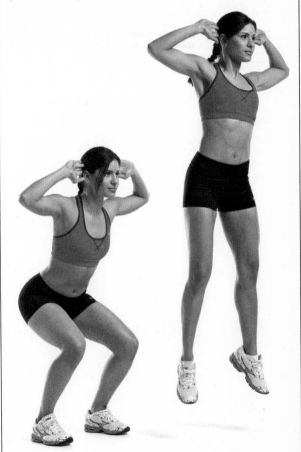

FORWARD LUNGE

Stand with your feet hip-width apart and your hands on your hips. Step forward with your right leg and slowly lower your body until your right knee is bent at least 90 degrees. Push back to the starting position and repeat with your left leg. That's 1 rep.

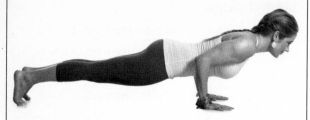

PUSHUP

Assume a pushup position with your feet hip-width apart and your hands slightly outside your shoulders. Your body should form a straight line from head to heels. Lower your body until your chest nearly touches the floor. Pause, then push back to the starting position as quickly as possible. That's 1 rep. (If the traditional pushup is too difficult, do a modified version by resting your knees on the floor.)

BEND AND THRUST

With your arms at your sides, stand with your feet hip-width apart. In one motion, bend your knees and place your hands on the floor on either side of your legs, then jump both feet back so you're in a pushup position with your back straight. Quickly reverse the motion to return to the starting position. That's 1 rep.

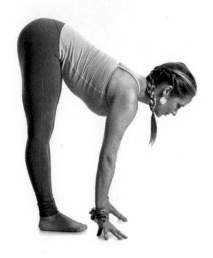

JUMPING JACK

Stand with your feet together and your arms at your sides, then simultaneously raise your arms out to the sides and over your head and jump your feet out so they are slightly more than shoulder-width apart. Without pausing, quickly reverse the movement. Repeat.

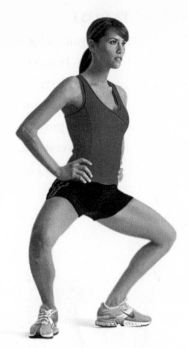

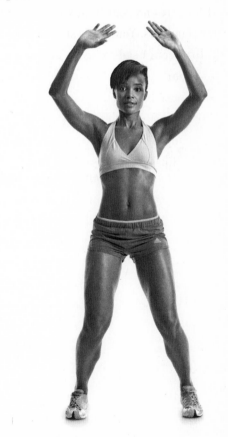

PLIÉ SQUAT

Stand with your legs 2 to 3 feet apart, toes turned out. Place your hands on your hips. Push your hips back and lower your body until your thighs are parallel to the floor. Pause, then slowly push yourself back to the starting position. That's 1 rep.

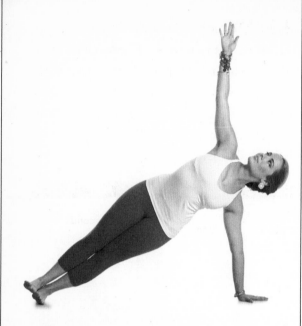

T-STABILIZATION

Start in a pushup position with your body in a straight line from your head to your heels. Keeping your arms straight and your core engaged, shift your weight onto your left arm, rotate your torso to the right, and raise your right arm toward the ceiling so that your body forms a T. Your right foot should now be on top of your left. Pause for 3 seconds, then return to the starting position and repeat on the other side. That's 1 rep.

SEATED ROTATION

Sit on the floor with your legs in front of you, your knees bent, and your heels lifted a few inches into the air. Lean back at a 45-degree angle and extend your arms straight in front of your chest, palms together. Slowly rotate your torso to the right, pause, then rotate to the left. Continue alternating.

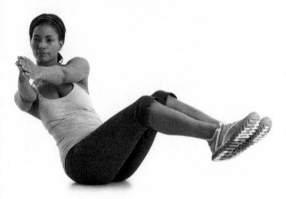

BELLY-BLAST DUMBBELL WORKOUT

Perform two sets of each exercise, resting a maximum of 60 seconds between sets. For the first set, use a dumbbell that you can lift for only 10 to 12 reps. For the second set, drop down to the next-lightest weight and complete as many reps as possible. If you can do more than 12, you need to use a heavier weight for the first set. Gradually increase your weight each week. After completing both sets of an exercise, move to the next lift.

EXERCISE	SETS	REPS	REST
Dumbbell squat	2	10–12 (first set) As many as possible (second set)	45–60 seconds
Chest press	2	10–12 (first set) As many as possible (second set)	45–60 seconds
Bent-over row	2	10–12 (first set) As many as possible (second set)	45–60 seconds
Overhead press	2	10–12 (first set) As many as possible (second set)	45–60 seconds
Reverse fly	2	10–12 (first set) As many as possible (second set)	45–60 seconds
Biceps curl	2	10–12 (first set) As many as possible (second set)	45–60 seconds
Triceps press-back	2	10–12 (first set) As many as possible (second set)	45–60 seconds
Dumbbell split squat	2	10–12 (first set) As many as possible (second set)	45–60 seconds

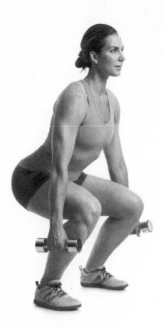

DUMBBELL SQUAT

Stand tall with your feet shoulder-width apart, holding dumbbells down at your sides, palms facing in. Shift your body weight back into your heels, bend your hips and then your knees, and lower your body, sticking your butt out as if sitting in a chair. Keep your head up, shoulders back, abs tight, and back straight as you lower until your thighs are almost parallel to floor. Make sure your knees stay behind your toes (if you look down, you should be able to see your toes). Pause, then slowly push back to the starting position.

CHEST PRESS

Holding dumbbells, lie faceup on the floor (or a bench), knees bent, feet flat. Position the weights on either side of your chest with your elbows bent and pointing out to the sides, your palms facing your legs. Push the weights straight up over your chest. Pause, then slowly lower them to the starting position. Repeat.

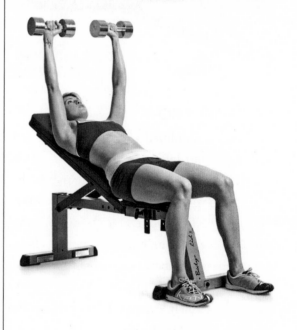

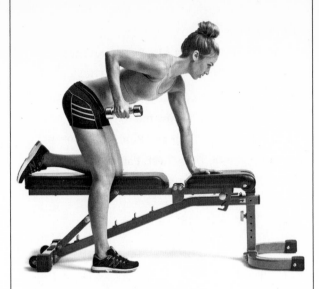

BENT-OVER ROW

Grasp a dumbbell with your right hand and place your left knee and left hand on a chair (or bench) so your back is parallel to the floor. Keep your head in line with your spine, abs tight. Allow your right arm to hang straight down, your palm facing the chair. Bend your right elbow toward the ceiling and pull the dumbbell up toward your chest. Pause, then slowly lower the weight. Complete a full set, then repeat with your left arm.

OVERHEAD PRESS

Holding dumbbells, stand with your feet hip-width apart. Bend your arms so the dumbbells are just above your shoulders, your palms facing forward. Press the dumbbells straight up overhead without arching your back. Pause, then slowly lower them to shoulder height.

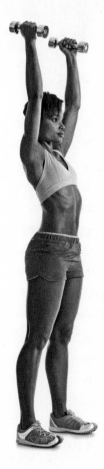

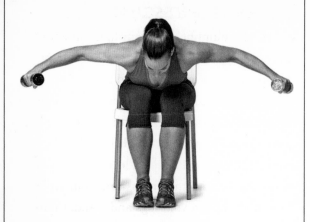

REVERSE FLY

Sit on the edge of a chair, feet together, and hold a dumbbell in each hand. Lean forward from the hips so your arms hang down next to your calves, with your elbows bent slightly and your palms facing each other. Squeeze your shoulder blades together and raise the weights out to the sides in an arcing motion until your arms are about parallel to floor. Keep your elbows slightly bent throughout the move. Pause, then slowly lower the dumbbells.

BICEPS CURL

Stand with your feet hip-width apart, holding dumbbells at your sides, your palms facing in. Keeping your elbows at your sides, bend your arms, rotate your wrists so your palms face up, and raise the dumbbells toward your shoulders. Pause, then slowly lower the weights, rotating your palms toward your thighs at the bottom position.

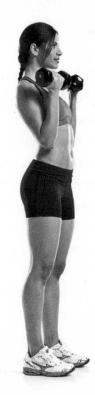

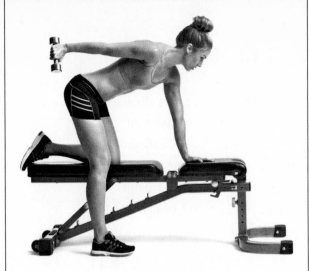

TRICEPS PRESS-BACK

Hold a dumbbell in your right hand and place your left knee and left hand on a chair (or bench) so your back is parallel to the floor. Bend your right arm so that your elbow is at your side and your forearm is perpendicular to the floor. Straighten your right arm, raising the weight back toward your butt. Pause and slowly return to the starting position. Complete a full set, then repeat the exercise with your left arm.

DUMBBELL SPLIT SQUAT

Hold a dumbbell in each hand down at your sides, your palms facing your thighs. Stand with your right foot 2 to 3 feet in front of the left, your toes pointing forward, left heel slightly off the floor. Bend both knees, slowly lowering the left knee toward the floor. Keep your right knee over your ankle; don't lean forward. Pause, and then press into your front foot to straighten your legs and stand. Complete a full set, then repeat the exercise with the opposite leg forward.

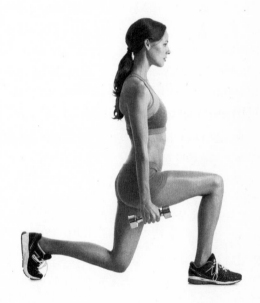

Track Your Progress

Your food and workout log

Why bother assessing your level of hunger? Simple: It helps you determine whether you're eating often enough and at the right times of day. Ideally, you'll chow down when you're in the 3 to 4 range. When you're at a 1 or 2, you don't need to eat, and by 5 or 6, you're so famished that you're likely to overeat or make poor food choices.

THE SCALE

1 You don't feel hungry.

2 Food sounds good, but you couldn't eat an entire apple.

3 Your stomach feels empty.

4 Your stomach is growling.

5 Your stomach and head hurt.

6 You are irritable and can't focus. Eating feels like an emergency.

Tracking your meals, snacks, and hunger is a proven tool for weight-loss success. "A food diary is a window into your habits," says Hale Deniz-Venturi, RD, owner of FitHealth Consulting in Chicago. By making you keenly aware of what you are consuming, the diary is a powerful motivational tool that can help you cut back even further than you thought possible.

Using the format opposite, write down everything you eat and drink—even the tiniest bite of cake—rate your hunger, and consider how you feel before you eat. You'll learn the whys and hows of your eating, which can help you stop mindless and emotional eating.

Don't stop there: Logging your workouts can help reinforce the other half of your weight-loss equation: exercise. Seeing your accomplishments on paper will help motivate you to sweat—especially after a few weeks into your program, when you start seeing fitness gains.

SAMPLE FOOD LOG

Date: **Weight:**   **Waist Circumference:**

MEAL	ITEMS & AMOUNT CONSUMED	CALORIES	HUNGER RATING	HOW I FEEL
Breakfast 7:25 a.m.	¼ cup steel-cut oats, prepared with water ¼ cup blueberries 1 slice ham ½ cup 1% milk 1 cup coffee	320	1 2 (3) 4 5 6	I feel happy and in control.
Lunch				

FRUIT	WHOLE GRAINS	NONSTARCHY VEGETABLES	LEAN PROTEIN	STARCHY VEGETABLES	LOW-FAT DAIRY	LEGUMES	HEALTHY FATS	TOTAL CALORIES
⊗ ○	⊗ ○	○ ○	⊗ ○	○ ○	⊗ ○	○ ○	⊗ ○	
○ ○	○ ○	○ ○	○ ○	○ ○	○ ○	○ ○	○ ○	
○ ○	○ ○	○ ○	○ ○	○ ○	○ ○	○ ○	○ ○	

SAMPLE EXERCISE LOG

Date: **Weight:**   **Waist Circumference:**

EXERCISE	SETS	REPS	WEIGHT USED	DURATION	DISTANCE	PERSONAL NOTES
Running				23 min.	2 miles	Felt great! Only had to rest once!

FOOD LOG

Date: *Weight:*   *Waist Circumference:*

MEAL	ITEMS & AMOUNT CONSUMED	CALORIES	HUNGER RATING	HOW I FEEL
Breakfast			1 2 3 4 5 6	
Lunch			1 2 3 4 5 6	
Dinner			1 2 3 4 5 6	
Optional Snack			1 2 3 4 5 6	
Optional Snack			1 2 3 4 5 6	
Optional Snack			1 2 3 4 5 6	

FRUIT	WHOLE GRAINS	NONSTARCHY VEGETABLES	LEAN PROTEIN	STARCHY VEGETABLES	LOW-FAT DAIRY	LEGUMES	HEALTHY FATS	TOTAL CALORIES
○ ○ ○ ○ ○ ○	○ ○ ○ ○ ○ ○	○ ○ ○ ○ ○ ○	○ ○ ○ ○ ○ ○	○ ○ ○ ○ ○ ○	○ ○ ○ ○ ○ ○	○ ○ ○ ○ ○ ○	○ ○ ○ ○ ○ ○	

EXERCISE LOG

Date: **Weight:**   **Waist Circumference:**

EXERCISE	SETS	REPS	WEIGHT USED	DURATION	DISTANCE	PERSONAL NOTES

15 Ways to Maintain Your New Body for Life!

It's one thing to lose the weight—it's quite another to keep it off. In a UCLA analysis of 31 long-term diet studies, researchers found that about two-thirds of dieters regained more weight than they initially lost within 4 to 5 years. A depressing statistic, no?

Well, you don't have to become one of those people who watch all their hard work go to potbelly if you understand how your body changes after it has shed pounds and if you develop a simple maintenance strategy.

First, it's crucial to recognize what happens internally when your body has lost weight. Without the extra energy stored in the form of fat, your body will attempt to compensate by slowing your resting metabolism, which results in reduced calorie burn 24/7. At the same time, your body naturally ramps up levels of the hunger hormone ghrelin, according to Israeli researchers. These metabolic changes, experts say, can persist even a year after you shed the weight.

All this means that in the weeks and months following any significant weight loss, you need to be extradiligent about maintaining the healthy habits that got you here in the first place. You may even have to work a bit harder at it. Here are some ways you can do that:

1 STAY ACTIVE

This sounds obvious, but it's important: To keep weight off, you have to keep moving. A 2006 study from the Centers for Disease Control and Prevention (CDC) found that people who successfully maintained weight loss were significantly more likely to exercise at least 30 minutes a day than those who regained. It can be as simple as taking a fast-paced walk around the block every night or committing to regular visits to the gym. A study in the journal *Obesity* found that people who lost weight and exercised 80 minutes a week didn't regain dangerous visceral fat after a year.

2 RETHINK YOUR WORKOUT

Dieters who struggled to stick to an exercise routine were 74 percent more likely to experience regain, the CDC study found. If you find any excuse to avoid the gym, you may need to rework your routine. Planning to perform your favorite exercise first can decrease your workout dread, according to 2011 Canadian research. So if you love Swiss-ball exercises, do those first. Or read a magazine on the elliptical to start, if that's what you enjoy.

3 TRACK CALORIES

Yes, counting calories may be laborious. But it's also one of the most foolproof forms of accountability (and yet another strategy used by successful maintainers in the CDC study).

Fortunately, you don't have to go it alone. Tools like MyFitnessPal.com or prevention.com/healthtracker will calculate your intake for you.

4 PRIORITIZE PRODUCE

Don't think of fruits and vegetables as "diet" foods. They're healthy-living foods—which means you need to keep eating them long after you've lost the weight! In a 2011 Penn State study, dieters who kept the pounds off continued eating lots of produce even after they reached their goal. Work produce into every meal: Have a piece of fruit with breakfast, a salad with lunch, and steamed vegetables with dinner, and munch on berries for dessert or a snack.

5 PLAN YOUR MEALS

When you're famished, it's all too easy to stuff your face with pizza and wings. But if you plan your meals ahead of time, as the successful maintainers in the CDC study did, you're much more likely to stay on track (and less likely to resort to junk when you're hungry). Make it a ritual: One night a week, jot down your battle plan, then fill your grocery cart accordingly.

6 CONTROL YOUR PORTIONS

Trimming your portions—another successful maintenance strategy in the Penn State study—allows you to eat the foods you love, without the risk of weight gain. Scientists estimate that people eat 92 percent of what they serve themselves. Which means if you dish out smaller portions, you'll eat less! A simple place to start: Downsize your plates and bowls. In a 2006 Cornell University study, nutrition experts—not just regular folks—served themselves 31 percent more ice cream when given a 34-ounce bowl versus a 17-ounce bowl. Try switching to salad plates, and use soup cups instead of cereal bowls.

7 PLAY IRON CHEF

A homemade pan of brownies sounds like a nightmare for a weight-conscious person. But, surprisingly, the CDC scientists found that dieters who cooked and baked for fun were actually less likely to regain weight. One reason: Amateur chefs may eat meals at home more often, thus avoiding calorie-dense restaurant foods. Just make sure to practice portion control when you do bake those brownies—limit yourself to one, then take the rest into the office!

8 REWARD YOURSELF

Watching what you eat shouldn't be torturous. Rather, it should be a way to earn an indulgence. People who reward themselves for sticking to their eating or exercise plans are more than twice as likely to maintain weight loss, the Penn State scientists found. Your reward doesn't have to involve food: Buy yourself a new outfit, take a day trip, or book a manicure.

9 STAY POSITIVE

If you gain a few pounds, don't freak out. A 2011 British study found that long-term weight maintainers refuse to see small weight gains as automatic failure. (This "failure" attitude only encourages you to give up or, worse, soothe yourself with food.) Instead, the successful losers acknowledged the extra couple of pounds, then renewed their weight-loss efforts. Likewise, if you slip up and scarf an extra cookie, don't beat yourself up. Simply tell yourself you'll do better tomorrow.

10 WEIGH YOURSELF DAILY

Research consistently shows that people who step on the scale most often are best at catching new pounds before they stick for good. In fact, in the CDC study, successful maintainers were 85 percent more likely to weigh themselves daily than dieters who regained weight. Make it part of your routine: Weigh yourself at the same time every day to most accurately track your progress.

11 RELIVE YOUR SUCCESS

Flip through photos of yourself before you lost the weight. This will remind you of how far you've come, which can be incredibly motivating, and will remind you why you lost the weight—and why you want to keep it off!

12 MONITOR YOUR CLOTHING

Don't upgrade to your "fat pants" when you feel the squeeze. Instead, use your body-hugging waistband as a signal to get back on track. In the British study, dieters who maintained their losses reported using "shrinking" clothing as a gauge of weight gain. Another subtle sign: Your wedding band becomes too tight.

13 DON'T MAX OUT

To keep weight off, establish an upper weight limit. British researchers found that weight maintainers set an "allowable" weight range. The top of this range should act as a trigger point—a signal to change your diet and activity level before you've packed on significant weight. Your changes don't have to be drastic: Try cutting out a snack or a glass of wine until you're back in your comfortable weight range, the scientists say.

14 PACK IN THE PROTEIN

During the weight-loss phase, it's easy to prioritize calorie cutting at the expense of nutrition. (Not a good idea, by the way.) But to meet your long-term goals, you need to control your calorie intake *and* satisfy your nutritional needs. Otherwise, you'll never be able to sustain your new diet. Lean protein—chicken breast, fish, eggs—has been shown to promote weight loss since it takes longer to digest than other nutrients and helps you feel fuller longer. In the Penn State study, dieters who regularly ate lean protein were 76 percent more likely to maintain their losses.

15 READ NUTRITION LABELS

Ignore the claims—low fat! heart healthy! all natural!—on the front of the box. Learn to decode the nutrition panel on the back, a strategy used by successful maintainers in the Penn State study. What to focus on: calories, fat (look for healthy monounsaturated fat), sodium (avoid foods with higher sodium counts than calories), fiber, and protein.

Index

Underscored page references indicate sidebars and tables. **Boldface** references indicate illustrations and photographs.

Wine (*cont.*)
    mixers with, 94
    red, <u>256</u>
        health benefits of, 211–12
    serving size of, 117, 224
Workout partner, 83, 84
Workouts. *See* Exercise(s)
Workplace fitness programs, 84
Wraps. *See also* Tortillas
    carbohydrates in, 129
    spinach, <u>275</u>
    substitute for, <u>130</u>

Y

Yams, for hunger prevention, 37
Yoga
    beginners, tips for, <u>345</u>
    benefits of, 52, 340
    morning, <u>340</u>
    poses
        boat pose, 341, **341**
        bridge, 341, **341**

    cat cow, 342, **342**
    chair, 342, **342**
    child's pose, 343, **343**
    downward-facing dog, 343, **343**
    forward fold, 344, **344**
    hero pose, 344, **344**
    warrior 1, 345, **345**
    styles of, <u>346–47</u>
Yogurt
    frozen, <u>145</u>, 147
    Greek
        for breakfast, 106, <u>108</u>, 110, <u>133</u>, <u>140</u>, 141,
            154, 158
        for dessert, 147–48
        in smoothie, 173, 242
        as snack, <u>163</u>
    high-fructose corn syrup in, 182
    as high-volume food, 185
    low-fat, 158, 168
    sugar-packed, avoiding, 143, 178,
        262
    vitamin D in, 280
Yohimbe, as weight-loss supplement, 267